ATS-29   ADMISSION TEST SERIES

This is your
PASSBOOK for...

Veterinary College Admission Test (VCAT)

Test Preparation Study Guide
Questions & Answers

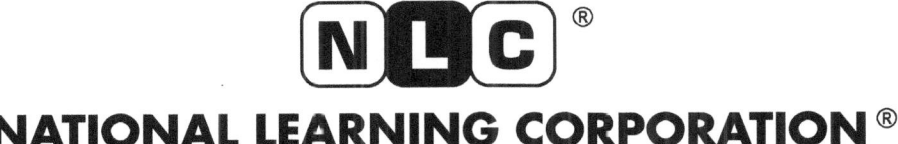

NATIONAL LEARNING CORPORATION®

COPYRIGHT NOTICE

This book is SOLELY intended for, is sold ONLY to, and its use is RESTRICTED to individual, bona fide applicants or candidates who qualify by virtue of having seriously filed applications for appropriate license, certificate, professional and/or promotional advancement, higher school matriculation, scholarship, or other legitimate requirements of education and/or governmental authorities.

This book is NOT intended for use, class instruction, tutoring, training, duplication, copying, reprinting, excerption, or adaptation, etc., by:

1) Other publishers
2) Proprietors and/or Instructors of "Coaching" and/or Preparatory Courses
3) Personnel and/or Training Divisions of commercial, industrial, and governmental organizations
4) Schools, colleges, or universities and/or their departments and staffs, including teachers and other personnel
5) Testing Agencies or Bureaus
6) Study groups which seek by the purchase of a single volume to copy and/or duplicate and/or adapt this material for use by the group as a whole without having purchased individual volumes for each of the members of the group
7) Et al.

Such persons would be in violation of appropriate Federal and State statutes.

PROVISION OF LICENSING AGREEMENTS – Recognized educational, commercial, industrial, and governmental institutions and organizations, and others legitimately engaged in educational pursuits, including training, testing, and measurement activities, may address request for a licensing agreement to the copyright owners, who will determine whether, and under what conditions, including fees and charges, the materials in this book may be used them. In other words, a licensing facility exists for the legitimate use of the material in this book on other than an individual basis. However, it is asseverated and affirmed here that the material in this book CANNOT be used without the receipt of the express permission of such a licensing agreement from the Publishers. Inquiries re licensing should be addressed to the company, attention rights and permissions department.

All rights reserved, including the right of reproduction in whole or in part, in any form or by any means, electronic or mechanical, including photocopying, recording, or by any information storage and retrieval system, without permission in writing from the Publisher.

Copyright © 2025 by
National Learning Corporation

212 Michael Drive, Syosset, NY 11791
(516) 921-8888 • www.passbooks.com
E-mail: info@passbooks.com

PASSBOOK® SERIES

THE *PASSBOOK® SERIES* has been created to prepare applicants and candidates for the ultimate academic battlefield – the examination room.

At some time in our lives, each and every one of us may be required to take an examination – for validation, matriculation, admission, qualification, registration, certification, or licensure.

Based on the assumption that every applicant or candidate has met the basic formal educational standards, has taken the required number of courses, and read the necessary texts, the *PASSBOOK® SERIES* furnishes the one special preparation which may assure passing with confidence, instead of failing with insecurity. Examination questions – together with answers – are furnished as the basic vehicle for study so that the mysteries of the examination and its compounding difficulties may be eliminated or diminished by a sure method.

This book is meant to help you pass your examination provided that you qualify and are serious in your objective.

The entire field is reviewed through the huge store of content information which is succinctly presented through a provocative and challenging approach – the question-and-answer method.

A climate of success is established by furnishing the correct answers at the end of each test.

You soon learn to recognize types of questions, forms of questions, and patterns of questioning. You may even begin to anticipate expected outcomes.

You perceive that many questions are repeated or adapted so that you can gain acute insights, which may enable you to score many sure points.

You learn how to confront new questions, or types of questions, and to attack them confidently and work out the correct answers.

You note objectives and emphases, and recognize pitfalls and dangers, so that you may make positive educational adjustments.

Moreover, you are kept fully informed in relation to new concepts, methods, practices, and directions in the field.

You discover that you are actually taking the examination all the time: you are preparing for the examination by "taking" an examination, not by reading extraneous and/or supererogatory textbooks.

In short, this PASSBOOK®, used directedly, should be an important factor in helping you to pass your test.

VETERINARY COLLEGE ADMISSION TEST (VCAT)

The Veterinary College Admission Test (VCAT) was designed to measure achievement in areas critical for success in the basic veterinary medicine curriculum. Surveys of colleges of veterinary medicine were used to determine the content areas needed for the test.

Veterinary colleges now accept the Medical College Admission Test (MCAT) or Graduate Record Examination (GRE) for admission. There are five content areas measured by the Medical College Admission Test:

- The **Verbal Ability** section measures general vocabulary and verbal reasoning.

- The **Biology** section measures knowledge of principles and concepts from elementary college biology courses.

- The **Chemistry** section measures knowledge of principles and concepts from elementary college chemistry courses including organic and inorganic chemistry.

- The **Quantitative Ability** section measures ability to reason through and understand concepts and relationships.

- The **Reading Comprehension** section measures ability to read and understand college-level reading passages.

SAMPLE TEST QUESTIONS AND ANSWERS

SAMPLE QUESTIONS
The following sample questions are similar to those found in the test.

Verbal Ability

DIRECTIONS: Choose the word that means the **opposite** or most nearly the opposite to the word in capitals.

1. IMPUDENT   1._____
    A. Wise
    B. Cautious
    C. Respectful
    D. Destructive

2. ASSUAGE   2._____
    A. Harm
    B. Oppress
    C. Motivate
    D. Intensify

DIRECTIONS: Choose the word that **best** completes the analogy in capital letters.

3. PLANE : AIRPORT :: SHIP :   3._____
    A. Pier
    B. Berth
    C. Depot
    D. Station

4. INEPT : SKILL :: FLIMSY :   4._____
    A. Power
    B. Weight
    C. Strength
    D. Thickness

Biology

DIRECTIONS: Choose the **best** answer to each of the following questions.

5. RNA and DNA are alike in that both   5._____
    A. contain uracil.
    B. contain deoxyribose.
    C. are double-stranded.
    D. have codons consisting of 3 nucleotides.

6. The hormone usually secreted when an animal senses danger and which causes the "fight or flight" reaction is
   A. insulin.
   B. thyroxine.
   C. adrenaline.
   D. parathormone.

6._____

Chemistry

DIRECTIONS: Choose the best answer to each of the following questions.

7. If a solution of H_3PO_4 is 0.90 molar, what is its normality?
   A. 0.30
   B. 0.45
   C. 1.80
   D. 2.70

7._____

8. Isotopes of the same element differ with respect to
   A. mass numbers.
   B. atomic numbers.
   C. electron configuration.
   D. number of protons in the nucleus.

8._____

Quantitative Ability

DIRECTIONS: Choose the correct answer to each of the following questions.

9. If $2x + y = 10$ and $x - 2 = y$, then $x =$
   A. 2
   B. 4
   C. 8
   D. 12

9._____

10. If (4,2) and (2,-2) describe two points on a straight line, what is the slope of that line?
    A. −2
    B. −1/2
    C. +1/2
    D. +2

10._____

11. $Z^{3x}/Z^{6x} =$
    A. Z^{-3x}
    B. Z^{-2x}
    C. $Z^{x/2}$
    D. Z^{-3}

11._____

Reading Comprehension

DIRECTIONS: Read the following passage and answer the questions following it.

Thallium sulfate, an inexpensive salt of a metal akin to lead, is one of the most potent poisons that man has developed to combat insects and rodents. Vermin are highly attracted to it; they continue nibbling doughnut-shaped baits containing the poison until they have absorbed a fatal dose. Children, however, are likely to do the same. Cases of this fatal poisoning have been reported in every state, but they are most common in the South, where the use of pesticides is most widespread. In 1957, Texas reduced the legal dosage of thallium sulfate in a rat poison mixture from three percent to one percent; in 1960, the federal government did the same. But even the weaker mixture is dangerous and can be deadly. Children who survive accidental poisoning may, months or years later, suffer from convulsions, severe mental illness, or retardation.

12. Cases of thallium sulfate poisoning in children are more common in the South than in other regions of the United States because Southern children
    A. are more exposed to the poison.
    B. are more attracted to the poison.
    C. are more susceptible to the poison.
    D. have developed less immunity to the poison.

12.____

13. According to the passage, one symptom of thallium sulfate poisoning is
    A. vomiting
    B. paralysis.
    C. uncontrolled movements.
    D. difficulty in breathing.

13.____

KEY (CORRECT ANSWERS)

1. C
2. D
3. A
4. C
5. D
6. C
7. D
8. A
9. B
10. D
11. A
12. A
13. C

HOW TO TAKE A TEST

You have studied long, hard and conscientiously.

With your official admission card in hand, and your heart pounding, you have been admitted to the examination room.

You note that there are several hundred other applicants in the examination room waiting to take the same test.

They all appear to be equally well prepared.

You know that nothing but your best effort will suffice. The "moment of truth" is at hand: you now have to demonstrate objectively, in writing, your knowledge of content and your understanding of subject matter.

You are fighting the most important battle of your life—to pass and/or score high on an examination which will determine your career and provide the economic basis for your livelihood.

What extra, special things should you know and should you do in taking the examination?

I. YOU MUST PASS AN EXAMINATION

A. WHAT EVERY CANDIDATE SHOULD KNOW
Examination applicants often ask us for help in preparing for the written test. What can I study in advance? What kinds of questions will be asked? How will the test be given? How will the papers be graded?

B. HOW ARE EXAMS DEVELOPED?
Examinations are carefully written by trained technicians who are specialists in the field known as "psychological measurement," in consultation with recognized authorities in the field of work that the test will cover. These experts recommend the subject matter areas or skills to be tested; only those knowledges or skills important to your success on the job are included. The most reliable books and source materials available are used as references. Together, the experts and technicians judge the difficulty level of the questions.
Test technicians know how to phrase questions so that the problem is clearly stated. Their ethics do not permit "trick" or "catch" questions. Questions may have been tried out on sample groups, or subjected to statistical analysis, to determine their usefulness.
Written tests are often used in combination with performance tests, ratings of training and experience, and oral interviews. All of these measures combine to form the best-known means of finding the right person for the right job.

II. HOW TO PASS THE WRITTEN TEST

A. BASIC STEPS

1) Study the announcement

How, then, can you know what subjects to study? Our best answer is: "Learn as much as possible about the class of positions for which you've applied." The exam will test the knowledge, skills and abilities needed to do the work.

Your most valuable source of information about the position you want is the official exam announcement. This announcement lists the training and experience qualifications. Check these standards and apply only if you come reasonably close to meeting them. Many jurisdictions preview the written test in the exam announcement by including a section called "Knowledge and Abilities Required," "Scope of the Examination," or some similar heading. Here you will find out specifically what fields will be tested.

2) Choose appropriate study materials

If the position for which you are applying is technical or advanced, you will read more advanced, specialized material. If you are already familiar with the basic principles of your field, elementary textbooks would waste your time. Concentrate on advanced textbooks and technical periodicals. Think through the concepts and review difficult problems in your field.

These are all general sources. You can get more ideas on your own initiative, following these leads. For example, training manuals and publications of the government agency which employs workers in your field can be useful, particularly for technical and professional positions. A letter or visit to the government department involved may result in more specific study suggestions, and certainly will provide you with a more definite idea of the exact nature of the position you are seeking.

3) Study this book!

III. KINDS OF TESTS

Tests are used for purposes other than measuring knowledge and ability to perform specified duties. For some positions, it is equally important to test ability to make adjustments to new situations or to profit from training. In others, basic mental abilities not dependent on information are essential. Questions which test these things may not appear as pertinent to the duties of the position as those which test for knowledge and information. Yet they are often highly important parts of a fair examination. For very general questions, it is almost impossible to help you direct your study efforts. What we can do is to point out some of the more common of these general abilities needed in public service positions and describe some typical questions.

1) General information

Broad, general information has been found useful for predicting job success in some kinds of work. This is tested in a variety of ways, from vocabulary lists to questions about current events. Basic background in some field of work, such as sociology or economics, may be sampled in a group of questions. Often these are principles which have become familiar to most persons through exposure rather than through formal training. It is difficult to advise you how to study for these questions; being alert to the world around you is our best suggestion.

2) Verbal ability

An example of an ability needed in many positions is verbal or language ability. Verbal ability is, in brief, the ability to use and understand words. Vocabulary and grammar tests are typical measures of this ability. Reading comprehension or paragraph interpretation questions are common in many kinds of civil service tests. You are given a paragraph of written material and asked to find its central meaning.

IV. KINDS OF QUESTIONS

1. Multiple-choice Questions

Most popular of the short-answer questions is the "multiple choice" or "best answer" question. It can be used, for example, to test for factual knowledge, ability to solve problems or judgment in meeting situations found at work.

A multiple-choice question is normally one of three types:
- It can begin with an incomplete statement followed by several possible endings. You are to find the one ending which best completes the statement, although some of the others may not be entirely wrong.
- It can also be a complete statement in the form of a question which is answered by choosing one of the statements listed.
- It can be in the form of a problem – again you select the best answer.

Here is an example of a multiple-choice question with a discussion which should give you some clues as to the method for choosing the right answer:

When an employee has a complaint about his assignment, the action which will best help him overcome his difficulty is to
- A. discuss his difficulty with his coworkers
- B. take the problem to the head of the organization
- C. take the problem to the person who gave him the assignment
- D. say nothing to anyone about his complaint

In answering this question, you should study each of the choices to find which is best. Consider choice "A" – Certainly an employee may discuss his complaint with fellow employees, but no change or improvement can result, and the complaint remains unresolved. Choice "B" is a poor choice since the head of the organization probably does not know what assignment you have been given, and taking your problem to him is known as "going over the head" of the supervisor. The supervisor, or person who made the assignment, is the person who can clarify it or correct any injustice. Choice "C" is, therefore, correct. To say nothing, as in choice "D," is unwise. Supervisors have and interest in knowing the problems employees are facing, and the employee is seeking a solution to his problem.

2. True/False

3. Matching Questions

Matching an answer from a column of choices within another column.

V. RECORDING YOUR ANSWERS

Computer terminals are used more and more today for many different kinds of exams.

For an examination with very few applicants, you may be told to record your answers in the test booklet itself. Separate answer sheets are much more common. If this separate answer sheet is to be scored by machine – and this is often the case – it is highly important that you mark your answers correctly in order to get credit.

VI. BEFORE THE TEST

YOUR PHYSICAL CONDITION IS IMPORTANT

If you are not well, you can't do your best work on tests. If you are half asleep, you can't do your best either. Here are some tips:

1) Get about the same amount of sleep you usually get. Don't stay up all night before the test, either partying or worrying—DON'T DO IT!
2) If you wear glasses, be sure to wear them when you go to take the test. This goes for hearing aids, too.
3) If you have any physical problems that may keep you from doing your best, be sure to tell the person giving the test. If you are sick or in poor health, you relay cannot do your best on any test. You can always come back and take the test some other time.

Common sense will help you find procedures to follow to get ready for an examination. Too many of us, however, overlook these sensible measures. Indeed, nervousness and fatigue have been found to be the most serious reasons why applicants fail to do their best on civil service tests. Here is a list of reminders:

- Begin your preparation early – Don't wait until the last minute to go scurrying around for books and materials or to find out what the position is all about.
- Prepare continuously – An hour a night for a week is better than an all-night cram session. This has been definitely established. What is more, a night a week for a month will return better dividends than crowding your study into a shorter period of time.
- Locate the place of the exam – You have been sent a notice telling you when and where to report for the examination. If the location is in a different town or otherwise unfamiliar to you, it would be well to inquire the best route and learn something about the building.
- Relax the night before the test – Allow your mind to rest. Do not study at all that night. Plan some mild recreation or diversion; then go to bed early and get a good night's sleep.
- Get up early enough to make a leisurely trip to the place for the test – This way unforeseen events, traffic snarls, unfamiliar buildings, etc. will not upset you.
- Dress comfortably – A written test is not a fashion show. You will be known by number and not by name, so wear something comfortable.
- Leave excess paraphernalia at home – Shopping bags and odd bundles will get in your way. You need bring only the items mentioned in the official notice you received; usually everything you need is provided. Do not bring reference books to the exam. They will only confuse those last minutes and be taken away from you when in the test room.

- Arrive somewhat ahead of time – If because of transportation schedules you must get there very early, bring a newspaper or magazine to take your mind off yourself while waiting.
- Locate the examination room – When you have found the proper room, you will be directed to the seat or part of the room where you will sit. Sometimes you are given a sheet of instructions to read while you are waiting. Do not fill out any forms until you are told to do so; just read them and be prepared.
- Relax and prepare to listen to the instructions
- If you have any physical problem that may keep you from doing your best, be sure to tell the test administrator. If you are sick or in poor health, you really cannot do your best on the exam. You can come back and take the test some other time.

VII. AT THE TEST

The day of the test is here and you have the test booklet in your hand. The temptation to get going is very strong. Caution! There is more to success than knowing the right answers. You must know how to identify your papers and understand variations in the type of short-answer question used in this particular examination. Follow these suggestions for maximum results from your efforts:

1) Cooperate with the monitor

The test administrator has a duty to create a situation in which you can be as much at ease as possible. He will give instructions, tell you when to begin, check to see that you are marking your answer sheet correctly, and so on. He is not there to guard you, although he will see that your competitors do not take unfair advantage. He wants to help you do your best.

2) Listen to all instructions

Don't jump the gun! Wait until you understand all directions. In most civil service tests you get more time than you need to answer the questions. So don't be in a hurry. Read each word of instructions until you clearly understand the meaning. Study the examples, listen to all announcements and follow directions. Ask questions if you do not understand what to do.

3) Identify your papers

Civil service exams are usually identified by number only. You will be assigned a number; you must not put your name on your test papers. Be sure to copy your number correctly. Since more than one exam may be given, copy your exact examination title.

4) Plan your time

Unless you are told that a test is a "speed" or "rate of work" test, speed itself is usually not important. Time enough to answer all the questions will be provided, but this does not mean that you have all day. An overall time limit has been set. Divide the total time (in minutes) by the number of questions to determine the approximate time you have for each question.

5) Do not linger over difficult questions

If you come across a difficult question, mark it with a paper clip (useful to have along) and come back to it when you have been through the booklet. One caution if you do this – be sure to skip a number on your answer sheet as well. Check often to be sure that you have not lost your place and that you are marking in the row numbered the same as the question you are answering.

6) Read the questions

Be sure you know what the question asks! Many capable people are unsuccessful because they failed to read the questions correctly.

7) Answer all questions

Unless you have been instructed that a penalty will be deducted for incorrect answers, it is better to guess than to omit a question.

8) Speed tests

It is often better NOT to guess on speed tests. It has been found that on timed tests people are tempted to spend the last few seconds before time is called in marking answers at random – without even reading them – in the hope of picking up a few extra points. To discourage this practice, the instructions may warn you that your score will be "corrected" for guessing. That is, a penalty will be applied. The incorrect answers will be deducted from the correct ones, or some other penalty formula will be used.

9) Review your answers

If you finish before time is called, go back to the questions you guessed or omitted to give them further thought. Review other answers if you have time.

10) Return your test materials

If you are ready to leave before others have finished or time is called, take ALL your materials to the monitor and leave quietly. Never take any test material with you. The monitor can discover whose papers are not complete, and taking a test booklet may be grounds for disqualification.

VIII. EXAMINATION TECHNIQUES

1) Read the general instructions carefully. These are usually printed on the first page of the exam booklet. As a rule, these instructions refer to the timing of the examination; the fact that you should not start work until the signal and must stop work at a signal, etc. If there are any special instructions, such as a choice of questions to be answered, make sure that you note this instruction carefully.

2) When you are ready to start work on the examination, that is as soon as the signal has been given, read the instructions to each question booklet, underline any key words or phrases, such as least, best, outline, describe and the like. In this way you will tend to answer as requested rather than discover on reviewing your paper that you listed without describing, that you selected the worst choice rather than the best choice, etc.

3) If the examination is of the objective or multiple-choice type – that is, each question will also give a series of possible answers: A, B, C or D, and you are called upon to select the best answer and write the letter next to that answer on your answer paper – it is advisable to start answering each question in turn. There may be anywhere from 50 to 100 such questions in the three or four hours allotted and you can see how much time would be taken if you read through all the questions before beginning to answer any. Furthermore, if you

come across a question or group of questions which you know would be difficult to answer, it would undoubtedly affect your handling of all the other questions.

4) If the examination is of the essay type and contains but a few questions, it is a moot point as to whether you should read all the questions before starting to answer any one. Of course, if you are given a choice – say five out of seven and the like – then it is essential to read all the questions so you can eliminate the two that are most difficult. If, however, you are asked to answer all the questions, there may be danger in trying to answer the easiest one first because you may find that you will spend too much time on it. The best technique is to answer the first question, then proceed to the second, etc.

5) Time your answers. Before the exam begins, write down the time it started, then add the time allowed for the examination and write down the time it must be completed, then divide the time available somewhat as follows:
   - If 3-1/2 hours are allowed, that would be 210 minutes. If you have 80 objective-type questions, that would be an average of 2-1/2 minutes per question. Allow yourself no more than 2 minutes per question, or a total of 160 minutes, which will permit about 50 minutes to review.
   - If for the time allotment of 210 minutes there are 7 essay questions to answer, that would average about 30 minutes a question. Give yourself only 25 minutes per question so that you have about 35 minutes to review.

6) The most important instruction is to read each question and make sure you know what is wanted. The second most important instruction is to time yourself properly so that you answer every question. The third most important instruction is to answer every question. Guess if you have to but include something for each question. Remember that you will receive no credit for a blank and will probably receive some credit if you write something in answer to an essay question. If you guess a letter – say "B" for a multiple-choice question – you may have guessed right. If you leave a blank as an answer to a multiple-choice question, the examiners may respect your feelings but it will not add a point to your score. Some exams may penalize you for wrong answers, so in such cases only, you may not want to guess unless you have some basis for your answer.

7) Suggestions
   a. Objective-type questions
      1. Examine the question booklet for proper sequence of pages and questions
      2. Read all instructions carefully
      3. Skip any question which seems too difficult; return to it after all other questions have been answered
      4. Apportion your time properly; do not spend too much time on any single question or group of questions
      5. Note and underline key words – all, most, fewest, least, best, worst, same, opposite, etc
      6. Pay particular attention to negatives
      7. Note unusual option, e.g., unduly long, short, complex, different or similar in content to the body of the question
      8. Observe the use of "hedging" words – probably, may, most likely, etc.

9. Make sure that your answer is put next to the same number as the question
10. Do not second-guess unless you have good reason to believe the second answer is definitely more correct
11. Cross out original answer if you decide another answer is more accurate; do not erase until you are ready to hand your paper in
12. Answer all questions; guess unless instructed otherwise
13. Leave time for review

b. Essay questions
  1. Read each question carefully
  2. Determine exactly what is wanted. Underline key words or phrases.
  3. Decide on outline or paragraph answer
  4. Include many different points and elements unless asked to develop any one or two points or elements
  5. Show impartiality by giving pros and cons unless directed to select one side only
  6. Make and write down any assumptions you find necessary to answer the questions
  7. Watch your English, grammar, punctuation and choice of words
  8. Time your answers; don't crowd material

8) Answering the essay question

Most essay questions can be answered by framing the specific response around several key words or ideas. Here are a few such key words or ideas:

M's: manpower, materials, methods, money, management
P's: purpose, program, policy, plan, procedure, practice, problems, pitfalls, personnel, public relations

a. Six basic steps in handling problems:
  1. Preliminary plan and background development
  2. Collect information, data and facts
  3. Analyze and interpret information, data and facts
  4. Analyze and develop solutions as well as make recommendations
  5. Prepare report and sell recommendations
  6. Install recommendations and follow up effectiveness

b. Pitfalls to avoid
1. Taking things for granted – A statement of the situation does not necessarily imply that each of the elements is necessarily true; for example, a complaint may be invalid and biased so that all that can be taken for granted is that a complaint has been registered
2. Considering only one side of a situation – Wherever possible, indicate several alternatives and then point out the reasons you selected the best one
3. Failing to indicate follow up – Whenever your answer indicates action on your part, make certain that you will take proper follow-up action to see how successful your recommendations, procedures or actions turn out to be
4. Taking too long in answering any single question – Remember to time your answers properly

EXAMINATION SECTION

ANTONYMS/OPPOSITES
EXAMINATION SECTION
TEST 1

DIRECTIONS: Each question below consists of a word printed in capital letters, followed by five words or phrases lettered A through E. Choose the lettered word or phrase that is *most nearly* OPPOSITE in meaning to the word in capital letters. *PRINT THE LETTER OF THE CORRECT ANSWER IN THE SPACE AT THE RIGHT.*

1. ACRID
    - A. smoky
    - B. withered
    - C. sharp
    - D. mild
    - E. acerb

2. ALLERGY
    - A. extreme sensitivity
    - B. distaste
    - C. sleepiness
    - D. suppressed desire
    - E. unsusceptibility

3. AMBIGUOUS
    - A. acoustic
    - B. ambivalent
    - C. equivocal
    - D. imitating
    - E. succinct

4. AMELIORATE
    - A. bring together
    - B. settle a dispute
    - C. worsen
    - D. improve
    - E. amend

5. AUGMENT
    - A. sever
    - B. disperse
    - C. increase
    - D. diminish
    - E. argue

6. BANAL
    - A. sarcastic
    - B. trite
    - C. novel
    - D. futuristic
    - E. sagacious

7. BEATIFY
    - A. make lovely
    - B. desecrate
    - C. make happy
    - D. restore
    - E. hallow

8. BOURGEOIS
    - A. middle-class citizen
    - B. capital letters
    - C. swollen streams
    - D. nobility
    - E. peasant

9. BROMIDE
    - A. vegetable
    - B. petty bribe
    - C. pamphlet
    - D. skin abrasion
    - E. epigram

10. BRING
    A. fetch B. transfer C. relate
    D. suggest E. dispatch

11. CAPRICIOUS
    A. fickle B. fault-finding C. sneering
    D. dominating E. resolve

12. CASUAL
    A. watery B. fated C. fortuitous
    D. aromatic E. moving

13. CHOLERIC
    A. dignified B. high-tempered C. gloomy
    D. unexcitable E. caustic

14. CIRCULAR
    A. muscular B. oblique C. grouped
    D. pivotal E. incongruous

15. CIRCUMVENT
    A. succor B. reserve C. fortify
    D. surround E. delude

16. COMPASSIONATE
    A. pitiful B. merciful C. ruthless
    D. reluctant E. pietistic

17. COMPLIANCE
    A. violation B. regulation C. attendance
    D. submission E. conformance

18. CONDIGN
    A. punishable B. scheming C. undeserved
    D. merited E. condemn

19. CONDONE
    A. demand payment B. express sympathy C. forget
    D. revenge E. forgive

20. COPE
    A. fail in striving B. contend on equal terms
    C. plug with soft material D. crown with laurel
    E. compare with others

21. DECOROUS
    A. unseemly B. proper C. low cut
    D. in groups of ten E. deteriorating

22. DESPONDENT

    A. powdery   B. bent   C. optional
    D. artificial   E. elated

23. DESULTORY

    A. pompous   B. methodical   C. rambling
    D. oppressively hot   E. cursory

24. DETONATE

    A. explode   B. deafen   C. muffle
    D. fizzle out   E. destroy

25. DISCIPLE

    A. impostor   B. follower   C. antagonist
    D. paragon   E. colleague

KEYS (CORRECT ANSWERS)

1.	D	11.	E
2.	E	12.	B
3.	E	13.	D
4.	C	14.	B
5.	D	15.	A
6.	C	16.	C
7.	B	17.	A
8.	E	18.	C
9.	E	19.	D
10.	E	20.	A

21. A
22. E
23. B
24. C
25. C

TEST 2

DIRECTIONS: Each question below consists of a word printed in capital letters, followed by five words or phrases lettered A through E. Choose the lettered word or phrase that is *most nearly* OPPOSITE in meaning to the word in capital letters. *PRINT THE LETTER OF THE CORRECT ANSWER IN THE SPACE AT THE RIGHT.*

1. DISCREET 1.____
   - A. cautious
   - B. chary
   - C. prudent
   - D. distinct
   - E. temerarious

2. DISINTER 2.____
   - A. dig up from a grave
   - B. lack interest
   - C. interrupt
   - D. inject between muscles
   - E. entomb

3. DOGGEREL 3.____
   - A. trivial verse
   - B. small canine species
   - C. stubborn behavior
   - D. sophisticated poetry
   - E. manger

4. DOLE OUT 4.____
   - A. squander
   - B. distribute piecemeal
   - C. control
   - D. deny alms
   - E. hoard

5. DOMINEERING 5.____
   - A. dictatorial
   - B. pliant
   - C. considerate
   - D. unsympathetic
   - E. recreant

6. ELEGY 6.____
   - A. inheritance
   - B. burnt offering
   - C. violin obbligato
   - D. dirge
   - E. paean

7. ELICIT 7.____
   - A. concoct with alcohol
   - B. draw out
   - C. compel approval
   - D. request sharply
   - E. ignite

8. EMOLLIENT 8.____
   - A. salve
   - B. monument
   - C. tariff charge
   - D. extra tip
   - E. abrasive

9. ENCORE 9.____
   - A. intermission
   - B. termination
   - C. heart of the matter
   - D. repetition
   - E. variation

10. ENERVATE 10.____
    - A. stumble
    - B. devitalize
    - C. stimulate
    - D. rejoice
    - E. impede

11. EXPIATION 11._____
    A. reprobation   B. clarification   C. failure
    D. atonement   E. interpretation

12. FABULOUS 12._____
    A. wealthy   B. impressionistic   C. realistic
    D. legendary   E. fictional

13. FAIRWAY 13._____
    A. airplane landing field   B. golf greensward   C. captain's private quarters
    D. entrance to ferry slip   E. coppice

14. FEASIBLE 14._____
    A. garish   B. festive   C. theoretical
    D. practicable   E. pertinent

15. FIERY 15._____
    A. vehement   B. irritable   C. restive
    D. gay   E. indifferent

16. FLORID 16._____
    A. flowing   B. livid   C. blotchy
    D. ruddy   E. over-heated

17. FLOUT 17._____
    A. move   B. mock   C. obey
    D. defy   E. flog

18. FOREGO 18._____
    A. prosecute   B. align   C. renounce
    D. look forward E. over-heated

19. FURTIVE 19._____
    A. fleeing   B. hairy   C. glancing
    D. stealthy   E. ingenuous

20. GARBLE 20._____
    A. substantiate B. garnish   C. mutilate
    D. unravel   E. embroider

21. GARRULOUS 21._____
    A. talkative   B. quarrelsome   C. snarling
    D. laconic   E. ungainly

22. GOSSAMER 22._____
    A. sleezy   B. dusty   C. gauzy
    D. unbreakable   E. zephyr-like

23. GOURMAND 23.____
   A. greedy eater   B. epicure   C. hungry person
   D. ascetic   E. fried pumpkin shell

24. GRIEVOUS 24.____
   A. rutty   B. gratifying   C. sorrowful
   D. vicious   E. unmentionable

25. GRIMACE 25.____
   A. happy smile   B. fruit sherbet   C. twisting of the countenance
   D. fine quality silk   E. sneer

KEYS (CORRECT ANSWERS)

1.	E	11.	A
2.	E	12.	C
3.	D	13.	E
4.	A	14.	C
5.	B	15.	E
6.	E	16.	B
7.	D	17.	C
8.	E	18.	A
9.	B	19.	E
10.	C	20.	A

21. D
22. D
23. D
24. B
25. A

TEST 3

DIRECTIONS: Each question below consists of a word printed in capital letters, followed by five words or phrases lettered A through E. Choose the lettered word or phrase that is *most nearly* OPPOSITE in meaning to the word in capital letters. *PRINT THE LETTER OF THE CORRECT ANSWER IN THE SPACE AT THE RIGHT.*

1. HEINOUS
    - A. criminal
    - B. elevated
    - C. inhuman
    - D. flagrant
    - E. moderate

2. HUE
    - A. tint
    - B. shade
    - C. tone
    - D. tinge
    - E. etiolation

3. IMMUNITY
    - A. protection against accident
    - B. exemption
    - C. freedom from disease
    - D. dispensation
    - E. tendency

4. IMPLICIT
    - A. directly stated
    - B. understood though not expressed
    - C. omitted entirely by chance
    - D. stated but not for publication
    - E. inherent

5. IMPUTE
    - A. insult
    - B. contradict
    - C. ascribe
    - D. question
    - E. refer

6. INCIPIENT
    - A. tasteless
    - B. criminal
    - C. beginning
    - D. diseased
    - E. terminal

7. INGENUOUS
    - A. guileful
    - B. naive
    - C. frank
    - D. uncertain
    - E. jealous

8. INIQUITOUS
    - A. awesome
    - B. unequal
    - C. wicked
    - D. present everywhere
    - E. exemplary

9. INTERMITTENT
    - A. continuing without break
    - B. occurring at intervals
    - C. persistently noisy
    - D. gradually subdued
    - E. intermediate

10. INTRANSIGENT   10.____
    A. utterly fearless   B. irreconcilable   C. invalid
    D. not transferable   E. tractable

11. INTREPID   11.____
    A. fearful   B. uneasy   C. dauntless
    D. stumbling   E. insistent

12. INURE   12.____
    A. maim   B. entice   C. deplete
    D. toughen   E. endure

13. INVOKE   13.____
    A. provoke   B. denounce   C. slanderous
    D. address in prayer   E. evoke

14. NOSTALGIA   14.____
    A. homesickness   B. inertia   C. gloominess
    D. nasal catarrh   E. wanderlust

15. OCCULT   15.____
    A. abstract   B. manifest   C. secret
    D. oriental   E. acute

16. ONEROUS   16.____
    A. unwanted   B. impossible   C. delicate
    D. burdensome   E. facile

17. OPULENT   17.____
    A. expensive   B. oily   C. crafty
    D. profuse   E. jejune

18. ORDINANCE   18.____
    A. excess weight   B. anarchy   C. law
    D. military supplies   E. mound of filth

19. ORTHOGRAPHY   19.____
    A. correct accent   B. choice of words   C. misspelling
    D. derivation of words   E. clear enunciation

20. PAROCHIAL   20.____
    A. limited in range   B. sacred   C. stubborn
    D. objective   E. easily manageable

21. PEREMPTORY   21.____
    A. trifling   B. compliant   C. arbitrary
    D. binding   E. camouflaged

22. PERVADE

    A. pass along
    B. escape quietly
    C. convince at length
    D. to be diffused throughout
    E. confine

23. PERVERSITY

    A. cruelty
    B. miserliness
    C. conformity
    D. adherent
    E. frugality

24. PHLEGMATIC

    A. stolid
    B. figurative
    C. aphasic
    D. sentient
    E. substantial

25. POIGNANT

    A. melancholy
    B. soothing
    C. doubtful
    D. keen
    E. reluctant

KEYS (CORRECT ANSWERS)

1.	B	11.	A
2.	E	12.	C
3.	E	13.	B
4.	A	14.	E
5.	B	15.	B
6.	E	16.	E
7.	A	17.	E
8.	E	18.	B
9.	A	19.	C
10.	E	20.	D

21. B
22. E
23. C
24. D
25. B

TEST 4

DIRECTIONS: Each question below consists of a word printed in capital letters, followed by five words or phrases lettered A through E. Choose the lettered word or phrase that is *most nearly* OPPOSITE in meaning to the word in capital letters. *PRINT THE LETTER OF THE CORRECT ANSWER IN THE SPACE AT THE RIGHT.*

1. PRODIGIOUS
   A. extraordinary   B. commonplace   C. profound
   D. prehistoric   E. infinitesmal
1._____

2. PUERILE
   A. childish   B. mature   C. feverish
   D. immaculate   E. pusillanimous
2._____

3. PUNCTILIOUS
   A. offensively frank   B. willing to admit blame   C. sarcastically polite
   D. precise in conduct   E. indiscriminate
3._____

4. RAZE
   A. torture   B. erect   C. salvage
   D. destroy   E. prorogue
4._____

5. RECESSIVE
   A. inclined to go back   B. relating to slavery   C. moving forward
   D. modest   E. allemorphic
5._____

6. RENEGADE
   A. turncoat   B. loyalist   C. habitual drunkard
   D. confirmed criminal   E. one who kills a king
6._____

7. RENASCENCE
   A. unwinding   B. restoration   C. unscrewing
   D. detraining   E. perdition
7._____

8. RESPITE
   A. pardon   B. re-trial   C. stay
   D. vengeance   E. continuation
8._____

9. SALIENT
   A. hidden   B. salty   C. floating
   D. prominent   E. flagrant
9._____

10. SATELLITE
   A. falling star   B. attentive follower   C. adversary
   D. flint spark   E. fellow captive
10._____

11. SCRUPULOUS
    - A. niggardly
    - B. abusive
    - C. conscientious
    - D. unprincipled
    - E. guilty

12. SINEWY
    - A. callused
    - B. enervated
    - C. springy
    - D. slimy
    - E. brawny

13. SKEPTIC
    - A. agnostic
    - B. suave
    - C. ingenious
    - D. credulous
    - E. faithful

14. SPARE
    - A. forbear
    - B. forego
    - C. reserve
    - D. control
    - E. squander

15. SPORADIC
    - A. isolated
    - B. incessant
    - C. dissipated
    - D. involuntary
    - E. discrete

KEYS (CORRECT ANSWERS)

1. E
2. B
3. E
4. B
5. C
6. B
7. E
8. E
9. A
10. C
11. D
12. B
13. D
14. E
15. B

ANTONYMS/OPPOSITES
EXAMINATION SECTION
TEST 1

DIRECTIONS: Each question below consists of a word printed in capital letters, followed by five words or phrases lettered A through E. Choose the lettered word or phrase that is *most nearly* OPPOSITE in meaning to the word in capital letters. *PRINT THE LETTER OF THE CORRECT ANSWER IN THE SPACE AT THE RIGHT.*

1. CELERITY
   - A. torpor
   - B. felicity
   - C. fame
   - D. acrimony
   - E. temerity

2. APATHETIC
   - A. stoical
   - B. amative
   - C. lissome
   - D. finical
   - E. redolent

3. FLACCID
   - A. cold
   - B. sterile
   - C. brave
   - D. stiff
   - E. whimsical

4. INGENUOUS
   - A. foolish
   - B. intelligent
   - C. wily
   - D. indigent
   - E. native

5. AMENABLE
   - A. prayerful
   - B. conciliatory
   - C. pliant
   - D. truculent
   - E. mendacious

6. PARSIMONIOUS
   - A. benevolent
   - B. worldly
   - C. scoffing
   - D. ungrammatical
   - E. grudging

7. INDIGENOUS
   - A. caustic
   - B. factitious
   - C. exotic
   - D. opulent
   - E. sophisticated

8. SAPIENT
   - A. distasteful
   - B. animalistic
   - C. ignorant
   - D. jejune
   - E. zestful

9. TENUOUS
   - A. substantial
   - B. decadent
   - C. salubrious
   - D. illogical
   - E. slender

10. ZENITH
    - A. acme
    - B. nadir
    - C. pentacle
    - D. azimuth
    - E. apogee

2 (#1)

11. RESTIVE
    - A. overactive
    - B. refractory
    - C. compliant
    - D. uneasy
    - E. listless

12. ADAMANT
    - A. primeval
    - B. laudatory
    - C. polite
    - D. yielding
    - E. intractable

13. DISCRETE
    - A. continuous
    - B. separate
    - C. foolish
    - D. tactful
    - E. serrated

14. SANGUINE
    - A. bloody
    - B. diffident
    - C. happy
    - D. pale
    - E. confident

15. PLACATE
    - A. retaliate
    - B. confuse
    - C. wander
    - D. nettle
    - E. condone

16. FATUOUS
    - A. inane
    - B. stout
    - C. witty
    - D. empty
    - E. vacuous

17. INNOCUOUS
    - A. toxic
    - B. guileful
    - C. gullible
    - D. criminal
    - E. culpable

18. DEARTH
    - A. demise
    - B. copiousness
    - C. nativity
    - D. distaste
    - E. lack

19. RESPITE
    - A. affirmation
    - B. intermission
    - C. continuance
    - D. colloquy
    - E. fairness

20. LACONIC
    - A. turgid
    - B. replete
    - C. tearful
    - D. negligent
    - E. draconic

21. ANIMADVERSION
    - A. censure
    - B. distaste
    - C. spirituality
    - D. bestiality
    - E. approbation

22. NOISOME
    - A. boisterous
    - B. beneficial
    - C. villous
    - D. pallid
    - E. noxious

23. EXPURGATE 23._____

    A. cleanse   B. harden   C. improve
    D. deflect   E. smirch

24. ATAVISM 24._____

    A. progression   B. favoritism   C. inclination
    D. cannibalism   E. reversion

25. ATTRITION 25._____

    A. appeasement   B. capitulation   C. wearing away
    D. calming down   E. aggrandizement

KEYS (CORRECT ANSWERS)

1. A	11. C
2. B	12. D
3. D	13. A
4. C	14. B
5. D	15. D
6. A	16. C
7. C	17. A
8. C	18. B
9. A	19. C
10. B	20. A

21. E
22. B
23. E
24. A
25. E

TEST 2

DIRECTIONS: Each question below consists of a word printed in capital letters, followed by five words or phrases lettered A through E. Choose the lettered word or phrase that is *most nearly* OPPOSITE in meaning to the word in capital letters. *PRINT THE LETTER OF THE CORRECT ANSWER IN THE SPACE AT THE RIGHT*

1. FABRICATE
   - A. consume
   - B. furrow
   - C. construct
   - D. materialize
   - E. delete

2. COMMAND
   - A. mandate
   - B. consummation
   - C. correlation
   - D. commitment
   - E. supplication

3. DISSIPATE
   - A. sip
   - B. amass
   - C. disturb
   - D. outdistance
   - E. disperse

4. UNBIASED
   - A. unfair
   - B. unreasonable
   - C. uniform
   - D. equitable
   - E. disquieting

5. SATURNINE
   - A. buoyant
   - B. gloomy
   - C. aspiring
   - D. incongruous
   - E. splenetic

6. PROFITABLE
   - A. preferable
   - B. chagrined
   - C. ruinous
   - D. lucrative
   - E. profligate

7. GENERATING
   - A. generous
   - B. originating
   - C. degenerating
   - D. terminating
   - E. ingenuous

8. SANCTION
   - A. safety
   - B. performance
   - C. injunction
   - D. sanctuary
   - E. permission

9. PROBABLE
   - A. perchance
   - B. imprudent
   - C. unlikely
   - D. perilous
   - E. unsavory

10. FRUITION
    - A. exposure
    - B. harvest
    - C. frustration
    - D. neglect
    - E. attainment

2 (#2)

11. RANCOROUS 11.____
    A. benign   B. confusing   C. satiated
    D. complex   E. malicious

12. AVARICIOUS 12.____
    A. munificent B. rapacious   C. analogous
    D. perverse   E. atonal

13. UNIQUE 13.____
    A. uniform   B. single   C. utilitarian
    D. senescent   E. unitary

14. PROCURE 14.____
    A. decline   B. reap   C. forfeit
    D. effect   E. contrive

15. RAVENOUS 15.____
    A. birdlike   B. hungry   C. rancid
    D. venial   E. sated

16. INNOCUOUS 16.____
    A. mixed   B. pernicious   C. defiled
    D. harmless   E. diffused

17. PERMEATE 17.____
    A. smooth   B. pulverize   C. obstruct
    D. pollute   E. penetrate

18. AXIOM 18.____
    A. adage   B. proof   C. precept
    D. dictum   E. hearsay

19. RELEVANT 19.____
    A. immaterial B. pertinent   C. relenting
    D. capable   E. released

20. POTENT 20.____
    A. secretive   B. powerful   C. restive
    D. puissant   E. enervated

21. AMELIORATE 21.____
    A. improve   B. embitter   C. alter
    D. mellow   E. impair

22. IMPENDING 22.____
    A. pendulous   B. impeding   C. fortuitous
    D. imminent   E. looming

3 (#2)

23. LATENT

   A. tricky B. hidden C. pompous
   D. overt E. hateful

24. DISCERNMENT

   A. concern B. obtuseness C. distance
   D. sickness E. acumen

25. SUAVE

   A. genuine B. captive C. gauche
   D. bland E. captious

KEYS (CORRECT ANSWERS)

1.	A	11.	A
2.	E	12.	A
3.	B	13.	A
4.	A	14.	C
5.	A	15.	E
6.	C	16.	B
7.	D	17.	C
8.	C	18.	E
9.	C	19.	A
10.	C	20.	E

21. B
22. C
23. D
24. B
25. C

TEST 3

DIRECTIONS: Each question below consists of a word printed in capital letters, followed by five words or phrases lettered A through E. Choose the lettered word or phrase that is *most nearly* OPPOSITE in meaning to the word in capital letters. *PRINT THE LETTER OF THE CORRECT ANSWER IN THE SPACE AT THE RIGHT.*

1. WORLDLY 1.____
   - A. trifling
   - B. secular
   - C. mundane
   - D. unworthy
   - E. impractical

2. BEG 2.____
   - A. seek
   - B. implore
   - C. convert
   - D. vaunt
   - E. donate

3. ERUDITE 3.____
   - A. impolite
   - B. learned
   - C. correct
   - D. illiterate
   - E. contrite

4. CURSORY 4.____
   - A. protracted
   - B. persistent
   - C. evanescent
   - D. superficial
   - E. gentle

5. ENIGMATIC 5.____
   - A. evident
   - B. enormous
   - C. lucid
   - D. abstruse
   - E. sphinxlike

6. PROSCRIBE 6.____
   - A. banish
   - B. condemn
   - C. diagnose poorly
   - D. transcend
   - E. prescribe

7. TURBID 7.____
   - A. limpid
   - B. muddy
   - C. moody
   - D. settled
   - E. turgid

8. PERSPICACITY 8.____
   - A. keenness
   - B. penetration
   - C. rudeness
   - D. discernment
   - E. insensibility

9. CONTIGUOUS 9.____
   - A. contagious
   - B. adjoining
   - C. intolerant
   - D. unconnected
   - E. uncontaminated

10. ASSUAGE 10.____
    - A. intensify
    - B. coagulate
    - C. alleviate
    - D. congeal
    - E. molest

11. PROTAGONIST
    A. enemy   B. participant   C. champion
    D. protector   E. patron

12. VIRULENT
    A. vehement   B. virtuous   C. deadly
    D. reparatory   E. virile

13. PROLIX
    A. tiresome   B. exciting   C. wordy
    D. terse   E. pompous

14. LEVITY
    A. lengthiness   B. glumness   C. lenience
    D. frivolity   E. lewdness

15. METICULOUS
    A. careful   B. approximate   C. untrue
    D. metallic   E. indiscriminate

16. ANALOGOUS
    A. tantamount   B. extracurricular C. distinctive
    D. presumptuous   E. cavernous

17. VICARIOUS
    A. inconsiderate B. direct   C. fraudulent
    D. substitute   E. prestigious

18. ABROGATION
    A. promulgation   B. repeal   C. extension
    D. investigation E. postponement

19. HOMOGENEOUS
    A. manly   B. assorted   C. creamy
    D. similar   E. parallel

20. ARRAIGN
    A. accuse   B. convict   C. disentangle
    D. disarrange   E. discharge

21. ABJURE
    A. remove   B. disavow   C. acknowledge
    D. imagine   E. entreat

22. INTESTATE
    A. relating to inner parts   B. legally devised   C. shipped from one place to another
    D. subject to taxation   E. not disposed of by will

23. ANCILLARY

    A. deterrent   B. temporary   C. auxiliary
    D. approved   E. additional

24. EXTRANEOUS

    A. foreign   B. accidental   C. mixed
    D. indigenous   E. adventitious

25. DISPARAGE

    A. divide   B. dismiss   C. depreciate
    D. discourage   E. dignify

KEYS (CORRECT ANSWERS)

1.	E	11.	A
2.	E	12.	D
3.	D	13.	D
4.	A	14.	B
5.	C	15.	E
6.	E	16.	C
7.	A	17.	B
8.	E	18.	A
9.	D	19.	B
10.	A	20.	E

21. C
22. B
23. A
24. D
25. E

TEST 4

DIRECTIONS: Each question below consists of a word printed in capital letters, followed by five words or phrases lettered A through E. Choose the lettered word or phrase that is *most nearly* OPPOSITE in meaning to the word in capital letters. *PRINT THE LETTER OF THE CORRECT ANSWER IN THE SPACE AT THE RIGHT.*

1. FUGACIOUS
    - A. pugnacious
    - B. tenacious
    - C. mendacious
    - D. settled
    - E. migratory

   1.____

2. THRASONICAL
    - A. treasonable
    - B. gingival
    - C. vainglorious
    - D. unassuming
    - E. lyrical

   2.____

3. PELAGIC
    - A. terrestrial
    - B. aquatic
    - C. noncontagious
    - D. polemical
    - E. epigrammatic

   3.____

4. FUSCOUS
    - A. importunate
    - B. chaste
    - C. radiant
    - D. fractious
    - E. amenable

   4.____

5. CREPUSCULAR
    - A. glimmering
    - B. crackling
    - C. pussy
    - D. mutable
    - E. distinct

   5.____

6. NOISOME
    - A. attractive
    - B. noxious
    - C. inoffensive
    - D. winsome
    - E. noiseless

   6.____

7. PEJORATIVE
    - A. appreciative
    - B. acceding
    - C. ultimate
    - D. alliterative
    - E. conceding

   7.____

8. JEJUNE
    - A. valiant
    - B. vital
    - C. graceful
    - D. senile
    - E. incipient

   8.____

9. FULGENT
    - A. divergent
    - B. lambent
    - C. unresplendent
    - D. cogent
    - E. indigent

   9.____

10. LENITIVE
    - A. laxative
    - B. provocative
    - C. menial
    - D. incursive
    - E. malevolent

    10.____

2 (#4)

11. IRREFRAGABLE 11._____
    A. breakable   B. desirable   C. tractable
    D. inconclusive E. refutable

12. INCHOATE 12._____
    A. chaotic   B. disclosed   C. coherent
    D. infatuated E. complete

13. MINATORY 13._____
    A. vanishing B. nugatory   C. myriad
    D. malignant E. propitious

14. AMBIENT 14._____
    A. wandering B. pandering   C. transient
    D. remote   E. hostile

15. EUPHEMISTIC 15._____
    A. euphuistic B. grating   C. masochistic
    D. palpable   E. insolent

16. FACTIOUS 16._____
    A. fractious B. fictitious C. scrupulous
    D. seemly   E. disinterested

17. FRIABLE 17._____
    A. unseasoned   B. palatable   C. renascent
    D. indestructible E. adhesive

18. HEGEMONY 18._____
    A. thraldom   B. testimony   C. followership
    D. necromancy E. obligation

19. IMMANENT 19._____
    A. illative   B. imminent   C. emanating
    D. unessential E. clement

20. INDEFEASIBLE 20._____
    A. defensible B. abrogable   C. disputable
    D. deferential E. execrable

21. EQUIVOCAL 21._____
    A. ambiguous B. ambivalent C. equitable
    D. esoteric   E. unquestionable

22. LIVID 22._____
    A. lurid   B. discolored C. unrestrained
    D. rubicund   E. ghastly

3 (#4)

23. MOIETY

   A. impiety   B. notoriety   C. unity
   D. harmony   E. inconsistency

23.____

24. PEREMPTORY

   A. dogmatic   B. authoritarian   C. indecisive
   D. conciliatory   E. whimsical

24.____

25. VENIAL

   A. mercenary   B. venous   C. purulent
   D. aberrant   E. loathsome

25.____

KEYS (CORRECT ANSWERS)

1.	D	11.	E
2.	D	12.	E
3.	A	13.	E
4.	C	14.	D
5.	E	15.	B
6.	C	16.	E
7.	A	17.	D
8.	B	18.	A
9.	C	19.	D
10.	B	20.	B

21. E
22. D
23. C
24. C
25. E

VERBAL ANALOGIES – 2 BLANKS
EXAMINATION SECTION
TEST 1

DIRECTIONS: Each question in this part consists of two capitalized words which have a certain relationship to each other, followed by five lettered pairs of words in small letters. Choose the letter of the pair of words which are related to each other in the SAME way as the words of the capitalized pair are related to each other. *PRINT THE LETTER OF THE CORRECT ANSWER IN THE SPACE AT THE RIGHT.*

1. DOOR : KEY : : _____ : _____ 1.____
    - A. crossword puzzle : design
    - B. frame : window
    - C. problem : solution
    - D. suitcase : handle
    - E. password : sentry

2. STORM WINDOW : COLD :: _____ : _____ 2.____
    - A. Dr. Salk : polio
    - B. roof : rain
    - C. disease : vaccination
    - D. thermos : heat
    - E. vitamin D : rickets

3. ACORN : OAK : : _____ : _____ 3.____
    - A. pistil : stamen
    - B. tree : leaf
    - C. bulb : tulip
    - D. root : grass
    - E. rose : thorn

4. SICKNESS : DOCTOR :: _____ : _____ 4.____
    - A. dividends : stocks
    - B. salary : laborer
    - C. robbery : thief
    - D. wind : sail
    - E. leak : plumber

5. FRICTION/ : HEAT :: _____ : _____ 5.____
    - A. eating : appendicitis
    - B. grass : lawn mower
    - C. typewriter : ribbon
    - D. match : flame
    - E. night : day

6. MODERATE : EXTREMIST ::_____ : _____ 6.____
    - A. scribe : inscribe
    - B. spiritual : material
    - C. agnostic : prognosis
    - D. noticeable : flagrant
    - E. heathen : pagan

7. AGGRESSION : WAR :: _____ : _____ 7.____
    - A. fear : dread
    - B. neurosis : psychosis
    - C. nervousness : reaction
    - D. demise : disease
    - E. illness : treatment

8. BILL : AMENDMENT : : _____ : _____ 8.____
    - A. introduction : theme
    - B. antithesis : synthesis
    - C. stanza : poem
    - D. letter : postscript
    - E. summary : report

9. SPHERE : HEMISPHERE :: _____ : _____ 9.____

    A. polygon : hexagon   B. circle : quadrant
    C. duality : modality   D. acute angle : obtuse angle
    E. triangle : rectangle

10. TOP : STRING :: _____ : _____ 10.____

    A. hoof : horse   B. runner : sled
    C. wheel : axle   D. ramrod : rifle
    E. propeller : wing

11. AQUARIUM : FISH :: _____ : _____ 11.____

    A. jungle : monkeys   B. estuary : monkeys
    C. nest : birds   D. museum : monkeys
    E. aviary : birds

12. MOTH : LARVA :: _____ : _____ 12.____

    A. accomplishment : plan   B. accomplishment : community
    C. community : plan   D. populace : community
    E. train : community

13. HERESY : CHURCH :: _____ : _____ 13.____

    A. treason : institution   B. institution : state
    C. orthodoxy : atheism   D. atheism : agnosticism
    E. treason : state

14. RANSOM : CAPTIVE :: _____ _____ 14.____

    A. death : suffer   B. money : prisoner
    C. war : prisoner   D. money : kidnapper
    E. blackmail : victim

15. ROCK : EROSION :: _____ : _____ 15.____

    A. signature : forgery   B. landscape : flatness
    C. food : fasting   D. character : dissipation
    E. task : fatigue

16. FIBER : FABRIC :: _____ : _____ 16.____

    A. appurtenance : object   B. obstinate : deadlock
    C. nucleus : cell   D. leverage : aggregate
    E. member : league

17. REST : FATIGUE :: _____ : _____ 17.____

    A. relaxation : recreation   B. precipice : mountain
    C. laziness : obesity   D. diploma : graduate
    E. praise : dejection

18. RULES : BASEBALL :: _____ : 18.____

    A. law : jury   B. law : society
    C. jury : sentence   D. prisoner : cell
    E. prisoner : law

19. TORTOISE : HARE :: _____ : _____   19._____

    A. letter : telegram   B. truth : lie
    C. essay : thesis   D. word : number
    E. modesty : egotism

20. CANNON : CATAPULT :: _____ : _____   20._____

    A. matter : mind   B. church : temple
    C. oak : scorn   D. clock : hourglass
    E. temple : foundation

21. HOOF : HORSE :: _____ : _____   21._____

    A. wing : robin   B. egg : chicken
    C. paw : cat   D. hole : chipmunk
    E. purr : kitten

22. CLUB : SWORD :: _____ : _____   22._____

    A. pound : pierce   B. cut : parry
    C. thrust : pierce   D. cut : break
    E. break : crack

23. BIRD : EGG :: _____ : _____   23._____

    A. vegetable : earth   B. oak : acorn
    C. muscle : cell   D. flight : motion
    E. crime : implication

24. OBJECTIVE : CAMPAIGN :: _____ : _____   24._____

    A. success : talent   B. goal : motivation
    C. triumph : victory   D. consequence : misdeed
    E. destination : voyage

25. LOSE : POSSESS :: _____ : _____   25._____

    A. supply : produce   B. advance : hesitate
    C. perform : undertake   D. desist : continue
    E. recur : cease

KEY (CORRECT ANSWERS)

1.	C	11.	E
2.	B	12.	A
3.	C	13.	E
4.	E	14.	E
5.	D	15.	D
6.	D	16.	E
7.	B	17.	E
8.	D	18.	B
9.	B	19.	A
10.	C	20.	D

21. C
22. A
23. B
24. E
25. D

TEST 2

DIRECTIONS: Each question in this part consists of two capitalized words which have a certain relationship to each other, followed by five lettered pairs of words in small letters. Choose the letter of the pair of words which are related to each other in the SAME way as the words of the capitalized pair are related to each other. *PRINT THE LETTER OF THE CORRECT ANSWER IN THE SPACE AT THE RIGHT.*

1. METAL : ALLOY :: _____ : _____

    A. mixture : blend
    B. species : hybrid
    C. plant : flower
    D. rock : metal
    E. block : chip

2. INSULT : SENSITIVE :: _____ : _____

    A. cheat : unassuming
    B. convince : gullible
    C. steal : starved
    D. suffer : fatigued
    E. fear : frightened

3. APPROBATION : APPLAUSE :: _____ : _____

    A. retaliation : injury
    B. superiority : scorn
    C. understanding : praise
    D. contempt : snub
    E. amusement : grimace

4. BLAME : EXCULPATE :: _____ : _____

    A. honor : retract
    B. debt : regain
    C. duty : resent
    D. position : retract
    E. obligation : absolve

5. PERJURE : RELATE :: _____ : _____

    A. examine : glance
    B. sprawl : recline
    C. gorge : eat
    D. destroy : mar
    E. trespass : wander

6. TORPID : TEMPERATE :: _____ : _____

    A. lethargic : abstemious
    B. pusillanimous : absent
    C. militant : irascible
    D. dogmatic : truculent
    E. latent : gregarious

7. HEADLONG : DEJECTED :: _____ : _____

    A. melancholy : unhappy
    B. askew : explicit
    C. nebulous : credulous
    D. intrinsic : fatuous
    E. precipitous : disconsolate

8. APPLAUSE : RIDICULE :: _____ : _____

    A. amnesia : oblivion
    B. felon : miscreant
    C. constantly : bow
    D. encore : catcall
    E. generosity : lechery

9. PARSIMONY : MAGNANIMITY :: _____ : _____

   A. urgency : exigency
   B. ribaldry : prodigality
   C. profession : avocation
   D. unselfish . selfish
   E. bigotry : tolerance

10. TROPICAL. : LUXURIANT : : _____ : _____

    A. penicillin : cure
    B. invigoration : exhilaration
    C. arctic : gelid
    D. cold : muddy
    E. disturbed : halcyon

11. ISLAND : ARCHIPELAGO _____ : _____

    A. cerebrum : nucleus
    B. strait : peninsula
    C. nucleus : cell
    D. Africa : Australia
    E. individual : multitude

12. DOWNCAST : EXUBERANT : : _____ : _____

    A. melancholy : effusive
    B. beaver : eager
    C. lavish : exultant
    D. abundant : parsimonious
    E. dispersal : congregation

13. OBELISK : HIEROGLYPHIC :: _____ : _____

    A. statue : sphinx
    B. masterpiece : signature
    C. geography : cartography
    D. medicine : cardiograph
    E. blackboard : penmanship

14. CAVIAR : GOURMET :: _____ : _____

    A. art : artificer
    B. edition : critic
    C. patrician : plebeian
    D. seance : clairvoyant
    E. masterpiece : connoisseur

15. GRACEFUL : GAUCHE :: _____ : _____

    A. wealthy : indigent
    B. poised : sad
    C. secretive : clandestine
    D. melancholy : lugubrious
    E. thoughtless : inadvertent

16. DYNAMO : SWITCH :: _____ : _____

    A. ambition : aspiration
    B. lamp : light
    C. spur : horse
    D. man : stimulus
    E. dynamo : switch

17. RAGE : RED : : _____ : _____

    A. depressed : yellow
    B. envy : green
    C. fright : chalk
    D. red : henna
    E. cadaverous : ashen

18. STUDY : DIPLOMA :: _____ : _____

    A. ambition : honor
    B. examination : marks
    C. diligence : bonus
    D. labor : wages
    E. course : promotion

19. FEDERATION : UNION :: _____ :_____

    A. league : team
    B. city : borough
    C. gender : girls
    D. congregation : sect
    E. organization : club

20. BULLDOG : PUGNACITY :: _____ :_____

    A. bloodhound : odor
    B. hen : cowardice
    C. truck : commodious
    D. Pekingese : affectation
    E. greynound : fleetness

21. DEJECTION : FAILED :: _____ :_____

    A. disapproval : approved
    B. emotion: success
    C. dejected : failed
    D. angry : rejected
    E. elation : passed

22. HAZE : LABYRINTH :: _____ :_____

    A. string : labyrinth
    B. matador : bull
    C. alternative : dilemma
    D. riddle : enigma
    E. ancient : sphinx

23. WINE : DREGS :: _____ : _____

    A. wheat : chaff
    B. dress : ore
    C. lead : gold
    D. humanity : dregs
    E. wisdom : cunning

24. WARLIKE : PEACEFUL :: _____ : _____

    A. belligerent : growling
    B. martial : halcyon
    C. warlike : mournful
    D. Mars : sun
    E. worried : soothed

25. SAVAGE : BARBARIAN :: _____ : _____

    A. belief : peaceful
    B. charm : talisman
    C. superstition : talisman
    D. ritual : savage
    E. experiment : antitoxin

KEY (CORRECT ANSWERS)

1.	B	11.	D
2.	B	12.	A
3.	D	13.	E
4.	E	14.	E
5.	E	15.	A
6.	A	16.	E
7.	E	17.	B
8.	D	18.	D
9.	E	19.	A
10.	C	20.	E

21. E
22. D
23. A
24. B
25. C

TEST 3

DIRECTIONS: Each question in this part consists of two capitalized words which have a certain relationship to each other, followed by five lettered pairs of words in small letters. Choose the letter of the pair of words which are related to each other in the SAME way as the words of the capitalized pair are related to each other. *PRINT THE LETTER OF THE CORRECT ANSWER IN THE SPACE AT THE RIGHT.*

1. FLOOD : LEVEE : : _____ : _____   1._____

   A. money : miser   B. stoic : emotion
   C. humility : arrogant   D. dilemma : solution
   E. disorder : police

2. RECONDITE : BULKY :: _____ : _____   2._____

   A. remote : ponderous   B. protracted : laden
   C. distant : momentous   D. hence : pensive
   E. yonder : onerous

3. MATURITY : INFANCY :: _____ : _____   3._____

   A. lamb : cub   B. pod : seed
   C. senility : puerility   D. novice : fundamental
   E. culmination : inception

4. VERSE : POET :: _____ : _____   4._____

   A. art : sculptor   B. statue : sculptor
   C. prelude : musician   D. house : architect
   E. chisel : craftsman

5. FOUNDER : SHIP :: _____ : _____   5._____

   A. fame : disgrace   B. illness : woman
   C. collapse : regime   D. incarcerate : criminal
   E. holocaust : earthquake

6. OBTUSE : ACUTE :: _____ : _____   6._____

   A. knife : blade   B. dull : shrewd
   C. chisel : hammer   D. opaque : transparent
   E. perspicuous : perspicacious

7. CARAT : WEIGHT :: _____ : _____   7._____

   A. fathom : depth   B. rod : farm
   C. speed : knot   D. acre : distance
   E. pennyweight : diamond

8. COMMUNISTS : FASCISTS :: _____ : _____   8._____

   A. Fascists : Nazis   B. red : black
   C. Liberals : Blackshirts D. Whites : Brownshirts
   E. subversive : patriotic

33

9. CARBINE : SOLDIER :: _____ : _____   9.____
   A. marine : sailor   B. pirate : ship
   C. book : writer   D. spear : knight
   E. test tube : chemist

10. HORSE : CARRIAGE : : _____ :_____   10.____
    A. teacher : prodigy   B. coolie : rickshaw
    C. ass : Ford   D. Shetland : pony
    E. hen : egg

11. PROBABLY : PERHAPS ::_____: _____   11.____
    A. rarely : generally   B. necessity : invention
    C. certainly : surely   D. surely : accidentally
    E. incidentally : fortuitous

12. HARDIHOOD : HARDY :: _____ : _____   12.____
    A. egotism : selfish   B. fortitude : force
    C. solitude : indifference D. friendship : friends
    E. great : greater

13. UNTRUTH : LIE :: _____ :_____   13.____
    A. weakness : act   B. prevaricate : deny
    C. homicide : murder   D. accident : assault
    E. hallucination : nightmare

14. MINISTER : CONGREGATION ::_____ : _____   14.____
    A. guide : tourists   B. doctor : patients
    C. scientists : knowledge   D. dean : students
    E. leader : paratroop team

15. PRAISE : DEPRESSION :: _____ : _____   15.____
    A. steam : engine   B. apathy : despair
    C. ulcer : cancer   D. bicarbonate : gastric acidity
    E. hope : despair

16. BROOK : RIVER : : _____ :_____   16.____
    A. island : peninsula   B. cove: bay
    C. lagoon : bay   D. ocean : gulf
    E. stream : outlet

17. BRASS: COPPER : : _____ : _____   17.____
    A. pewter : lead   B. tin : foil
    C. urn : copper   D. zinc : iron
    E. coin : silver

18. ENGINE : CABOOSE : : _____ : _____   18.____
    A. motor : housing   B. introduction : conclusion
    C. cabin : train   D. power : freight
    E. beginning : commencement

19. DIAMOND : CARAT :: _____ : _____   19._____
    A. bullion : silver   B. ring : gold
    C. gold : ore   D. potato : peck
    E. bushel : oat

20. WOODMAN : AXE :: _____ : _____   20._____
    A. mason : awl   B. reader : novel
    C. ploughman : scythe   D. teacher : quadrant
    E. pilot : sextant

21. ARCHEOLOGIST : ANTIQUITY :: _____ : _____   21._____
    A. philologist : stamps   B. entomologist : words
    C. theologian : astronomy   D. ornithologist : horticulture
    E. ichthyologist : marine life

22. SERFDOM : FEUDALISM :: _____ : _____   22._____
    A. taxation : totalitarianism B. independence : agriculture
    C. entrepreneur : laissez-faire D. nationalization : socialism
    E. reedom : dictatorship

23. RAISIN PRUNE :: _____ : _____   23._____
    A. apricot : fig   B. grape : raisin
    C. wine : alcohol   D. privet : barberry
    E. cherry : wine

24. PYRAMID : CUBE :: _____ : _____   24._____
    A. triangle : square   B. square : parallelogram
    C. triangle : cone   D. hexagon : pentagon
    E. cone : cylinder

25. COKE : COAL :: _____ : _____   25._____
    A. steel : iron   B. oxygen : nitrogen
    C. bread : yeast   D. charcoal : wood
    E. skeleton : body

KEY (CORRECT ANSWERS)

1.	E	11.	C
2.	A	12.	A
3.	E	13.	C
4.	B	14.	D
5.	C	15.	D
6.	B	16.	C
7.	A	17.	A
8.	B	18.	B
9.	D	19.	D
10.	B	20.	E

21. E
22. D
23. A
24. A
25. D

TEST 4

DIRECTIONS: Each question in this part consists of two capitalized words which have a certain relationship to each other, followed by five lettered pairs of words in small letters. Choose the letter of the pair of words which are related to each other in the SAME way as the words of the capitalized pair are related to each other. *PRINT THE LETTER OF THE CORRECT ANSWER IN THE SPACE AT THE RIGHT.*

1. EACH : EVERYBODY :: _____ : _____   1.____
   - A. solo : ensemble
   - B. ocean : wave
   - C. ball of wool : skein
   - D. spool : thread
   - E. house : beams

2. NEXT : BY :: _____ : _____   2.____
   - A. wit : approach
   - B. off : from
   - C. contiguous : close
   - D. warmth : glow
   - E. adjacent : sequence

3. TOO : VERY :: _____ : _____   3.____
   - A. potion : beverage
   - B. of : off
   - C. approach : accost
   - D. overdose : heaping measure
   - E. copious : scanty

4. REVEREND : REVERENT :: _____ : _____   4.____
   - A. intend : pretend
   - B. proud : haughty
   - C. respected : respectful
   - D. kneeling : pious
   - E. sycophant : king

5. HEADLONG : IMPETUOSITY :: _____ : _____   5.____
   - A. dry : moderation
   - B. degenerate : perversity
   - C. accident : recklessness
   - D. phlegmatic : stolidity
   - E. quiet : tacit

6. TRULY : FORSOOTE :: _____ : _____   6.____
   - A. really : consequently
   - B. statement : hyperbole
   - C. average : extraordinary
   - D. in fact : indeed
   - E. reality : fiction

7. ON CONDITION THAT : ACCEPTANCE :: _____ : _____   7.____
   - A. granted that : nevertheless
   - B. except : consent
   - C. relying upon : enmity
   - D. provided that : agreement
   - E. in accordance with : depending

8. NAMELY : FOR EXAMPLE :: _____ : _____   8.____
   - A. like : i.e.
   - B. that is : such as
   - C. for instance : especially
   - D. to wit : thus
   - E. viz. : ibid.

2 (#4)

9. NECESSITY : INVENTION :: _____ : _____   9. _____
   A. because : out   B. emergency : effect
   C. luxury : lethargy   D. hardship : luck
   E. opulence : affluence

10. PARAPHRASE : VERBATIM :: _____ : _____   10. _____
    A. imitate : lampoon   B. quotation : allusion
    C. caricature : portrait   D. similarity : likeness
    E. likeness : sketch

11. MAN : CONSCIENCE :: _____ : _____   11. _____
    A. imitate : lampoon   B. quotation : allusion
    C. caricature : portrait   D. similarity : likeness
    E. likeness : sketch

12. PICTURE : PAINTER :: _____ : _____   12. _____
    A. cement : bricklayer   B. friendship : stranger
    C. cure : doctor   D. magic : magician
    E. wall : mason

13. CANARY : CAGE :: _____ : _____   13. _____
    A. pugilist : ring   B. poodle : kennel
    C. tiger : zoo   D. bird : nest
    E. fish : tackle

14. MOUNTAIN : VALLEY :: _____ : _____   14. _____
    A. lake:river   B. country:state
    C. order:cancel   D. peak:gorge
    E. pla eap:plain

15. MACHINE : JAM :: _____ : _____   15. _____
    A. stone : crack   B. pain : throb
    C. order : cancel   D. muscle : cramp
    E. lightning : flash

16. TOUCH : GRASP :: _____ : _____   16. _____
    A. watch : search   B. Took : see
    C. ponder : examine   D. eye : sight
    E. glance : scrutinize

17. TAX : EXEMPTION :: _____ : _____   17. _____
    A. obligation : debt   B. custom : conformity
    C. disease : immunity   D. change : adaptation
    E. transgression : pardon

18. IRREGULAR : SYMMETRICAL :: _____ : _____   18. _____
    A. oblong : square   B. trapezoid : parallel
    C. coastline : statue   D. area : perimeter
    E. solid : sphere

19. EVENT : PROPHECY :: _____ : _____   19._____
    A. disaster : premonition   B. fact : opinion
    C. religion : faith   D. life : dream
    E. expectation : hope

20. CURRENT : SWITCH :: _____ : _____   20._____
    A. rope : pulley   B. drawer : handle
    C. light : bulb   D. bullet : trigger
    E. gun : holster   F.

21. ALWAYS : NEVER :: _____ : _____   21._____
    A. happy : sad   B. frequently : seldom
    C. never : always   D. intermittently : occasionally
    E. constantly : ubiquitously

22. NEVADA : JAVA :: _____ : _____   22._____
    A. clever : shrewd   B. bald : stupid
    C. obtuse : acute   D. California : New York
    E. sparse : dense

23. LIBERAL : CONSERVATIVE :: _____ : _____ 23._____
    A. Socialist : Monarchist   B. Whig : Tory
    C. Democrat : Republican   D. patriot : traitor
    E. Republican : Conservative

24. SPEAKER : HECKLER :: _____ : _____   24._____
    A. song : vocalist   B. cow : matador
    C. bull : picador   D. victim : executioner
    E. E. eye : mote

25. PIG : PORK :: _____ : _____   25._____
    A. youth : age   B. sheep : lamb
    C. beef : steer   D. beef : veal
    E. sheep : mutton

KEY (CORRECT ANSWERS)

1.	A	11.	D
2.	C	12.	E
3.	D	13.	B
4.	C	14.	E
5.	D	15.	D
6.	D	16.	E
7.	D	17.	C
8.	B	18.	C
9.	C	19.	A
10.	C	20.	D

21. B
22. E
23. B
24. C
25. E

TEST 5

DIRECTIONS: Each question in this part consists of two capitalized words which have a certain relationship to each other, followed by five lettered pairs of words in small letters. Choose the letter of the pair of words which are related to each other in the SAME way as the words of the capitalized pair are related to each other. *PRINT THE LETTER OF THE CORRECT ANSWER IN THE SPACE AT THE RIGHT.*

1. BIRDS : AVIARY :: _____ : _____ 1.____
   - A. apiary : bees
   - B. grain : barn
   - C. bus : depot
   - D. subway : kiosk
   - E. ships : drydock

2. BULLION : COIN :: _____ : _____ 2.____
   - A. wool : suit
   - B. voice : words
   - C. mint : money
   - D. soup : dessert
   - E. print : periodical

3. PROGNOSIS : DISEASE :: _____ : _____ 3.____
   - A. medicine : illness
   - B. cause : disaster
   - C. hypothesis : problem
   - D. forecast : humidity
   - E. warning : detour

4. CONDEMN : COMPLAIN :: _____ : _____ 4.____
   - A. laugh : titter
   - B. jail : sentence
   - C. sigh : weep
   - D. laughter : anger
   - E. brightness : fancy

5. WEEPING : PUNISHMENT :: _____ : _____ 5.____
   - A. grief : sadness
   - B. dying : grave
   - C. peace : lose
   - D. evil : chastisement
   - E. self-satisfaction : praise

6. FROM : TO :: _____ : _____ 6.____
   - A. hardship : emergency
   - B. apparently : really
   - C. by : of
   - D. angrily : satirically
   - E. off : down

7. RATHER : QUITE :: _____ : _____ 7.____
   - A. apparently : secretly
   - B. fault : guilt
   - C. more : less
   - D. nearly : hardly
   - E. guilt : punishment

8. IRRETRIEVABLE : MISLAID :: _____ : _____ 8.____
   - A. smashed : cracked
   - B. mend : break
   - C. found : lost
   - D. present : gone
   - E. invisible : seen

9. ARCHITECT : HOUSE :: _____ : _____   9.____
   A. general : army   B. farm : produce
   C. priest : religion   D. conspirators : plot
   E. government : people

10. WHEEL : CIRCLE :: _____ : _____   10.____
   A. sphere : triangle   B. square : house
   C. orange : sphere   D. round : sphere
   E. round : orange

KEY (CORRECT ANSWERS)

1. C   6. B
2. A   7. B
3. C   8. A
4. A   9. D
5. E   10. C

VERBAL ANALOGIES 2 BLANKS

EXAMINATION SECTION
TEST 1

DIRECTIONS: Each question in this part consists of two capitalized words which have a certain relationship to each other, followed by five lettered pairs of words in small letters. Choose the letter of the pair of words which are related to each other in the SAME way the words of the capitalized pair are related to each other. *PRINT THE LETTER OF THE CORRECT ANSWER IN THE SPACE AT THE RIGHT.*

1. DISCRETE : ABRIDGED :: _____ : _____   1._____

    A. quotes : parentheses B. decimal : fraction
    C. separation : partition D. hyphenated : abbreviated
    E. separated : slang

2. COURT : DESERT :: _____ : _____   2._____

    A. boar : camel B. diversion : pachyderm
    C. fig : forest D. droll : dromedary
    E. plant : person

3. RECORDS : FILE :: _____ : _____   3._____

    A. stipend : income B. wall : plug
    C. socket : bulb D. stocks : bonds
    E. savings : bank

4. FURROW : PLOW :: _____ : _____   4._____

    A. sign : street B. route : avenue C. orbit : earth
    D. ring : bull E. crash : aeroplane

5. FAMILY : CHILDREN :: _____ : _____   5._____

    A. party : guests B. clan : crest C. flag : country
    D. club : members E. feline : cat

6. RECIDIVISTIC : PRUDENT :: _____ : _____   6._____

    A. period : proper B. cadence : credo
    C. impoverished : wealthy D. depraved : respectful
    E. decadent : circumspect

7. PARTITION : SERIES :: _____ : _____   7._____

    A. enclosing : parieta B. division : rescission
    C. septum : spectrum D. wall : ghastly
    E. fencing : parading

8. SEISMOGRAPH : EARTHQUAKE :: _____ : _____   8._____

    A. barometer : temperature B. thermometer : pressure
    C. fluoroscope : tuberculosis D. lubritorium : laboratory
    E. x-ray : pulsation

9. ELECTRICITY : ILLUMINATION :: _____ : _____

    A. gravity : force
    B. water : power
    C. sieve : straining
    D. stroke : brush
    E. atomic : bomb

10. DEMEANOR : CHARACTER :: _____ : _____

    A. innate : temperament
    B. distinguished : personified
    C. singer : song
    D. tenor : type
    E. aspect : acuity

11. INSTINCT : BEAST :: _____ : _____

    A. reason : rationale
    B. mind : brain
    C. thought : process
    D. intelligence : man
    E. rattle : snake

12. ROMANTIC : PRACTICAL :: _____ : _____

    A. weak : strong
    B. inspired : clumsy
    C. quixotic : realistic
    D. light : heavy
    E. surface : depth

13. REPRESSION : AWARENESS :: _____ : _____

    A. passivity : activity
    B. sleep : dream
    C. forget : remember
    D. coma : comatose
    E. unconscious ; conscious

14. PREDISPOSITION : RELATIONSHIP :: _____ : _____

    A. prepossession : prediction
    B. atom : combination
    C. impartiality : partiality
    D. predilection : affinity
    E. affiliation : preponderance

15. STORM : HURRICANE :: _____ : _____

    A. disease : germ
    B. fear : panic
    C. ship : sank
    D. courage : hero
    E. solitude : hermit

16. SUPPLY : DEMAND :: _____ : _____

    A. cost : market
    B. price : value
    C. wholesale : retail
    D. net : worth
    E. tax : article

17. CAMOUFLAGE : GUERRILLA :: _____ : _____

    A. radar : instrument
    B. painter : anonymity
    C. cocoon : butterfly
    D. costume : masquerader
    E. color : ship

18. LENS : CAMERA :: _____ : _____

    A. toe : foot
    B. beacon : lighthouse
    C. eye : mind
    D. head : body
    E. vision : thought

19. CRUTCHES : MOVEMENT :: _____ : _____   19.____

    A. windows : houses   B. defect : myopic
    C. glasses : vision   D. teeth : braces
    E. telescope : astronomer

20. MILES : AUTOMOBILES :: _____ : _____   20.____

    A. sea : fathoms   B. suits : divers   C. knots : ships
    D. gasoline : aeroplane E. milligram : gram

21. NOMINATION : CONVENTION :: _____ : _____   21.____

    A. judge : sentence   B. panel : member   C. verdict : jury
    D. criminal : crime   E. policeman : arrest

22. FACET : GEM :: _____ : _____   22.____

    A. intelligence : test   B. father : son
    C. brilliance : genius   D. heredity : environment
    E. constellation : star

23. ABSTRUSE : OBTUSE :: _____ :   23.____

    A. concave : convex   B. erudition : profundity
    C. dull : translucent   D. abstract : realistic
    E. recondite : opaque

24. TURNSTILE : SUBWAY :: _____ : _____   24.____

    A. ticket : aeroplane B. price : goods   C. desk : office
    D. door : taxicab   E. porthole : ship

25. CAGE : CANARY :: _____ : _____   25.____

    A. walls : jail   B. warden : prison   C. cell : inmate
    D. jungle : lion   E. patient : hospital

KEY (CORRECT ANSWERS)

1.	D	11.	D
2.	D	12.	C
3.	E	13.	E
4.	C	14.	D
5.	D	15.	B
6.	E	16.	B
7.	C	17.	D
8.	C	18.	C
9.	B	19.	C
10.	D	20.	C

21. C
22. C
23. E
24. D
25. C

TEST 2

DIRECTIONS: Each question in this part consists of two capitalized words which have a certain relationship to each other, followed by five lettered pairs of words in small letters. Choose the letter of the pair of words which are related to each other in the SAME way as the words of the capitalized pair are related to each other. *PRINT THE LETTER OF THE CORRECT ANSWER IN THE SPACE AT THE RIGHT.*

1. PSEUDONYM : ASSUMED NAME :: _____ : _____   1._____
    - A. nomenclature : title
    - B. appellation : given name
    - C. nom de plume : pen name
    - D. surname : first name
    - E. title : aristocrat

2. PECK : BUSHEL :: _____ : _____   2._____
    - A. dram : ton
    - B. rod : pound
    - C. gill : fathom
    - D. gallon : cord
    - E. ounce : inch

3. ABDICATE : KING :: _____ : _____   3._____
    - A. track : train
    - B. derail : engineer
    - C. execute : warden
    - D. crash : aeroplane
    - E. revolution : anarchist

4. SECURE : WITHDRAW :: _____ : _____   4._____
    - A. anchor : anchorite
    - B. ship : mausoleum
    - C. sailor : salacious
    - D. secrete : drop
    - E. article : manufacturer

5. MATHEMATICAL : VERBAL :: _____ : _____   5._____
    - A. numbers : equation
    - B. quotient : proportion
    - C. ratio : analogy
    - D. fraction : word
    - E. computation : anagram

6. SEASONING : THYME :: _____ : _____   6._____
    - A. space : season
    - B. hybrid : herb
    - C. measure : mite
    - D. predict : plant
    - E. time : season

7. VOLATILE : TACITURN :: _____ : _____   7._____
    - A. planet : position
    - B. mercurial : saturnine
    - C. Mercury : Saturn
    - D. mood : fluid
    - E. undependable : stolid

8. HEAD : AX :: _____ : _____   8._____
    - A. pine : cone
    - B. close : call
    - C. cylinder : engine
    - D. chair : rung
    - E. angle : line

9. BEAM : SEARCHLIGHT :: _____ : _____   9._____
    - A. tank : oil
    - B. flame : welder
    - C. torch : fire
    - D. film : projector
    - E. forest : timber

10. CONSPIRE : CABAL :: _____ : _____   10._____
    - A. scheme : expedite
    - B. contrivance : contrive
    - C. machinate : plot
    - D. conspiracy : intrigue
    - E. object : plan

47

11. LAW : PROMULGATION :: _____ : _____
    A. voting : election
    B. interview : census
    C. decision : declaration
    D. battle : war
    E. idea : action

12. MEMBER : SOCIETY :: _____ : _____
    A. molecule : amoeba
    B. growth : osmosis
    C. cell : organism
    D. disease : parasite
    E. leg : foot

13. HIPPOCRATIC OATH : PHYSICIAN :: _____ : _____
    A. fealty : fief
    B. citizenship : alien
    C. allegiance : citizen
    D. contract : marriage
    E. covenant : treaty

14. SKIS : SNOW :: _____ : _____
    A. cork : water
    B. rain : umbrellas
    C. clouds : sky
    D. shoes : feet
    E. parachutes : air

15. TASTE : SMELL :: _____ : _____
    A. touch : hand
    B. sight : hearing
    C. ears : eyes
    D. hearing aid : eye-glasses
    E. aural : oral

16. SORCERY : PRESTIDIGITATOR :: _____ : _____
    A. magic : demonology
    B. witchcraft : entomologist
    C. conjure : spirit
    D. astrology : astrologist
    E. fetishism : palmist

17. YOUTH : IMPULSIVE :: _____ : _____
    A. juvenile : puerile
    B. characteristic : degree
    C. adolescence : childhood
    D. soil : erosion
    E. age : senile

18. SATISFACTION : DISQUIETUDE :: _____ : _____
    A. chaos : satisfaction
    B. doubt : security
    C. dissatisfaction : friction
    D. civilization : jungle
    E. complacent : restive

19. GASLIGHT : ELECTRICITY :: _____ : _____
    A. jet : aeroplane
    B. fiction : science
    C. loud : gift
    D. obsolete : extant
    E. horse : carriage

20. HYPOTHETICAL : FORMULATED :: _____ : _____
    A. method : science
    B. irrational : deranged
    C. insanity : sanity
    D. vagary : rationality
    E. animal : machine

21. OATH : PERJURY :: _____ : _____
    A. truth : oath
    B. perfidy : imposture
    C. promise : renege
    D. inviolability : swear
    E. inaccuracy : falsity

22. PROSAIC : AESTHETIC :: _____ : _____
    A. dull : beautiful
    B. lethargic : ambitious
    C. behavior : feeling
    D. humorous : brilliant
    E. judicious : sensitivity

23. OPERATION : SURGEON :: _____ : _____
    A. philately : necromancer
    B. student : study
    C. pyromaniac : fire
    D. embezzlement : thief
    E. murderer : homicide

24. BEIGE : BROWN : : _____ : _____
    A. primary : secondary
    B. hue : value
    C. shade : color
    D. yellow : gold
    E. red : pink

25. CLOTH : DESIGNER :: _____ : _____
    A. clay : model
    B. statue : sculptor
    C. brush : palette
    D. paint : artist
    E. painting : canvas

KEY (CORRECT ANSWERS)

1. C
2. A
3. B
4. A
5. C

6. E
7. B
8. C
9. D
10. C

11. C
12. C
13. C
14. E
15. B

16. D
17. E
18. E
19. D
20. D

21. C
22. A
23. D
24. C
25. D

TEST 3

DIRECTIONS: Each question in this part consists of two capitalized words which have a certain relationship to each other, followed by five lettered pairs of words in small letters. Choose the letter of the pair of words which are related to each other in the SAME way the words of the capitalized pair are related to each other. *PRINT THE LETTER OF THE CORRECT ANSWER IN THE SPACE AT THE RIGHT.*

1. RUPEE : INDIA :: _____ : _____
   A. peseta : Cuba
   B. drachma : Hong Kong
   C. escudo : Spain
   D. franc : France
   E. krona : Czechoslavakia

   1. ___

2. REDUCTION : REMOVAL :: _____ : _____ .
   A. abate : abstruse
   B. dwindle : inattentive
   C. decree : summarize
   D. diminution : difficult
   E. contraction : abstraction

   2. ___

3. STYLIZED : FACTUAL :: _____ : _____
   A. question : fact
   B. abstract : equation
   C. rhetorical : pragmatical
   D. florid : dogma
   E. doctrinaire : philosophy

   3. ___

4. REFLECTOR : SIGHT :: _____ : _____
   A. color wheel : rotation
   B. vision : eyeglasses
   C. mirror : image
   D. compendium : exhibit
   E. spectrum : spectacles

   4. ___

5. GENE : GENDER :: _____ : _____
   A. corporeal : body
   B. paper : wood
   C. factor : characteristic
   D. composition : author
   E. ventricle : heart

   5. ___

6. STRONGHOLD : MUNICIPALITY :: _____ : _____
   A. state : capital
   B. citadel : city
   C. fortress : command
   D. protected : protector
   E. strategic : locale

   6. ___

7. HYDROGEN : WATER :: _____ : _____
   A. organic : compound
   B. dextrose : glucose
   C. coal : carbon
   D. liquid : solid
   E. pure : impure

   7. ___

8. ARRAY : MEDITATION :: _____ : _____
   A. image : idea
   B. spectrum : speculation
   C. varying : thought
   D. sequence : continuous
   E. reflecting : reflect

   8. ___

9. BUDDHISM : MOHAMMEDANISM :: _____ : _____
   A. Islamic : Utopia
   B. Hindu : Arabian
   C. heaven : center
   D. nirvana : mecca
   E. fantasy : reality

   9. ___

10. NOTICE : APPEASE :: _____ : _____
    A. pacific : pacify
    B. placard : placate
    C. poster : propaganda
    D. agreement : compromise
    E. place : please

    10. ___

11. WEEK : MONTH :: _____ : _____
    A. month : day   B. foot : inch   C. hour : clock
    D. vacation : holiday E. Sunday : July

12. CANOE : RIVER :: _____ : _____
    A. element : vehicle B. ride : winter   C. ice : skate
    D. sleigh : snow   E. hounds : ranger

13. MINERAL : REPTILE :: _____ : _____
    A. lizard : lair   B. ocean : amphibian C. stone : snake
    D. mummy : body   E. water : goldfish

14. MAN : BEE :: _____ : _____
    A. domestic : habitat   B. abode : hiatus
    C. domicile : hive   D. ant : hill
    E. sanctuary : wilderness

15. PATIENT : PHYSICIAN :: _____ : _____
    A. jury : judge   B. audience : actor   C. client : attorney
    D. customer : store   E. adviser : advised

16. PIANO : SCALE :: _____ : _____
    A. violin : music   B. range : singer
    C. instrument : octave   D. one : seven
    E. stanza : poem

17. MAN : BROTHER :: _____ : _____
    A. death : dishonor   B. homicide : fratricide
    C. father : son   D. murder : man
    E. child : murder

18. ARM : HEAD :: _____ : _____
    A. leg : temple   B. brain : foot   C. hole : bullet
    D. head : neck   E. break : concussion

19. SEW : CLOTH :: _____ : _____
    A. staple : machine   B. sharpener : pencil
    C. stamp : letter   D. clip : paper
    E. stamp : mail

20. PAPER : BODY :: _____ : _____
    A. break : crack   B. arm cast
    C. bruise : heal   D. tear : wound
    E. rip mend

21. PLUCK : CHICKEN :: _____ : _____
    A. wood : fire   B. goat : milk   C. skin : snake
    D. fur : bear   E. feather : ostrich

22. SAIL : BOAT : : _____ : _____ 22._____

    A. pinwheel : toy B. pilot : controls C. wing : aeroplane
    D. fender : automobile E. ski shoes : skis

23. VIBRATION : LIGHT :: _____ : _____ 23._____

    A. sound : reflection B. symphony : color wheel
    C. intensity : pitch D. music : color
    E. rhyme : harmony

24. REBELLION : GOVERNMENT :: _____ : _____ 24._____

    A. motion : meeting B. discord : partisan
    C. dissent : group D. disbanding : party
    E. commitment : withdrawl

25. GREGARIOUSNESS : ASCETICISM :: _____ : _____ 25._____

    A. denial : acceptance B. austere : sensuous
    C. monastery : monk D. conviviality : seclusion
    E. secluded : remote

KEY (CORRECT ANSWERS)

1.	D	11.	E
2.	E	12.	D
3.	C	13.	C
4.	E	14.	C
5.	C	15.	C
6.	B	16.	C
7.	B	17.	B
8.	B	18.	E
9.	D	19.	D
10.	B	20.	D

21. C
22. C
23. D
24. C
25. D

TEST 4

DIRECTIONS: Each question in this part consists of two capitalized words which have a certain relationship to each other, followed by five lettered pairs of words in small letters. Choose the letter of the pair of words which are related to each other in the SAME way the words of the capitalized pair are related to each other. *PRINT THE LETTER OF THE CORRECT ANSWER IN THE SPACE AT THE RIGHT.*

1. BURY : DISINTER :: _____ : _____   1.____
   - A. inhale : exhale
   - B. inhume : exhume
   - C. corporeal : spirit
   - D. autopsy : funeral
   - E. burial : cremation

2. INVOLUNTARY : VOLUNTARY :: _____ : _____   2.____
   - A. criminal : soldier
   - B. export : import
   - C. illegal : legal
   - D. deportation : expatriation
   - E. punishment : crime

3. IGNITE : FIRE :: _____ : _____   3.____
   - A. water : flood
   - B. ax : tree
   - C. incite : revolt
   - D. mass : riot
   - E. flame : gasoline

4. LEDGER : BOOKKEEPER _____ : _____   4.____
   - A. fort : cavalry
   - B. compass : direction
   - C. log : captain
   - D. deck : crew
   - E. biography : historian

5. SPACE : TIME :: _____ : _____   5.____
   - A. locale : situation
   - B. geography : history
   - C. navigation : course
   - D. individual : ancestry
   - E. dimension : depth

6. STRAITS : GIBRALTAR :: _____ : _____   6.____
   - A. island : coast
   - B. ocean : Atlantic
   - C. peninsula : Malta
   - D. cape : Africa
   - E. Danube : river

7. HERD : CATTLE :: _____ : _____   7.____
   - A. sled : snow
   - B. team : dogs
   - C. race : horse
   - D. people : group
   - E. sheep : flock

8. ELECT : GOVERNOR :: _____ : _____   8.____
   - A. office : appoint
   - B. administer : administration
   - C. position : order
   - D. inauguration : president
   - E. deputize : deputy

9. COMBINATION : SAFE :: _____ : _____   9.____
   - A. raise : window
   - B. key : door
   - C. nail : picture
   - D. hanger : coat
   - E. latch : key

10. SALT : SHAKER :: _____ : _____   10.____
    - A. minute : time
    - B. bottle : milk
    - C. sand : hourglass
    - D. sun dial : sun M
    - E. ship : ocean

11. STORY : SENTENCE :: _____ : _____   11.____
    - A. poem : rhyme
    - B. chant : paean
    - C. hymn : note
    - D. brushstroke : painting
    - E. song : music

2 (#4)

12. LOOSE : DISCIPLINE :: _____ : _____   12.____
    A. lazy : perfect   B. individual : political
    C. dinner : banquet   D. order : disorder
    E. lax : protocol

13. CREST : CLAN :: _____ : _____   13.____
    A. judge : robe   B. road : sign   C. insignia : army
    D. fairy : wand   E. king : scepter

14. PENULTIMATE : ULTIMATE :: _____ : _____   14.____
    A. among : between   B. first : second
    C. perfect : excellent   D. better : best
    E. more : many

15. WORSEN : WITHDRAW :: _____ : _____   15.____
    A. regress : egress   B. down : up   C. fantasy : reality
    D. swing : gate   E. retrogress : digress

16. CEREMONY : CORRECT :: _____ : _____   16.____
    A. manner : might   B. rite : right   C. kinsman : kind
    D. inauguration : irate   E. sworn : swerve

17. CHALLENGE : CONTEST :: _____ : _____   17.____
    A. sprint : pistol   B. fencing : sport   C. hat : ring
    D. insult : duel   E. sword : rapier

18. WORM : SNAKE :: _____ : _____   18.____
    A. shark : whale   B. lion : tamer   C. cat : mouse
    D. cat : panther   E. shark : carnivorous

19. INDIFFERENCE : UNDERSTANDING :: _____ : _____   19.____
    A. sympathy : identification   B. peasant : worker
    C. apathy : empathy   D. peon : peonage
    E. happiness : sadness

20. INCIPIENT : RUDIMENTARY :: _____ : _____   20.____
    A. disappearing : appearing   B. plant : seed
    C. inchoate : embryonic   D. unknown : unseen
    E. death : birth

21. SEASONING : HERB :: _____ : _____   21.____
    A. saccharine : sugar   B. candy : dextrose
    C. condiment : thyme   D. synthetic : genuine
    E. natural : manufactured

22. SIMULATED : GENUINE :: _____ : _____   22.____
    A. semi-precious : precious   B. bullion : gold
    C. pretense : fraud   D. rhinestone : diamond
    E. private : general

23. FLOWER : PETAL :: _____ : _____

   A. sprout : potato
   B. seed : plant
   C. tree : branch
   D. root : earth
   E. moss : stone

24. DESERT : OCEAN :: _____ : _____

   A. illness : death
   B. parch : thirst
   C. abundance : surfeit
   D. suffocation : evaporation
   E. dehydrate : drown

25. STANZA : CHAPTER :: _____ : _____

   A. art : fiction
   B. meter : rhyme
   C. narration : style
   D. poetry : prose
   E. clause : sentence

KEY (CORRECT ANSWERS)

1.	B	11.	C
2.	D	12.	E
3.	C	13.	C
4.	C	14.	D
5.	B	15.	A
6.	B	16.	B
7.	B	17.	D
8.	E	18.	D
9.	B	19.	C
10.	C	20.	C

21. C
22. D
23. C
24. E
25. D

TEST 5

DIRECTIONS: Each question in this part consists of two capitalized words which have a certain relationship to each other, followed by five lettered pairs of words in small letters. Choose the letter of the pair of words which are related to each other in the SAME way the words of the capitalized pair are related to each other. *PRINT THE LETTER OF THE CORRECT ANSWER IN THE SPACE AT THE RIGHT.*

1. DOGMATIC : VACILLATORY :: _____ : _____   1._____
    A. absolute relative   B. all : few   C. certain : decisive
    D. affinity infinity   E. pure : contaminated

2. LINE : CURVE : _____ : _____   2._____
    A. perimeter : parallel   B. hypotenuse : rectangle
    C. earth : equator   D. diameter : circumference
    E. semi-circle : circle

3. BOWL : BALL : : _____ : _____   3._____
    A. up : down   B. hemisphere : globe
    C. concave : convex   D. earth : cave
    E. bulging and curved : hollow and curved

4. WIND : CYCLONE :: _____ : _____   4._____
    A. river : ocean   B. exhaust : fume   C. suffocate : drown
    D. water : deluge   E. pressure : atmosphere

5. LION : JUNGLE :: _____ : _____   5._____
    A. faun : deer   B. plant : flower   C. fauna : flora
    D. seaweed : octopus   E. cow : milk

6. SUBTERRANEAN : SURFACE :: _____ : _____   6._____
    A. road : sea   B. league : fathom   C. ship : car
    D. depth : distance   E. diver : driver

7. IMPASSIVE : INFLATED :: _____ : _____   7._____
    A. pain : noise   B. enthusiasm : exuberance
    C. stoical : bombastic   D. mediocre : outstanding
    E. hermit : pedant

8. PRODUCT : MULTIPLICATION :: _____ : _____   8._____
    A. multiplication : table   B. add : arithmetic
    C. part : whole   D. words : sentence
    E. sum : addition

9. DECIMAL : COMMA : : _____ : _____   9._____
    A. sum : fraction   B. number : word   C. letter : fraction
    D. period : sentence   E. clause : ratio

10. ANARCHIST : PATRIOT :: _____ : _____   10._____
    A. iconoclast : chauvinist   B. agnostic : heretic
    C. soldier : revolutionary   D. topple : government
    E. Loyalist : Tory

56

2 (#5)

11. SPEED : SOUND :: _____ : _____ 11._____
    A. linear : dimension   B. fathom : ocean   C. time : hour
    D. velocity : light   E. force : gravity

12. SUBURB : CITY :: _____ : _____ 12._____
    A. peasant : peon   B. prince : pauper
    C. provincial : urban   D. capital : state
    E. town : country

13. VELOCITY : WIND :: _____ : _____ 13._____
    A. economy : gross national product   B. element : temperament
    C. variable : constant   D. same : change
    E. fluctuation : rate

14. WIRE : TELEPHONE :: _____ : _____ 14._____
    A. refrigerator : freezer   B. bookcase : book
    C. telephone : dial   D. bureau : drawer
    E. ribbon : typewriter

15. TRAIN : DEPOT :: _____ : _____ 15._____
    A. cow : barn   B. traveler : destination
    C. baseball : home plate   D. bus : terminal
    E. field : hangar

KEY (CORRECT ANSWERS)

1. A   6. E
2. D   7. C
3. C   8. E
4. D   9. B
5. C   10. A

11. D
12. C
13. C
14. E
15. D

EXAMINATION SECTION
TEST 1

DIRECTIONS: Each question or incomplete statement is followed by several suggested answers or completions. Select the one that BEST answers the question or completes the statement. *PRINT THE LETTER OF THE CORRECT ANSWER IN THE SPACE AT THE RIGHT.*

1. All of the following secrete digestive enzymes EXCEPT the   1.____

   A. pancreas
   B. salivary glands
   C. stomach
   D. small intestine
   E. liver

2. Soon after fertilization, the dividing zygote of the amphibian forms a hollow ball of cells surrounding a central cavity.   2.____
   This stage in development is called the

   A. morula
   B. blastula
   C. gastrula
   D. primitive streak
   E. fetus

3. The two products of the *light reactions* of photosynthesis that are required for the synthetic *dark reactions* are ATP and   3.____

   A. carbon dioxide
   B. the reduced form of coenzyme NADP
   C. oxygen
   D. glucose
   E. ribulose-1, 5-bisphosphate (RuBP)

4. Vertebrate skeletal muscle is able to contact as a result of muscle membrane depolarization due to the action of   4.____

   A. neurotransmitters
   B. Ca^{2+} ions
   C. actin and myosin
   D. phosphocreatine
   E. myoglobin

5. Assuming that all are of the same size, which of the following fishes would you expect to produce the *greatest* volume of urine per unit time?   5.____

   A. Bony fish living in freshwater
   B. Bony fish living in an estuary
   C. Bony fish living in the ocean
   D. Shark living in the ocean
   E. All about the same

6. One of the functions of light in the process of photosynthesis is to

    A. raise the energy level of electrons
    B. cause the formation of water
    C. cause the formation of ribulose-diphosphate
    D. fix CO_2
    E. oxidize NADP (nicotinamide adenine dinucleotide phosphate)

7. In mammalian embryonic development, the embryo proper develops from the

    A. trophoblast
    B. amnion
    C. inner cell mass
    D. primary yolk sac
    E. placenta

8. Hydrogen bonds

    A. have bond energy about equal to covalent bonds
    B. have bond energy much larger than covalent bonds
    C. are important in maintaining protein conformations
    D. are too weak to be of importance in biological molecules
    E. are any bonds between hydrogen and another atom

9. The MAIN function of the nucleolus is to

    A. direct the transcriptive activities of the nucleus
    B. coordinate the replication of chromosomal DNA
    C. synthesize components of the nuclear membrane
    D. synthesize ribosomal RNA
    E. regulate the condensation of chromosomes as the cell approaches metaphase

10. Which of the following would tend to shift a population out of Hardy-Weinberg equilibrium?

    A. Barriers to migration
    B. Prevention of mutation
    C. Population size increase
    D. Prevention of genetic drift
    E. Preferential mating

11. In the modern understanding of the concept of natural selection, the fittest individuals are those who

    A. produce the largest number of progeny
    B. are adapted to the widest diversity of environments
    C. produce most highly variable offspring
    D. survive for the largest number of years
    E. have the largest number of fertile offspring

12. Recombinant DNA technology uses which of the following to cleave DNA molecules into polynucleotide fragments?

    A. Reverse transcriptases
    B. DNA topoisomerases
    C. Restriction enzymes
    D. Plasmids or episomes
    E. Recombinases

13. During the development of a typical vertebrate embryo, the mesoderm germ layer produces the following series of structures: 13.____

    A. Epidermis, nails, and hair
    B. Dermis, blood vessels, and vertebrae
    C. Neural tube, brain and cranial nerves
    D. Lining of the gut, liver, and pancreas
    E. All of the above

14. The stem length of pea plants is genetically determined by a pair of alleles, *T* for tall and *t* for short. *T* is completely dominant over *t*.   14.____
    If the gene frequency for *T* is 0.9 in a given population, what will be the frequency of short-stemmed pea plants in the population?

    A. 0.1   B. 0.01   C. 0.5   D. 0.05   E. 0.15

15. The pituitary gland is attached to and secretes its hormones in response to neurahormonal stimulation from the   15.____

    A. thalamus   B. hypothalamus
    C. cerebrum   D. medullaoblongata
    E. cerebellum

16. To say that the genetic code is *degenerate* means that   16.____

    A. a given codon may specify more than one amino acid
    B. a given amino acid may be specified by more than one codon
    C. some of the codons are nonsense codons
    D. the code is nonoverlapping
    E. nonsense suppressor mutations occur in tRNA genes

17. When mammalian eyes become accommodated for close vision, the   17.____

    A. ciliary muscles are contracted and the lens becomes more convex
    B. ciliary muscles are relaxed and the lens becomes more convex
    C. ciliary muscles are contracted and the lens becomes flattened
    D. ciliary muscles are relaxed and the lens becomes flattened
    E. eyeball undergoes auteroposterior shortening

18. The movement of materials across a cell membrane from a region of low concentration to a region of high concentration   18.____

    A. is termed free diffusion
    B. occurs only in osmosis
    C. requires the expenditure of energy
    D. is termed faciliated diffusion
    E. none of the above

19. The liver of the mammal has many important functions. One function is the synthesis of a nitrogen waste product in the form of   19.____

    A. ammonia   B. urea   C. nitrates
    D. nitric acid   E. nitrous oxide

20. Which of the following organs plays a major role in the immune function?

    A. Thyroid   B. Pituitary   C. Pancreas
    D. Pineal   E. Thymus

21. The phylum chordata is usually judged to be *most closely* related to the

    A. Arthropoda   B. Annelida
    C. Echinodermata   D. Mollusca
    E. Coelenterata

22. The organelle MOST involved in the energy-producing functions of the cell is the

    A. nucleus   B. Golgi complex
    C. ER   D. mitochondrion
    E. ribosome

23. A feature common to the chromosomes of both prokaryotic and eukaryotic cells is the

    A. presence of DNA and histones in about equal amounts
    B. circularity of the DNA molecules
    C. involvement of DNA polymerase in chromosomal replication
    D. presence of the pyrimidines uracil and cytosine
    E. location of the chromosomes within a cell

24. Which of the following is homeothermic?

    A. Pisces   B. Amphibia   C. Aves
    D. Reptilia   E. Insects

25. Mammalian somatic motor neurons

    A. leave the spinal cord via the ventral root
    B. enter the spinal cord via the dorsal root
    C. innervate pressure receptors in muscle
    D. have their cell bodies outside the spinal cord
    E. innervate visceral organs

26. If a portion of a DNA base sequence is G-A-T, the complementary portion of a mRNA base sequence must be

    A. C-T-A   B. C-T-U   C. C-U-A
    D. G-A-T   E. C-U-U

27. The amylase present in saliva is *most likely* to be involved in the digestion of which component of a bacon, lettuce and tomato sandwich?

    A. Bacon   B. Lettuce   C. Tomato
    D. Bun   E. Butter

28. INITIAL SOLUTION CONCENTRATIONS

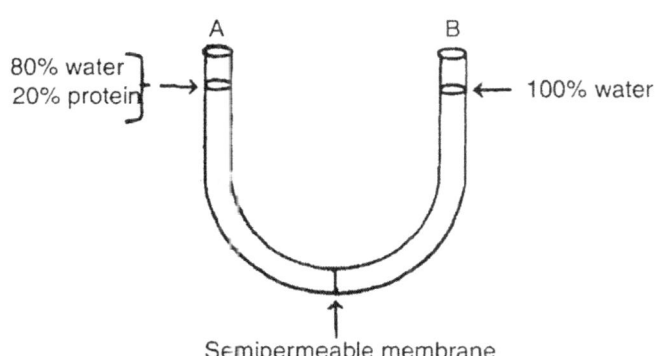

In the U-shaped tube with a semipermeable membrane separating Solution A from Solution B in the diagram on the preceding page, the water level will

A. rise inside A, because water will pass from the area of greater concentration of water to the area of lesser concentration of water
B. rise inside B, because water will pass from the area of lesser concentration of water to the area of greater concentration of water
C. rise inside B as the protein concentration equalizes on both sides
D. remain the same because atmospheric pressure is equal on both sides of the system

29. All of the solar energy that is converted by photosynthesis into the biomass of an ecosystem is ultimately lost from the ecosystem as

A. exports of biomass
B. organisms die
C. more biomass is produced
D. heat
E. decreased entropy

30. The majority of the known species of multicellular animals in the animal kingdom are characterized by

A. no skeleton
B. bony exoskeleton
C. chitinous endoskeleton
D. bony endoskeleton
E. chitinous exoskeleton

31. Which of the following is one of the morphogenetic movements that forms the gastrula of vertebrate embryos?

A. Differentiation   B. Cleavage
C. Metamorphosis   D. Induction
E. Invagination

32. In adult mammals, a blood vessel that carries deoxygenated blood is the

A. dorsal aorta   B. ventral aorta
C. pulmonary vein   D. pulmonary artery
E. coronary artery

33. Peptide linkages are found in

    A. enzymes
    B. nucleic acids
    C. nucleosides
    D. fatty acids
    E. carbohydrates

34. ATP is a chemical compound classified as a

    A. nucleoside
    B. nucleotide
    C. nucleic acid
    D. deoxyriboside
    E. nucleopeptide

35. When toxic nonbiodegradable fat-soluble organic chemicals, such as DDT, are introduced into an ecosystem, they become

    A. diluted and dispersed as they pass through the food chain
    B. harmless as organisms excrete them into the environment
    C. less toxic in higher trophic levels
    D. an energy source for tertiary consumers
    E. more concentrated in successive levels of the food chain

36. During contraction of vertebrate striated muscle cells,
    I. the thick filaments slide past the thin filaments in an energy-dependent process
    II. calcium ions are pumped rapidly into the sarcoplasmic reticulum
    III. the creatine phosphate concentration in the cell rises
    IV. the actin molecules of the thin filament contract
    V. the myosin molecules are replaced by tropomyosin

    The CORRECT answer is:

    A. I
    B. I, III
    C. I, IV
    D. I, II, III, IV
    E. IV only

37. A *basic* difference between all prokaryotic and all eukaryotic cells is that prokaryotic cells lack a

    A. cell wall
    B. plasma membrane
    C. centriole
    D. chlorophyll
    E. nuclear envelope

38. All flowering plants are classified as

    A. bryophytes
    B. phytoplankton
    C. gymnosperms
    D. angiosperms
    E. sea anemones

39. Escherichia coli is a common intestinal bacterium.
    One would expect a typical E. coli cell to be about the size of a(n)

    A. human liver cell
    B. polyribosome
    C. amoeba
    D. mitochondrion
    E. microfilament

40. Hemophilia is a sex-linked disease characterized by the inability of blood to clot. Prince Frederick was a hemophiliac.
    Which statement must be TRUE of Frederick's family? His

A. mother must have been a carrier
B. father must have been a hemophiliac
C. grandfather must have been a carrier
D. sister must have been a hemophiliac
E. uncle could have been a carrier

41. In the oxidation-reduction reaction $2MnO_4^- + 5C_2O_4^{2-} + 16H^+ \rightarrow 2Mn^{2+} + 10CO_2 + 8H_2O$ the oxidation number of each carbon atom changes from

    A. +2 to +4
    B. +3 to +6
    C. +3 to +4
    D. +4 to +2
    E. +3 to +2

42. Considering the nuclear reaction below, what is X?
    X + proton $\rightarrow$ ^{22}Mg + neutron

    A. ^{22}Na
    B. ^{23}Na
    C. ^{21}Mg
    D. ^{23}Mg
    E. ^{21}Ne

43. Which trend in the halogen family occurs with increasing atomic number?

    A. *Decreasing* ionic radius
    B. *Decreasing* melting points
    C. *Increasing* covalent radius
    D. *Increasing* electronegativity
    E. *Increasing* first ionization potential

44. In which of the following species does phosphorus exhibit its *highest* oxidation number?

    A. PCl_3
    B. P_4
    C. H_3PO_3
    D. PH_3
    E. P_2O_5

45. In which of the following solutions would CaF_2 be LEAST soluble?

    A. 0.01M $CaCl_2$
    B. 0.02M $CaCl_2$
    C. 0.01M NaF
    D. 0.02M NaF
    E. 0.02M NaCl

46. A mixture of gases containing CO_2 and SO_2 is allowed to effuse from one container through a pinhole into a second container which has been evacuated.

    A. The rate of effusion for CO_2 is faster because the molecules of CO_2 are lighter.
    B. The rate of effusion for SO_2 is faster because the molecules of SO_2 are lighter.
    C. The rate of effusion for CO_2 is slower because the molecules of CO_2 are lighter.
    D. The rate of effusion for SO_2 is faster because the molecules of SO_2 are heavier.
    E. Both compounds will effuse at the same rate since they are both at the same temperature.

47. The numbers of protons and neutrons, respectively, in $^{17}_{8}O^{2-}$ are

    A. 8, 17
    B. 8, 10
    C. 9, 8
    D. 6, 17
    E. 8, 9

48. The percent composition, by weight, of nitrogen in the compound $(NH_4)_2Cr_2O_7$ is (Atomic weights: H = 1, N = 14, O = 16, Cr = 52)

A. $\dfrac{14}{14 + 4(1) + 2(52) + 7(16)} \times 100$

B. $\dfrac{2(14)}{2(14) + 8(1) + 2(52) + 7(16)} \times 100$

C. $\dfrac{14}{14 + 1 + 52 + 16} \times 100$

D. $\dfrac{2(14)}{2(14) + 4(1) + 2(52) + 7(16)} \times 100$

E. $\dfrac{2(14)}{8(1) + 2(52) + 7(16)} \times 100$

49. How many unpaired electrons are in the ground state of a selenium atom (Z=34)?
    A. One B. Two C. Three D. Four E. Zero

50. The PRINCIPAL attractive force contributing to lattice energy in an ionic solid is
    A. coulombic repulsion
    B. electrostatic attraction
    C. London forces
    D. Van der Waals forces
    E. hydrogen bonding

KEY (CORRECT ANSWERS)

1. E	11. E	21. C	31. E	41. C
2. B	12. C	22. D	32. D	42. A
3. B	13. B	23. C	33. A	43. C
4. A	14. B	24. C	34. B	44. E
5. A	15. B	25. A	35. E	45. D
6. A	16. B	26. C	36. A	46. A
7. C	17. A	27. D	37. E	47. E
8. C	18. C	28. A	38. D	48. B
9. D	19. B	29. D	39. D	49. B
10. E	20. E	30. E	40. A	50. B

TEST 2

DIRECTIONS: Each question or incomplete statement is followed by several suggested answers or completions. Select the one that BEST answers the question or completes the statement. *PRINT THE LETTER OF THE CORRECT ANSWER IN THE SPACE AT THE RIGHT.*

1. Which gives the MOST basic solution when dissolved in water?   1._____

   A. H_3PO_4
   B. NaH_2PO_4
   C. P_2O_5
   D. $NaNO_3$
   E. $P_2O_5\ Na_3PO_4$

2. How many liters of 5.0 molar ethyl alcohol (C2H5OH) can be prepared by dissolving 460 grams of ethyl alcohol in water? (C_2H_5OH M.W. = 46)   2._____

   A. 0.5   B. 10   C. 2.0   D. 50   E. 5.0

3. What is the molarity of a solution resulting from the addition of 200 ml of 0.6M H_2SO_4 to 500 ml of 0.4M H_2SO_4 solution?   3._____

   A. $\dfrac{(0.6)(0.2) + (0.4)(0.5)}{0.7}$

   B. $\dfrac{(0.6) + (0.4)}{2}$

   C. $\dfrac{200/0.6 + 500/0.4}{700}$

   D. $\dfrac{(0.6)(200) + (0.4)(500)}{1000}$

   E. $(0.6)(200) + (0.4)(500)$

4. What is the geometry of SO_2 and the hybridization of the central atom?   4._____

   A. Linear, sp
   B. Linear, sp^2
   C. Bent, sp
   D. Bent, sp^2
   E. Triangular, sp^3

5. The data shown below were obtained for the reaction $A + 2B \rightarrow 2C + D$ 5._____

Experiment	Initial [A](M)	Initial [B](M)	Initial rate of appearance of D (M min^{-1})
1	1.0×10^{-4}	1.0×10^{-2}	0.65×10^{-6}
2	2.0×10^{-4}	1.0×10^{-2}	1.30×10^{-6}
3	2.0×10^{-4}	0.50×10^{-2}	0.65×10^{-6}
4	0.50×10^{-4}	2.0×10^{-2}	0.65×10^{-6}

   According to these data, the rate law for this system is rate =

A. $\dfrac{k[C]^2[D]}{[A][B]^2}$ B. $k[A][B]$ C. $k[A][B]^2$

D. $k[B]^2$ E. $k[A]$

6. The rate of most reactions tends to double with a 10C increase in temperature. This is thought to be due to a (n)

    A. *decrease* in the activation energy
    B. *increase* in the activation energy
    C. *increase* in the equilibrium constant
    D. *increase* in the fraction of molecules possessing at least the activation energy
    E. *decrease* in the fraction of molecules possessing at least the activation energy

7. Which reaction has the MOST positive value of ΔS?

    A. $2NO_{2(g)} \to N_2O_{4(l)}$
    B. $2NO_{2(g)} \to N_2O_{4(g)}$
    C. $N_2O_{4(l)} \to 2NO_{2(g)}$
    D. $N_2O_{4(g)} \to 2NO_{2(g)}$
    E. $N_2O_{4(l)} \to 2NO_{2(l)}$

8. The trigonal planar BCl_3 molecule is nonpolar. What is the explanation for this?

    A. Boron and chlorine have the same electro-negativity.
    B. The net polarity is zero due to the symmetry of the molecule.
    C. The polarity of each boron-chlorine bond is zero.
    D. Boron and chlorine have the same electron affinity.
    E. The electron density around the boron is the same as around the chlorine.

9. Which of the following will produce a change in the value of the equilibrium constant for a reaction?

    A. *Increase* the concentration of reactant
    B. *Decrease* the concentration of product
    C. Addition of a suitable catalyst
    D. *Increase* the temperature of the reaction
    E. All of the above

10. When 1.00 g of liquid water (M.W. = 18.0) is produced from H_2 and O_2 at a constant temperature (25°C) and pressure (1 atm), 15.8 kilojoules are produced. What is the molar heat of formation of liquid water, in kilojoules?

    A. -15.8×18.0
    B. 15.8×18.0
    C. $\dfrac{15.8}{18.0}$
    D. $\dfrac{-15.8}{18.0}$
    E. $\dfrac{-18.0}{15.8}$

11. Consider crystalline solids made from the following types of particles. Which type of particles gives the solid with the LOWEST melting point?

    A. Small non-polar molecules
    B. Small polar molecules
    C. Positive and negative ions
    D. Positive ions and mobile electrons
    E. Atoms covalently bonded in a continuous array

12. If the Group Numbers of elements x and z in the Periodic Table are VIA and VIIA, respectively, then what is the overall charge on the following Lewis dot formula?

    $$:\ddot{Z} - \ddot{X} - \ddot{Z}:$$
    $$\quad\quad |$$
    $$\quad :\ddot{Z}:$$

    A. +1   B. -1   C. +2   D. -2   E. +3

13. The equation for the Haber process for production of ammonia is $N_2 + 3H_2 \rightarrow 2NH_3$. What is the MAXIMUM number of moles of NH_3 which can be produced on reaction of a mixture containing 5 moles of N_2 and 6 moles of H_2?

    A. 9   B. 10   C. 6   D. 2   E. 4

14. A liter of solution contains 0.00001 moles of hydrochloric acid. What is the pH of this solution?

    A. 1.0   B. 4.0   C. -4.0   D. -5.0   E. 5.0

15. When solid NaOH is added to water, it dissolves and the solution becomes warm (sometimes even hot!). The signs of ΔG, ΔH, and ΔS, respectively, are

    A. +, +, +   B. +, -, +
    C. -, -, -   D. -, +, +
    E. -, -, +

16. The unbalanced equation for the oxidation of ammonia is:
    $$NH_3 + O_2 \rightarrow NO + H_2O$$
    After balancing the equation, which is the CORRECT set of coefficients for the substances from left to right?

    A. 2, 3, 2, 3   B. 3, 2, 3, 2
    C. 4, 5, 4, 6   D. 4, 6, 4, 6
    E. 2, 2, 2, 3

17. Which substance is oxidized in this reaction?
    $$3Cu + 8H^+ + 2NO_3^- \rightarrow 3Cu^{2+} + 2NO + 4H_2O$$

    A. NO   B. NO_3^- C. H^+ D. Cu   E. Cu^{2+}

18. Experimentally, it was found that 1.5×10^{-6} moles of $BaSO_4$ would dissolve in one liter of 0.001M Na_2SO_4 solution. Assuming ideal solution behavior, what is the solubility product constant for $BaSO_4$?

A. $(1.5 \times 10^{-6})^2$
B. $(1.5 \times 1^{-6})^2 (10^{-3})$
C. $\dfrac{(1.5 \times 10^{-6})^2}{10^{-3}}$
D. $(1.5 \times 10^{-6})(10^{-3})$
E. $\dfrac{10^3}{1.5 \times 10^{-6}}$

19. Which one of the following concentration terms is temperature dependent? 19.____

    A. % by weight
    B. Molality
    C. Molarity
    D. Mole fraction
    E. None of the above

20. What is the molecular weight of an ideal gas if a 15.0 g sample occupies 25.5 liters at 100C and 1 atmosphere of pressure? 20.____

    A. $\dfrac{(15)(0.082)(100)^5}{(1)(25.5)}$
    B. $\dfrac{(15)(0.082)(373)}{(1)(25.5)}$

    C. $\dfrac{(15)(82.0)(373)}{(760)(25.5)}$
    D. $\dfrac{(15)(82.0)(100)}{(1)(25.5)}$

    E. $\dfrac{(15)(0.082)(373)}{(760)(25.5)}$

21. Which compound gives the BEST yield of a *single* alkene on treatment with ethanolic KOH? 21.____

    A. $CH_3-\underset{\underset{OH}{|}}{\overset{\overset{CH_3}{|}}{C}}-CH_3$

    B. $CH_3-\underset{\underset{Br}{|}}{CH}-CH_2-CH_3$

    C. cyclohexane with CH$_3$ and Br substituents

    D. cyclohexanol

    E. $CH_3-CH_2-\underset{\underset{Br}{|}}{CH}-CH_2-CH_3$

22. Which of the following reactions would give 22.____

benzoic acid (COOH) with CH$_3$ substituent (p-methylbenzoic acid)

A. CH₃MgBr + [benzoic acid] →Δ

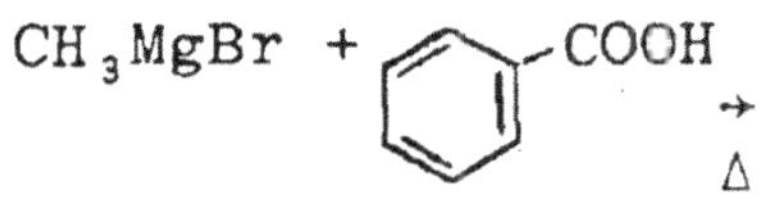

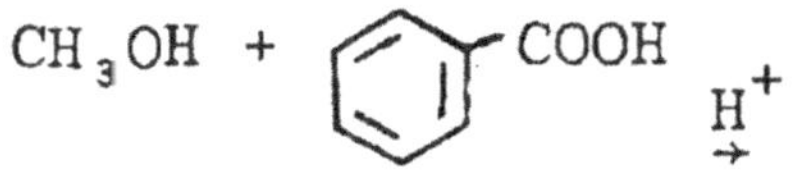

B. CH₃OH + [benzoic acid] →H⁺

C. [4-methylphenyl-MgBr] 1) CO₂ 2) H⁺ →

D. NaHCO₃ + [4-methylphenyl-N₂⁺,Cl] →

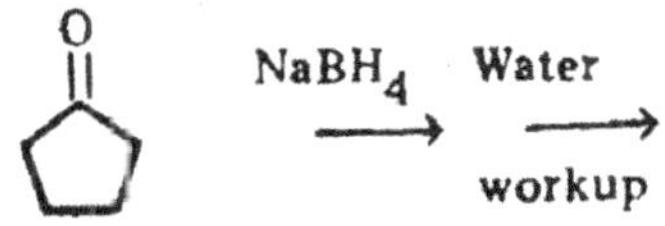

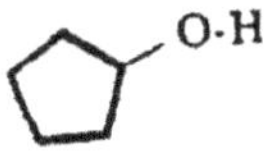

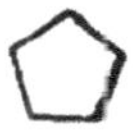

E. LiAlH₄ + [4-methylbenzaldehyde] →

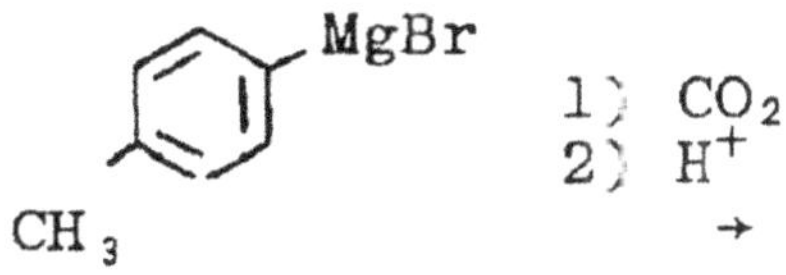

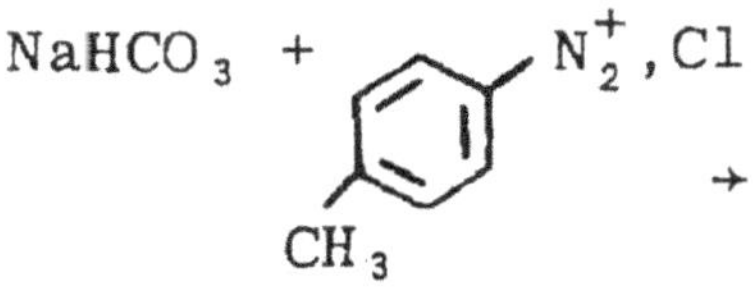

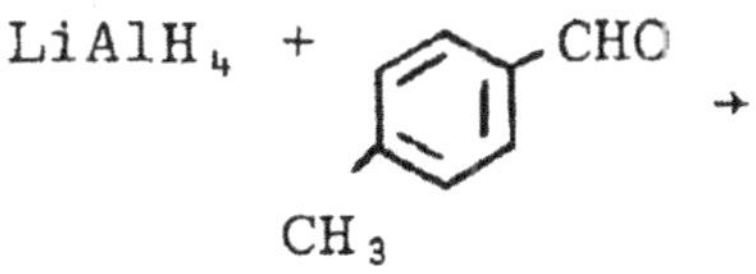

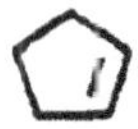

23. What is the product of the following reaction?

[cyclopentanone] —NaBH₄→ —Water workup→

A. [cyclopentanol]
B. [cyclopentane]
C. HO₂C-CH₂CH₂CH₂CO₂H
D. [cyclopentene]
E. [tetrahydropyran]

23._____

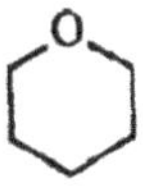

24. Which of the following is the STRONGEST acid?

A. ClCH₂CH₂CO₂H
B. Cl₂CHCO₂H
C. CH₃CHClCO₂H
D. ClCH₂CHClCO₂H
E. CH₃CH₂CO₂H

24._____

25. Which of the following reactions will proceed by an S_N2 reaction mechanism?

A. CH₃CH₂OH + K₂Cr₂O₇ → CH₃-C-OH
B. CH₄ + O₂ →heat CO₂ + H₂O
C. CH₃CH₂Br + NaNH₂ → CH₂=CH₂ + NaBr + NH
D. CH₃CH₂Br + NaCN → CH₃CH₂CN + NaBr
E. CH₃-CH=CH₂ + HBr → CH₃-CH-CH₃
                                    |
                                    Br

25._____

26. Which of the following statements is TRUE for the S_N2 reaction shown below?

$CH_3CH_2\text{—}\overset{H}{\underset{CH_3}{C}}\text{—}Br + CN^- \xrightarrow{acetone} Product$

(S) - 2 - bromobutane

A. The product will be a racemate.
B. A change in the concentration of the cyanide ion will not alter the rate of reaction.
C. A carbocation intermediate will be formed.
D. The reaction will occur with inversion of configuration.
E. The reaction will occur with retention of configuration.

27. What is the reagent and reaction condition that will bring about the conversion of benzoic acid to benzoyl chloride?

PhC(=O)OH $\xrightarrow{?}$ PhC(=O)Cl

A. HCl (in CCl_4)
B. CH_3Cl (reflux)
C. Fe, Cl_2
D. $SOCl_2$ (reflux)
E. $AlCl_3$

28. Which alcohol undergoes acid-catalyzed dehydration MOST readily when heated with concentrated sulfuric acid?

A. $CH_3CH_2CH_2CH_2CH_2OH$

B. $CH_3\underset{OH}{\overset{|}{CH}}CH_2CH_2CH_3$

C. cyclopentanol (with OH)

D. CH_3CH_2OH

E. $CH_3CH_2\underset{CH_3}{\overset{CH_3}{\underset{|}{\overset{|}{C}}}}OH$

29. (−)-Ribose shown below contains how many chiral centers?
    A. One
    B. Two
    C. Three
    D. Four
    E. None

    D-(−)-Ribose

29.____

30. Which of the following phenols is the STRONGEST acid?

    A.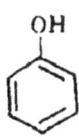
    B.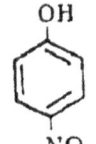
    C.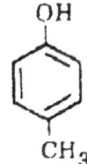

    D.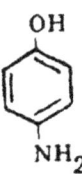
    E.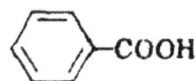

30.____

31. Reaction of 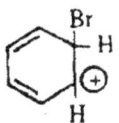 with a mixture of HNO_3 and H_2SO_4 would give predominately which of the following compounds?

    A.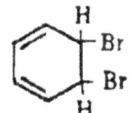
    B.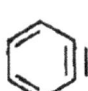

    C. ![] O_2N—〔 〕—OH
    D. ![] 〔 〕—CH_3 with O_2N

    E. ![] O_2N—〔 〕—CH_3

31.____

32. In the bromination of benzene (Br_2/$FeBr_3$), one of the reactive intermediates is:

    A. [Br, H on ring with +]
    B. [H, Br, Br on ring]
    C. [benzene–I]

32.____

D. 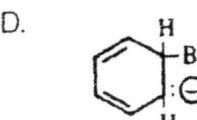 E.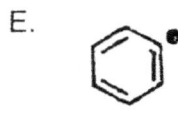

33. Which compound is *most likely* to have an infrared spectrum with a large peak between 1750-1700 cm⁻¹ (5.77-5.88?)?

    A. CH₃–O–CH₃

    B.
    $$CH_3-\underset{\underset{O}{\|}}{C}-CH_3$$

    C.
    $$CH_3-CH_2-\underset{\underset{H}{|}}{N}-CH_2-CH_3$$

    D. CH₃–CH₂–OH

    E. CH₃–CH₂–I

34. How many hydrogens in the compound below are exchangeable with the deuterium in D₂O under basic catalysis?

    CH₃-CH₂-O-C(=O)-CH₂-C(=O)-[cyclohexane with two CH₃ groups] $\xrightarrow{\text{NaOD}, D_2O}$

    A. Two B. Four C. Five
    D. Seven E. Thirteen

35. Propionaldehyde, CH₃CH₂CHO, is allowed to react with ethyl magnesium bromide, CH₃CH₂MgBr. Upon hydrolysis, compound A is formed. Oxidation of A by potassium dichromate-sulfuric acid gives compound B. What is B?

    A. $CH_3CH_2\overset{\overset{O}{\|}}{C}CH_3$

    B. $CH_3CH_2\overset{\overset{O}{\|}}{C}CH_2CH_3$

    C. $CH_3CH_2\overset{\overset{OH}{|}}{C}HCH_2CH_3$

    D. (CH₃CH₂)COH

    E. CH₃CH₂CH₂OCH₂CH₃

36. What is the product of the following sequence of reactions?

$$CH_3\text{-}CH_2\text{-}CH_2\text{-}\underset{O}{\overset{\|}{C}}\text{-}OH \xrightarrow{SOCl_2} A \xrightarrow[\text{excess}]{NH_3} B$$

A. $CH_3\text{-}CH_2\text{-}\underset{NH_2}{\overset{|}{CH}}\text{-}\underset{O}{\overset{\|}{C}}\text{-}OH$

B. $CH_3\text{-}CH_2\text{-}CH_2\text{-}CH_2\text{-}NH_2$

C. $CH_3\text{-}CH_2\text{-}CH_2\text{-}CH_2\text{-}Cl$

D. $CH_3\text{-}CH_2\text{-}CH_2\text{-}\underset{O}{\overset{\|}{C}}\text{-}NH_2$

E. (pyrrolidinone: 5-membered ring with C=O and NH)

37. Which of the following is NOT an ester?

A. $CH_3\text{-}\underset{O}{\overset{\|}{C}}\text{-}O\text{-}CH_3$

B. $H\text{-}\underset{O}{\overset{\|}{C}}\text{-}O\text{-}CH_2\text{-}CH_3$

C. $CH_3\text{-}\underset{H}{\overset{O\text{-}CH_3}{\underset{|}{\overset{|}{C}}}}\text{-}O\text{-}CH_3$

D. $CH_3\text{-}O\text{-}\underset{O}{\overset{\|}{C}}\text{-}H$

E. (benzene ring with O-CH₃ and C(O)-O-CH₃ substituents)

38. The correct hybridization state of the central carbon in neopentane,

$$CH_3\text{-}\underset{\underset{CH_3}{|}}{\overset{\overset{CH_3}{|}}{C}}\text{-}CH_3$$

and the approximate angles between the C-C bonds is

A. sp² and 120°
B. sp3 and 90°
C. sp and 180°
D. sp³ and 109°
E. sp and 109°

39. What is the product of the following reaction?

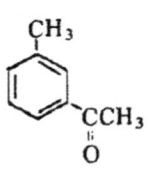 + CH₃CCl 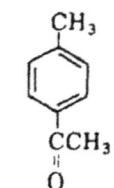 AlCl₃ →

A.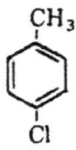

B. (structure: p-methyl acetophenone)

C. (structure: p-chlorotoluene)

D. (structure with CH₂CCl)

E. 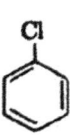 (structure: PhCH₂CCH₃)

40. Aniline (C₆H₅NH₂) will react most rapidly with

A. PhCH₂C(O)OCH₃

B. (indolinone structure)

C. (CH₃)₂CH–C(O)–Cl

D. dicyclopentyl ketone

E. chlorobenzene

41. In the reaction sequence

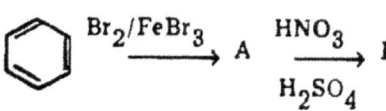

the MAJOR product is:

A. m-bromonitrobenzene (Br, NO₂)

B. p-bromonitrobenzene (Br, NO₂)

C. m-bromobenzenesulfonic acid (Br, SO₃H)

D. 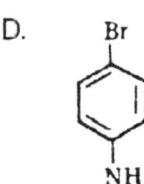 E.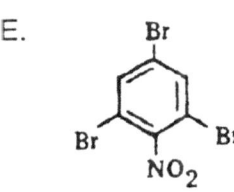

42. From the following compounds (which have similar molecular weights), select the one which has the *highest* boiling point.

    A. $CH_3CH_2\underset{\underset{O}{\|}}{C}CH_3$

    B. $CH_3CH_2OCH_2CH_3$

    C. $CH_3CH_2CO_2H$

    D. $CH_3CH_2CH_2CH_2OH$

    E. $CH_3CH_2CH_2CH_2CH_3$

43. Which of the following is a product of

    $CH_3\text{-}CH_2\text{-}ONa$ + -CH_2-Br $\longrightarrow$?

    A. cyclohexyl-CH_2-O-CH_2-CH_3

    B. cyclohexyl with CH_3 and OCH_2CH_3

    C. cyclohexyl-CH_2-CH_2-CH_2-OH

    D. methylcyclohexene + CH_3-CH_2OH

    E. cyclohexane with =CH_2 and O-CH_2-CH_3

44. Which of the following reactions listed below would have the *lowest* energy of activation (E act.)?

    A. $Cl\text{-}Cl \rightarrow Cl\cdot + Cl\cdot$
    B. $Cl\cdot + CH_3\text{-}H \rightarrow HCl + \cdot CH_3$
    C. $CH_3\text{-}CH_3 \rightarrow \cdot CH_3 + \cdot CH_3$
    D. $\cdot CH_3 + Cl\text{-}Cl \rightarrow CH_3\text{-}Cl + Cl\cdot$
    E. $\cdot CH_3 + \cdot CH_3 \rightarrow CH_3\text{-}CH_3$

45. Which of the following compounds will undergo nitration the *fastest* when treated with a mixture of concentrated H_2SO_4 and HNO_3?

    A. benzene   B. toluene   C.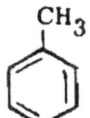

D. [benzene-NO2]   E. [benzene-OH]

46. Which of the following compounds is capable of intramolecular (internal) hydrogen bonding? 46.____

A. [2-hydroxybenzaldehyde]   B. [2-methoxybenzaldehyde]   C. [2-methylphenol]

D. [2-cyanobenzaldehyde]   E. [4-(hydroxymethyl)phenol]

47. Select the IUPAC name for

$$CH_3CHCH-C-CH_3$$ with OH, O (double bond), and CH_3 substituents

A. 3-hydroxy-2-hexanone
B. 3-hydroxy-4-hexanone
C. 3-hydroxy-2-methyl-4-pentanoate
D. 3-hydroxy-4-methyl-2-pentanal
E. 3-hydroxy-4-methyl-2-pentanone

47.____

48. Which of the following is achiral and, therefore, will NOT rotate plane polarized light? 48.____

A. [structure with CH3, H, Cl, CH2CH3]

B. an equimolar mixture of [two structures]

C. [structure with two stereocenters, both H/Cl same side]

D. [structure with two stereocenters, opposite]

E. [structure with CH3, H, Cl, CCl2CH3]

49. Which compound is chiral and, therefore, has a nonsuper-imposable mirror image?   49._____

A. $CH_3-CH(NH_2)-CH_2-CH_3$

B. $CH_3-CH_2-CH_2-CH_2-NH_2$

C. $CH_3-CH(CH_3)-CH_2-NH_2$

D. $CH_3-CH_2-CH(NH_2)-CH_2-CH_3$

E. cyclopentyl-NH_2

50. The fact that the allyl carbocation is more stable than primary carbocations such as can BEST be accounted for on the basis of   50._____

A. lack of steric hindrance in the allyl carbocation
B. tautomerism in the allyl carbocation
C. the electron withdrawing characteristic of the double bond in the allyl carbocation
D. resonance stabilization of the allyl carbocation
E. hydrogen bonding in the allyl carbocation

KEY (CORRECT ANSWERS)

1. E	11. A	21. E	31. E	41. B
2. C	12. A	22. C	32. A	42. C
3. A	13. E	23. A	33. B	43. A
4. D	14. E	24. B	34. A	44. E
5. B	15. E	25. D	35. B	45. E
6. D	16. C	26. D	36. D	46. A
7. C	17. D	27. D	37. C	47. E
8. B	18. D	28. E	38. D	48. C
9. D	19. C	29. C	39. B	49. A
10. A	20. B	30. B	40. C	50. D

EXAMINATION SECTION
TEST 1

DIRECTIONS: Each question or incomplete statement is followed by several suggested answers or completions. Select the one that BEST answers the question or completes the statement. *PRINT THE LETTER OF THE CORRECT ANSWER IN THE SPACE AT THE RIGHT.*

1. If a protein contains 80 amino acids, its corresponding gene must contain AT LEAST how many nucleotides?

   A. 40   B. 120   C. 240   D. 360   E. 480

   1.____

2. Which one of the following is characteristic ONLY of mitosis and NOT of meiosis?

   A. Synapsis occurs
   B. Cells with identical genotypes are produced
   C. Splitting of centromeres takes place
   D. Homologous chromosomes separate
   E. Spindle fibers are formed

   2.____

3. The PRIMARY role of oxygen in respiration is to

   A. yield energy in the form of ATP as it is passed down the respiratory chain
   B. act as an acceptor for electrons and hydrogen ions to form water
   C. combine with carbon to form CO_2
   D. combine with lactic acid to form pyruvic acid
   E. catalyze the reactions of glycolysis

   3.____

4. Fetal cells sloughed off into the amniotic fluid can be collected and cultured. The cultured cells CANNOT be used for prenatal diagnosis of

   A. identical twinning
   B. paternity
   C. genetic diseases whose metabolic basis is known
   D. the sex of the fetus
   E. aneuploidy

   4.____

5. The function of the Loop of Henle is to

   A. rid the body of excess urea and ammonia
   B. rid the body of excess hydrogen ions
   C. return reusable nutrients to the blood
   D. produce a sugar gradient capable of concentrating urine
   E. produce a salt gradient capable of concentrating urine

   5.____

6. The cells of the testis that are MOST like the follicle cells of the ovary in that they respond to the pituitary hormone LH by producing steroid hormones are

   A. spermatids   B. endometrial cells
   C. stem cells   D. interstitial cells
   E. germ cells

   6.____

7. Bacteriophages are

   A. organelles
   B. organisms
   C. prokaryotes
   D. bacteria
   E. viruses

8. When an aerobic organism is temporarily deprived of O_2, it obtains its chemical energy from

   A. the substrate level of ATP synthesis in glycolysis
   B. the oxidation of pyruvic acid to acetyl-CoA
   C. the respiratory electron transport chain
   D. chemiosmotic coupling
   E. metabolism of succinic acid in the TCA cycle

9. Examination of the eukaryotic cell surface by the electron microscope reveals that the plasma membrane

   A. is composed of a single layer of molecules approximately 75 Angstrom units in thickness
   B. is composed exclusively of phospholipids
   C. invaginates into the cellular cytoplasm to form canals and vesicles
   D. invaginates to form cristae on which are arranged the electron transport systems
   E. is composed exclusively of proteins

10. In a research project, a chemical was introduced to developing embryos that selectively destroyed the mesoderm germ layer.
    Which of the following structures would be absent in the fetus?

    A. Brain
    B. Pectoralis muscle
    C. Epidermis
    D. Intestinal mucosa
    E. Adrenal medulla

11. A restriction endonuclease produces a break in

    A. DNA at a specific base sequence
    B. tRNA at a specific base sequence
    C. any nucleic acid at the end of the molecule
    D. proteins at a specific amino acid sequence
    E. DNA at the 3' terminal end *only*

12. All chemosynthetic autotrophic prokaryotes belong to the

    A. bacteria
    B. fungi
    C. protozoa
    D. viruses
    E. tracheophytes

13. The carbon dioxide carried in the blood from the tissues to the lungs is MOST commonly found in the form of

    A. carbaminohemoglobin
    B. free carbon dioxide
    C. carbonic acid
    D. bicarbonate ions
    E. membrane-bound carbon dioxide

14. The regulation of body temperature, water balance, and appetite are a function of the

    A. thalamus
    B. hypothalamus
    C. medulla oblongata
    D. anterior lobe of pituitary
    E. cerebrum

15. In sex-linkage

    A. the recessive autosomal characters of the father are expressed in the sons
    B. X-linked characters of the mother must be expressed in the daughters
    C. the X-linked characters of the mother are never expressed in the daughters
    D. the primary sexual characteristics are determined by the sex hormones
    E. normal male fruitflies and humans always have a Y-chromosome

16. Assuming Hardy-Weinberg conditions, when 16 percent of a population is homozygous recessive for a trait, the percent that is heterozygous is

    A. 30   B. 25   C. 48   D. 24   E. 36

17. One of the evolutionary adaptations of reptiles for a terrestrial environment was

    A. a thin, pliable skin
    B. a four-chambered heart
    C. air breathing lung
    D. a shelled egg with extraembryonic membranes
    E. legs for rapid locomotion

18. According to the theory of natural selection, the environment *selects* ONLY those characteristics which

    A. fit the organism to future environmental change
    B. *increase* the life span of the individual
    C. *increase* the number of offspring which reach reproductive age
    D. result in stronger individuals
    E. affect social behavior

19. If acetylcholine were released at a synapse and acetyl-cholinesterase was inhibited, the

    A. postsynaptic neuron would not respond to the acetylcholine
    B. postsynaptic neuron would produce a single nerve impulse
    C. postsynaptic neuron would produce an abnormally long series of nerve impulses
    D. acetylcholine would not diffuse across the synapse
    E. acetylcholine would spontaneously decompose

20. Cystic fibrosis is inherited as a simple autosomal recessive. Suppose a woman who is heterozygous for this trait marries a man who is also heterozygous for it. What is the probability that they will have a child who is heterozygous for the trait?

    A. 0   B. 1/4   C. 1/2   D. 2/3   E. 3/4

KEY (CORRECT ANSWERS)

1.	C	11.	A
2.	B	12.	A
3.	B	13.	D
4.	A	14.	B
5.	E	15.	E
6.	D	16.	C
7.	E	17.	D
8.	A	18.	C
9.	C	19.	C
10.	B	20.	C

TEST 2

DIRECTIONS: Each question or incomplete statement is followed by several suggested answers or completions. Select the one that BEST answers the question or completes the statement. *PRINT THE LETTER OF THE CORRECT ANSWER IN THE SPACE AT THE RIGHT.*

1. Which of the following statements is TRUE of the archenteron? 1.____

   A. The cavity of the archenteron is called the blastocoel.
   B. The cavity of the archenteron represents the beginning of the primitive gut.
   C. The archenteron is formed during blastula formation.
   D. The cavity of the archenteron represents the first cavity of the developing heart.
   E. The archenteron is formed by a closing of the neural tube.

2. Which part of the cell is involved MOST directly with the synthesis of ribosomal subunits? 2.____

   A. Nucleolus   B. Microtubules
   C. Endoplasmic reticulum   D. Golgi apparatus
   E. Nuclear envelope

3. Which of the following substances is a nucleotide? 3.____

   A. Estrogen
   B. Growth hormone (somatotropin)
   C. Insulin
   D. Adenosine triphosphate (ATP)
   E. Amylose

4. Which of the following is NOT a function of microtubules? 4.____

   A. Maintaining or controlling the shape of the cell
   B. Movement of chromosomes during anaphase
   C. Temporary storage of proteins prior to secretion
   D. Forming the structural elements of the centrioles
   E. Activity of cells and flagella

5. The thymus gland is involved in 5.____

   A. the regulation of calcium metabolism
   B. the development of the immune response
   C. regulation of the activity of the thyroid gland
   D. endocrine and exocrine functions
   E. reproductive physiology

6. At different stages during the normal sequence of events in the menstrual cycle, there is an increase in progesterone, FSH, and estrogen. 6.____
   Which one of the following is the CORRECT sequence of *initial* increases in each substance, beginning with menstruation?

   A. Estrogen, FSH, progesterone
   B. FSH, estrogen, progesterone
   C. Estrogen, progesterone, FSH
   D. FSH, progesterone, estrogen
   E. Progesterone, estrogen, FSH

7. Suppose an individual is heterozygous for ten different independently assorting genes. How many genetically different gametes will be possible from this individual?

   A. 10   B. 20   C. 10^2 D. 200   E. 210

8. Viruses may not be considered true living organisms because they

   A. are too small
   B. can only reproduce in the cells of another living organism
   C. are not eukaryotes
   D. are extremely primitive organisms
   E. can only replicate in an anaerobic environment

9. One of the MAJOR advantages in using scanning electron microscopy as opposed to transmission electron microscopy is that

   A. greater magnification can be obtained
   B. greater resolving power can be obtained
   C. the specimen does not have to be treated with chemicals
   D. a three-dimensional image can be obtained
   E. there is no advantage

10. The following gland is both endocrine and exocrine in function.

    A. Thyroid   B. Liver   C. Adrenal
    D. Pancreas   E. Pituitary

11. Sucrose is

    A. a disaccharide of glucose and fructose
    B. a trisaccharide of galactose, glucose, and fructose
    C. the technical term for blood sugar
    D. the major subunit of cellulose
    E. the major subunit of starch

12. The intracellular ion that is PRIMARILY responsible for triggering muscle contraction is

    A. sodium   B. potassium   C. phosphorus
    D. calcium   E. magnesium

13. In which two of the following phyla do most biologists place the MOST primitive bilaterally symmetrical animals?

    A. Chordata and Hemichordata
    B. Coelenterata (Cnidaria) and Ctenophora
    C. Onycophora and Arthropoda
    D. Echinodermata and Chaetognatha
    E. Platyhelminthes and Nemertina

14. A classic example of primary embryonic induction is the induction by the vertebrate chordamesoderm of the

    A. vertebrae   B. axial musculature
    C. neural tube   D. heart
    E. liver primordium

15. In which of the following organelles is water synthesized from oxygen and hydrogen?   15._____

    A. Nucleus
    B. Mitochrondria
    C. Ribosomes
    D. Lysosomes
    E. Golgi apparatus

16. The biological significance of the evolution of fleshy fruits such as the apple and the   16._____
    peach is that such fruits are

    A. necessary for seed transpiration
    B. to protect the seeds from being eaten by animals
    C. exposed to rigorous natural selection because the matured ovary wall is triploid
    D. important sources of vitamin C for the plant
    E. adaptations to securing seed dispersal by animals

17. In a simple food chain, animals with the SMALLEST population *probably*   17._____

    A. are least likely to be an endangered species
    B. have a very high biotic potential
    C. are physically smaller than the others in the food chain
    D. are herbivorous
    E. are carnivorous

18. Which of the following enzymes acts on carbohydrates?   18._____

    A. Carboxypeptidase
    B. Trypsin
    C. Chymotrypsin
    D. Lipase
    E. Amylase

19. All of the following processes require energy input EXCEPT   19._____

    A. active transport
    B. muscle contraction
    C. DNA synthesis
    D. maintenance of the resting potential of neurons
    E. osmosis

20. The movement of fluid from the arteriole end of a mammalian capillary bed into the inter-   20._____
    stitial spaces is PRIMARILY due to

    A. hydrostatic pressure
    B. osmotic pressure
    C. active transport by the capillary walls
    D. contraction of skeletal muscles
    E. contraction of smooth muscle of the capillary walls

KEY (CORRECT ANSWERS)

1.	B	11.	A
2.	A	12.	D
3.	D	13.	E
4.	C	14.	C
5.	B	15.	B
6.	B	16.	E
7.	E	17.	E
8.	B	18.	E
9.	D	19.	E
10.	D	20.	A

EXAMINATION SECTION
TEST 1

DIRECTIONS: Each question or incomplete statement is followed by several suggested answers or completions. Select the one that *BEST* answers the question or completes the statement. *PRINT THE LETTER OF THE CORRECT ANSWER IN THE SPACE AT THE RIGHT.*

1. The structure in the corn seed that functions in the same way as does the cotyledon in a bean seed is the

   A. epicotyl B. endosperm C. pericarp D. plumule

2. The fleshy, edible part of an apple is derived mainly from the part of the flower called the

   A. pericarp B. pistil C. receptacle D. sepal

3. The placenta of a mammal is biologically MOST important because it

   A. is heavily vascularized and affords large surface area for interchange between separate vascular systems
   B. supports the foetus in a nourishing fluid
   C. protects the embryo from mechanical injury
   D. is a passageway for direct arterial connection from mother into the foetus

4. Of the following vertebrates, the one in which reproduction is characterized by internal fertilization of the ovum and external development of the embryo is the

   A. pigeon B. guppy C. rabbit D. whale

5. The Graafan follicle

   A. supports sebaceous glands necessary for keeping the skin soft
   B. produces the ovum during the menstrual cycle
   C. secretes the hormone, secretin
   D. stimulates the development of secondary sex characteristics in males

6. The process that takes place on or about the 14th day of the menstrual cycle in humans is

   A. breakdown of the uterus lining
   B. denigration
   C. ovulation
   D. parturition

7. In a breed of chickens that has 3 distinct colors in plumage (white; tan; brown) if 2 tan birds are bred, the offspring would be

   A. all tan
   B. 50% tan, 50% brown
   C. 25% tan, 50% brown, 25% white
   D. 25% brown, 50% tan, 25% white

8. If a tall, red-flowered pea plant (TtRr) is crossed with a tall, white-flowered pea plant (TTrr), the percentage of offspring that would be tall and white-flowered would be

   A. 25   B. 50   C. 75   D. 100

9. T. H. Morgan and his co-workers were the first to offer experimental proof that

   A. during formation of gametes there is separation of maternal and paternal factors
   B. genes are located on chromosomes in a linear arrangement
   C. a single phenotype may be the result of more than one gene
   D. non-allelomorphic factors segregate independently

10. Desoxyribonucleic acid (DNA) is believed to be the MOST important constituent of

    A. centrioles   B. centrosomes
    C. chromosomes   D. Golgi bodies

11. The Nobel prize winner who demonstrated that genes can be caused to mutate by x-rays is

    A. Correns   B. Dunn   C. Muller   D. Sturtevant

12. Of the following, the fossil of the MOST recent primate is called the

    A. Homo Neanderthalensis   B. Homarus Americanus
    C. Plesianthropus   D. Pithecanthropus

13. In an unfolded cliff of stratified rock the sequence of fossils from the bottom up would be expected to be

    A. mastodon, trilobite, archaeornis, Brontosaurus
    B. trilobite, Brontosaurus, archaeornis, mammoth
    C. Allosaurus, ammonite, Hesperornis, Homo
    D. ammonite, Hesperornis, trilobite, Sinanthropus

14. An animal with a water-vascular system, tube feet, and a spiny skin would belong to the phylum

    A. echinodermata   B. annelida
    C. molluscoidea   D. platyhelminthes

15. The organism that causes the disease trichinosis is a member of the phylum that includes

    A. annelids   B. flatworms   C. roundworms   D. fungi

16. Antheridia and archegonia are reproductive organs found in

    A. Angiosperms   B. Basidiomycetes
    C. Bryophytes   D. Schizophytes

17. The gametophyte generation is dominant in

    A. ferns   B. grains   C. legumes   D. mosses

18. The structures that transport water up the stem of woody plants are the

    A. bast fibers   B. parenchyma cells
    C. sieve tubes   D. tracheids

19. When the bark is stripped from a tree, the vital vascular tissue removed is the

    A. phloem   B. cork cambium   C. pith   D. vessels

20. Protein synthesis by green plants involves the combination of carbohydrate products with

    A. fats   B. minerals   C. steroids   D. vitamins

21. The cells in the chlorenchyma adapted to perform photosynthesis are called

    A. companion   B. fibrovascular   C. palisade   D. pith

22. Examination of soils in some areas have shown that what is now basswood and maple forestland was once occupied by lakes. The lake first choked up with water plants, and swamp vegetation appeared. Then spruce and pine grew. Finally maple and basswood became the dominant forms. The above process is best known as

    A. ecological succession   B. geological evidence
    C. natural selection   D. survival of the fittest

23. An insect that destroys a large number of plant lice is the

    A. hawkmoth
    B. ichneumon fly
    C. ladybird beetle (lady bug)
    D. robber fly

24. The Papanicolaou (PAP) test is used to discover early cases of

    A. cancer   B. typhoid   C. tuberculosis   D. syphilis

25. An anti-biotic derived from a soil mold is

    A. gramicidin   B. penicillin
    C. streptomycin   D. sulfaguanadine

26. An example of a wind-pollinated plant is

    A. dandelion   B. milkweed   C. ragweed   D. rose

27. The coronary artery supplies muscles of the

    A. crown of the skull   B. forearm
    C. heart   D. trachea

28. Of the following chromosome types, the one that would produce a female Drosophila fly is

    A. XY   B. XX   C. XO   D. OY

29. A disease characterized by a periodic fever produced by the destruction of red corpuscles by merozoites is

    A. malaria   B. typhus fever
    C. Q-fever   D. yellow fever

30. The sensory cells called rods and cones are found in the

    A. ear   B. eye
    C. olfactory organs   D. tactile organs

31. Nitrogen-fixing bacteria are MOST commonly found growing in the roots of

    A. corn B. wheat C. oats D. peas

32. Some plant lice are protected by certain ants that derive a sweet juice from the plant lice. This type of biological association is known as

    A. commensalism B. parasitism
    C. saprozoic nutrition D. symbiosis

33. The phrenic nerve regulates the contraction of the muscles of the

    A. diaphragm B. dorsal aorta
    C. pyloric sphincter D. stomach

34. Reserpine and meprobamate are forms of drugs known as

    A. narcotics B. stimulants C. tranquilizers D. vitamins

35. Urea is filtered from the blood as the blood flows through the

    A. glomeruli B. Haversian canals
    C. seminiferous tubules D. ureters

36. All malarial parasites belong to the genus

    A. Clostridium B. Plasmodium
    C. Rhizobium D. Spirillum

37. A toxoid, when introduced into the blood stream, acts as an anti-

    A. body B. coagulant C. gen D. toxin

38. A vector of a number of disease-producing trypanosomes is the

    A. body louse B. flea C. leech D. tsetse fly

39. A Rickettsial disease is

    A. tetanus B. trench mouth C. tularemia D. typhus

40. The usual portal of entry of the hookworm is

    A. exposed skin
    B. bite of an insect
    C. nasal passages
    D. ingestion of improperly cooked food

41. Bacteria are usually classified as plants because they

    A. are autotrophic
    B. produce extracellular enzymes
    C. have cell walls
    D. produce spores

42. The respiratory system of insects includes a complex network of air tubes called

    A. alveoli B. bronchial tubes C. spiracles D. tracheae

43. Sagittaria and myriophyllum would grow BEST in a(n)

    A. aquarium B. terrarium
    C. rock garden D. agar plate

44. The Douglas fir tree is native to

    A. Great Lakes forests B. Central hardwood forest
    C. Southern forest D. Pacific Coastal forest

45. A tree which has leaf venation similar to that of the maple is the

    A. chestnut B. ginkgo C. oak D. sycamore

46. The male gametophyte of a corn plant is the

    A. pollen tube B. anther C. stamen D. tassel

47. Root pressure is most responsible for

    A. abscission of leaves B. flow of sap in stems
    C. splitting of bark D. hydrotropism of roots

48. The micropyle

    A. activates the germination of a pollen grain
    B. allows the pollen tube to penetrate the ovule
    C. is the precursor of a pollen grain
    D. is the growing tip of a pollen grain

49. As a bean seed begins to germinate, it

    A. absorbs carbon dioxide B. digests starch
    C. synthesizes protein D. absorbs its embryo leaves

50. The structures found in all typical cells are

    A. cytoplasm, nucleus, cell membrane
    B. cytoplasm, nucleus, cell wall
    C. cytoplasm, nucleus, centrosome
    D. cytoplasm, nucleus, cell vacuole

KEY (CORRECT ANSWERS)

1. B	11. C	21. C	31. D	41. C
2. C	12. A	22. A	32. D	42. D
3. A	13. B	23. C	33. A	43. A
4. A	14. A	24. A	34. C	44. D
5. B	15. C	25. C	35. A	45. D
6. C	16. C	26. C	36. B	46. A
7. D	17. D	27. C	37. C	47. B
8. B	18. D	28. B	38. D	48. B
9. B	19. A	29. A	39. D	49. B
10. C	20. B	30. B	40. A	50. A

TEST 2

DIRECTIONS: Each question or incomplete statement is followed by several suggested answers or completions. Select the one that BEST answers the question or completes the statement. PRINT THE LETTER OF THE CORRECT ANSWER IN THE SPACE AT THE RIGHT.

1. The true cambium is

    A. meristematic tissue
    B. present in monocotyledenous plants
    C. located between the pith and heartwood
    D. responsible for the growth in height of a tree

2. A pigment found in the cell sap of plants is

    A. anthocyanin   B. carotene
    C. melanin   D. xanthophyll

3. Photoperiodism is associated with

    A. seasonal flights of birds
    B. limiting factors in photosynthesis
    C. flowering of plants at different seasons of the year
    D. reactions of lower animals to light

4. Bryophyllum and begonia are useful for demonstrating

    A. adventitious roots   B. bud scales
    C. leaf cuttings   D. lenticels

5. Zygospores of the spirogyra plant

    A. are asexual spores
    B. are produced in the wintertime
    C. germinate in the spring
    D. have the haploid number of chromosomes

6. Members of the genus Penicillium are most often found growing as

    A. fruit molds   B. pink molds
    C. powdery mildews   D. slime molds

7. Two breeds that have been crossed to produce a better variety of cattle are the Brahmin and

    A. Aberdeen-Angus   B. Ancon
    C. Plymouth rock   D. Poland China

8. The original seedless grape was produced by

    A. artificial pollination   B. hybridization
    C. inbreeding   D. mutation

9. With regard to human heredity the most accurate statement is

   A. Albinism is determined by several genes
   B. Hair color is determined by several genes
   C. Pure blue eyes are inherited as a simple recessive
   D. The inheritance of height and weight is better understood than the inheritance of skin color

10. The sea anemone and the hermit crab live in a relationship which is

    A. mutually destructive
    B. mutually helpful
    C. helpful to the anemone but destructive to the crab
    D. helpful to the crab but destructive to the anemone

11. The man who is correctly associated with a biological concept is

    A. DeVries - crossing over
    B. Lamarck - evolution by mutation
    C. Morgan - independent assortment
    D. Weisman - continuity of germplasm

12. Fossils are LEAST likely to be found in

    A. amber   B. granite   C. tarpits   D. limestone

13. Dinosaurs became extinct

    A. before the appearance of brachiopods
    B. before the disappearance of trilobites
    C. after the appearance of mammals
    D. after the disappearance of mastodons

14. Two insects that belong to different orders are

    A. cricket and grasshopper   B. butterfly and moth
    C. cicada and dragonfly   D. bee and ant

15. The forelimbs of a pterodactyl and a bat are said to be

    A. analogous   B. homologous   C. parallel   D. vestigial

16. A nutrient test for protein involves the use of nitric acid and

    A. acetic acid   B. ammonia
    C. sodium peroxide   D. sulfur dioxide

17. When carbon dioxide is bubbled through brom thymol blue the indicator turns

    A. colorless   B. pink   C. red   D. yellow

18. An example of a syncytium is seen in

    A. cardiac tissue   B. nerve tissue
    C. tendons   D. ligaments

19. The average composition of protoplasm in percent by weight is best represented by

   A. protein 15%; fats 3%; other substances 82%
   B. protein 20%; carbohydrates 18%; other substances 62%
   C. protein 25%; minerals 6%; other substances 69%
   D. protein 30%; water 60%; other substances 10%

20. A mycelium is MOST closely associated with

   A. algae   B. molds   C. rhizomes   D. root hairs

21. Desoxyribose is an example of a

   A. monosaccharide
   B. polysaccharide
   C. polypeptid
   D. phospholipid

22. A man who has recently succeeded in isolating mitotic spindles from living cells is

   A. Lipmann   B. Mazia   C. Sumner   D. Stern

23. Insufficient formation of the prothrombase will result from a deficiency in

   A. Vitamin B_2
   B. Vitamin P-P
   C. Vitamin B_{12}
   D. Vitamin K

24. The contractile vacuole of the paramecium functions in

   A. cell division
   B. digestion of carbohydrates
   C. formation of cytoplasm
   D. maintenance of water balance

25. A hanging drop slide would be used to

   A. detect motility of bacteria
   B. stain blood cells
   C. count red corpuscles
   D. make a permanent slide

26. A drop of fountain pen ink applied to a slide of living paramecia will enable one to demonstrate BEST

   A. the oral groove
   B. food vacuoles
   C. gullet
   D. trichocysts

27. Polar bodies are formed during

   A. budding   B. meiosis   C. sporulation   D. synapsis

28. A developmental stage associated with incomplete metamorphosis in insects is called

   A. larva   B. maggot   C. nymph   D. pupa

29. An example of a hermaphroditic animal is the

   A. centipede   B. earthworm   C. spider   D. stickleback

30. In the development of the embryo the correct sequence is

    A. blastula, gastrula, morula
    B. blastula, morula, gastrula
    C. gastrula, blastula, morula
    D. morula, blastula, gastrula

31. The euglena moves by means of

    A. cilia   B. flagella   C. myonemes   D. pseudopods

32. The witch hazel is an unusual shrub because it

    A. grows in an unusual habitat
    B. is saprophytic
    C. blooms in the fall
    D. shows marked thigmotropic responses

33. The cornea of the eye

    A. is comparable to the diaphragm of a camera
    B. is composed of connective tissue
    C. aids the lens in refracting light rays
    D. has the power of accommodation

34. The function of the green glands of a lobster is essentially

    A. circulatory   B. excretory   C. respiratory   D. reproductive

35. Adult birds normally possess only one functional

    A. kidney   B. ovary   C. testis   D. ureter

36. The primitive type of nervous system seen in a hydra is called

    A. autonomic   B. ganglion   C. nerve net   D. plexus

37. The function of the cerebellum is MOST closely associated with the function of the

    A. Eustachian tube   B. semi-circular canals
    C. cochlea   D. tympanic membrane

38. MOST vitamins are now known to function as

    A. antienzymes   B. apoenzymes   C. coenzymes   D. enzymes

39. The separation between right and left ventricles is generally incomplete among

    A. apes   B. birds   C. snakes   D. kangaroos

40. The MOST readily available source of quick energy in the cell is

    A. adenosine triphosphate   B. dehydrogenase
    C. hexosekinase   D. nucleoprotein

41. Afferent and efferent nerve fibres are respectively called

    A. motor and sensory   B. sensory and motor
    C. effector and receptor   D. receptor and effector

42. Peristaltic action is involved in

    A. contraction of the pupil
    B. flow of saliva
    C. movement of diaphragm
    D. passage of food through the esophagus

43. The aorta sends branches to all of the following EXCEPT to the

    A. kidney   B. liver   C. lungs   D. small intestine

44. The pancreas is stimulated to secrete pancreatic juice by

    A. pancreatin   B. renin   C. secretin   D. trypsin

45. The follicle stimulating hormone is produced by the

    A. anterior lobe of the pituitary gland
    B. posterior lobe of the pituitary gland
    C. adrenal cortex
    D. adrenal medulla

46. Contraction of the uterine wall during childbirth is aided by the injection of

    A. gonadotrophin   B. oxytocin   C. relaxin   D. sympathin

47. The blood vessel which brings blood to the liver is the hepatic

    A. artery   B. vein   C. portal artery   D. portal vein

48. The thoracic duct is part of the

    A. digestive system   B. lymphatic system
    C. nervous system   D. respiratory system

49. Oxygen debt is a factor involved in

    A. anaerobic fermentation   B. muscle metabolism
    C. photosynthesis   D. plant respiration

50. Addison's disease may result from tubercular infection of the

    A. adrenal glands   B. bones
    C. lymph nodes   D. spleen

KEY (CORRECT ANSWERS)

1. A	11. D	21. A	31. B	41. B
2. A	12. B	22. B	32. C	42. D
3. C	13. C	23. D	33. C	43. C
4. C	14. C	24. D	34. B	44. C
5. C	15. B	25. A	35. B	45. A
6. A	16. B	26. D	36. C	46. B
7. A	17. D	27. B	37. B	47. D
8. D	18. A	28. C	38. C	48. B
9. C	19. A	29. B	39. C	49. B
10. B	20. B	30. D	40. A	50. A

TEST 3

DIRECTIONS: Each question or incomplete statement is followed by several suggested answers or completions. Select the one that BEST answers the question or completes the statement. PRINT THE LETTER OF THE CORRECT ANSWER IN THE SPACE AT THE RIGHT.

1. In a nearsighted person the

    A. image is in focus behind the eyeball
    B. retina is too close to the lens
    C. lens is too concave
    D. eyeball is too long from lens to retina

2. The rods of the retina are MOST closely associated with

    A. the blind spot   B. bright light vision
    C. color vision   D. twilight vision

3. Plasmolysis refers to

    A. destruction of the plasma membrane
    B. increase of quantity of blood plasma
    C. loss of plasma from the blood
    D. shrinkage of protoplasm due to loss of water

4. The "anvil, hammer, and stirrup" refer to

    A. adaptations for pollination
    B. bones of the middle ear
    C. reflex arcs
    D. theory of immunity

5. Albinism in corn is an example of

    A. chimera   B. inversion
    C. lethal character   D. sex-linked character

6. The Archeopteryx possessed

    A. a toothless beak
    B. clawless wings
    C. tail feathers, but not a true tail
    D. a true tail with feathers on it

7. The stage in embryology at which the primitive gut is well-formed is called the

    A. blastula   B. fistula   C. gastrula   D. morula

8. Diabetes insipidus is caused by

    A. insufficient secretion of insulin
    B. oversecretion of insulin
    C. insufficient secretion of vasopressin
    D. insufficient secretion of renin

9. The MOST conclusive line of evidence that biological evolution has actually occurred is

   A. common ancestry of vertebrates
   B. fossil records
   C. geographic isolation
   D. comparative anatomy

10. Chlorophyll is found in the

    A. vacuole of a leaf cell
    B. nucleus of a leaf cell
    C. stomata of leaves
    D. plastids of leaf cells

11. Of the following, the one found in the Elodea cell, but NOT in a cheek lining cell is

    A. nucleus   B. cell wall   C. cytoplasm   D. cell membrane

12. Recently reported research on the common bread mold indicates the possible use of the mold in treating

    A. mental disorders
    B. fungal infections
    C. blood clots
    D. fatty deposits on arterial walls

13. Liquids are transported through stems and roots by the

    A. epidermis
    B. cortex
    C. vascular bundles
    D. pith

14. Root pressure is principally the result of

    A. capillarity   B. osmosis   C. adhesion   D. cohesion

15. A sliced piece of potato is placed into cold water. After several hours it becomes stiff and hard because

    A. new chemical substances have formed
    B. solid particles have formed because water has passed out of the cells
    C. water has passed into the cells to produce turgor
    D. additional cellulose has formed in the cell walls

16. The circulatory mechanism characteristic of all organisms is

    A. the xylem-phloem mechanism
    B. the gastrovascular mechanism
    C. the flame cell system
    D. diffusion

17. One similarity between reflexes and habits is that they are both

    A. inborn acts
    B. learned acts
    C. autonomic acts
    D. automatic

18. The number of glands in the group known as the parathyroids, is

    A. 1   B. 2   C. 3   D. 4

19. The vertebrate that could be MOST nearly described as a parasite is the

    A. eel   B. cowbird   C. lamprey   D. rodent

20. Nasal infection may spread through the Eustachian tubes to the

    A. esophagus
    B. lungs
    C. frontal sinuses
    D. middle ears

21. The relationship between cells and tissues is paralleled by that between

    A. organs and systems
    B. enzymes and the substrates
    C. carbohydrates and fats
    D. ectoderm and endoderm

22. In biology, the principle of "division of labor" involves

    A. the production of varied agricultural crops
    B. growth so that there are more cells to do the work
    C. differentiation of cells into tissues having different functions
    D. competition among organisms for the needs of life

23. A vitamin that contains cobalt as part of its chemical structure is vitamin

    A. A   B. B_2 C. B_{12} D. C

24. The term "differentially permeable" is used to describe the part of the living cell called the

    A. centrosome
    B. cytoplasm
    C. nucleus
    D. plasma membrane

25. The substances considered MOST important in the development of new protoplasm are the

    A. proteins   B. carbohydrates   C. fats   D. enzymes

26. In order that its underside be visible through a microscope, a material must possess the characteristic of being

    A. opaque
    B. light-colored
    C. stained
    D. able to transmit light

27. The word "control" as used in describing a scientific experiment is MOST closely defined as a

    A. preliminary trial experiment
    B. experiment with the variable factor
    C. repeat experiment
    D. comparison experiment

28. The study of the functioning of living organisms is called

    A. anatomy   B. pathology   C. ecology   D. physiology

29. The MOST nearly correct statement regarding osmosis is that it

    A. is essentially a diffusion process
    B. is essentially a process involving capillary action
    C. functions only in living organisms
    D. functions only in the presence of light

30. Elastic tissue is of the type known as

    A. connective   B. muscular   C. nerve   D. epithelial

31. Of the following terms, the one that includes all of the others is

    A. gametogenesis
    B. oogenesis
    C. spermatogenesis
    D. reduction division

32. Cutting away a complete ring of bark from a tree stops the passage of material through the

    A. xylem   B. tracheids   C. phloem   D. medullary rays

33. Independent assortment does NOT always occur in dihybrid crosses. This may be the result of

    A. recessiveness
    B. linkage
    C. dominance
    D. segregation

34. An example of a pair of homologous structures is

    A. the wing of a housefly and the wing of a bat
    B. the front leg of a cat and the wing of a bird
    C. the trunk of a tree and the trunk of an elephant
    D. the flipper of a whale and the tail of a fish

35. The relation between clover plants and nitrogen-fixing bacteria is a form of

    A. parasitism
    B. saprophytism
    C. commensalism
    D. symbiosis

36. Autumnal abscission of leaves benefits deciduous trees primarily in

    A. conserving water
    B. eliminating waste products
    C. allowing the tree to rest
    D. slowing respiration

37. A wire clothesline was tied six feet from the ground around an 18-foot elm tree. When the tree grew to a height of 36 feet, the height in feet of the line above the ground was

    A. six   B. nine   C. twelve   D. eighteen

38. The portions of the solar spectrum MOST effective as a source of energy for photosynthesis are the

    A. green and blue
    B. indigo and green
    C. yellow and blue
    D. red and violet

39. The role of chlorophyll in photosynthesis is similar to the role of

    A. an enzyme in digestion
    B. glucose in respiration
    C. carbon dioxide in respiration
    D. bile in fat digestion

40. In a given sample of blood, clumping occurred with both A serum and B serum. The blood type was

    A. A
    B. B
    C. AB
    D. O

41. Blood plasma from which the fibrinogen has been removed is known as

    A. blood concentrate
    B. serum
    C. hormone complement
    D. antibody component

42. A type of blood bank from which reserves of red blood corpuscles may be quickly mobilized when needed by the body is the

    A. liver
    B. bone marrow
    C. intestinal mesentery
    D. spleen

43. The lowest concentration of nitrogenous waste generally may be found in blood passing through the

    A. pulmonary artery
    B. renal artery
    C. hepatic vein
    D. renal vein

44. A drastic type of anemia, erythro blastosis fetalis, is caused by

    A. a deficiency of iron in the diet
    B. virus invasion of red blood corpuscles
    C. antibodies induced in the pregnant mother by fetal antigens
    D. a fetus that is Rh negative

45. Pleurococcus may most often be found

    A. on the moist shaded side of a tree trunk
    B. on the surface of a still pond
    C. in a running stream
    D. under a rock

46. The movement of raw materials and carbohydrates from one region to another within a plant is known as

    A. translocation
    B. transmutation
    C. transfusion
    D. transpiration

47. Oxygen enters the blood because

    A. there is a higher partial pressure of O_2 in the lungs
    B. there is a higher partial pressure of CO_2 in the lungs
    C. there is a higher partial pressure of O_2 in the blood
    D. blood contains hemoglobin

48. Failure of blood to clot readily when exposed to air may be due to a(n)

    A. oversupply of erythrocytes
    B. deficiency of leucocytes
    C. overabundance of fibrin
    D. inadequacy of thrombokinase

49. Acetylsalicylic acid retards the clotting of blood. This would be advantageous in

    A. an appendectomy   B. coronary thrombosis
    C. cancer   D. hemorrhage of the lungs

50. Failure of lymph to circulate would MOST directly affect

    A. fat digestion
    B. transport between the body cells and blood
    C. production of red blood cells
    D. circulation of blood platelets

KEY (CORRECT ANSWERS)

1. D	11. B	21. A	31. A	41. B
2. D	12. C	22. C	32. C	42. D
3. D	13. C	23. C	33. B	43. D
4. B	14. B	24. B	34. B	44. C
5. C	15. C	25. A	35. D	45. A
6. D	16. D	26. D	36. A	46. A
7. C	17. D	27. D	37. A	47. A
8. C	18. D	28. D	38. D	48. D
9. B	19. C	29. A	39. A	49. B
10. D	20. D	30. A	40. C	50. B

TEST 4

DIRECTIONS: Each question or incomplete statement is followed by several suggested answers or completions. Select the one that BEST answers the question or completes the statement. PRINT THE LETTER OF THE CORRECT ANSWER IN THE SPACE AT THE RIGHT.

1. The respiratory blood pigment found in mollusks is 1.___
   - A. hemoglobin
   - B. hemocyanin
   - C. hemerythrin
   - D. chlorocruorin

2. A rabbit sensitized to human blood gives the precipitin-clumping reaction LEAST promptly when its serum is added to the whole blood of a 2.___
   - A. lemur
   - B. human
   - C. chimpanzee
   - D. gorilla

3. The chemicals that cause clumping of the erythrocytes in the blood are found 3.___
   - A. platelets
   - B. red corpuscles
   - C. white corpuscles
   - D. plasma

4. In the human fetus, blood flows directly between the left and right auricles. This would indicate that 4.___
   - A. the pulmonary system does not function before birth
   - B. the heart does not function before birth
   - C. the heart of the fetus carries only unoxygenated blood
   - D. only the ventricles of the fetal heart are functional before birth

5. Many of the physical properties of protoplasm can be explained by considering it to be a(n) 5.___
   - A. solution
   - B. emulsion
   - C. colloidal suspension
   - D. mixture

6. If the pancreatic ducts of an experimental animal were tied off, the MOST probable consequence would be 6.___
   - A. a sudden increase in blood pressure and heart rate
   - B. a voracious appetite, with excessive thirst and urination
   - C. a derangement of the carbohydrate metabolism
   - D. stoppage of fat digestion and slowing of digestion of proteins and carbohydrates

7. A structure which normally serves as a common passageway for both food and air is the 7.___
   - A. pharynx
   - B. glottis
   - C. trachea
   - D. larynx

8. Deamination of proteins occurs mainly in the 8.___
   - A. small intestine
   - B. liver
   - C. pancreas
   - D. spleen

9. The products of fat digestion are absorbed by the 9.___
   - A. capillaries in the villi
   - B. lacteals in the villi
   - C. gall bladder
   - D. capillaries in the stomach walls

10. About 70 per cent of the energy from glucose oxidation is used

    A. as heat
    B. for contracting muscles
    C. to produce nerve impulses
    D. to cause gland cells to secrete

11. In the process of respiration in a plant,

    A. potential energy is stored
    B. chlorophyll is necessary
    C. stored food is utilized
    D. protein is synthesized

12. The glomeruli are MOST closely related to the system involved in

    A. reproduction
    B. support and movement
    C. digestion
    D. excretion

13. The liquid which collects in the cavity of Bowman's capsule is

    A. urine in concentrated form
    B. blood plasma minus plasma proteins
    C. freshly aerated blood
    D. used bile ready for excretion

14. Three of the following are chromosomal aberrations which are important in the origin of species. The one that is NOT is

    A. translocation
    B. inversion
    C. meiosis
    D. duplication

15. A trait determined by two identical alleles is said to be

    A. homologous
    B. analagous
    C. heterozygous
    D. homozygous

16. Three of the following responses in plants are brought about by the action of hormones. The response that is NOT brought about is the

    A. bending of a stem toward light
    B. inhibition of lateral bud development by a terminal bud
    C. growth of pollen tubes through the style
    D. movement of the specialized leaves of the Venusflytrap

17. The hormone that controls the use of calcium in the body is secreted by the

    A. thyroid   B. parathyroids   C. adrenals   D. pancreas

18. A "tropic" hormone is one that is secreted by an endocrine gland to

    A. regulate the temperature of the body
    B. regulate the metabolism of the body
    C. stimulate or inhibit the secretion of another endocrine gland
    D. produce a response to stress known as the general-adaptation syndrome

19. $C_{15}H_{11}O_4NI_4$ is the chemical formula of the hormone

   A. thyroxin   B. testosterone   C. insulin   D. adrenin

20. The animal phylum that numbers about 723,000 species is the

   A. mollusca   B. arthropoda   C. chordata   D. protozoa

21. Flatworms are usually found in ponds or streams

   A. on the underside of objects
   B. free-swimming
   C. on the upper side of objects
   D. on the north side of objects

22. Of the following, three are larval stages in the life history of the liver fluke. The one that is NOT is the

   A. redia   B. cercaria   C. trochophore   D. miracidium

23. The outer of the two membranes surrounding the embryo and fetus of mammals is the

   A. chorion   B. placenta   C. coelom   D. amnion

24. In the life cycle of the wheat rust the spores that settle and germinate on the leaves of barberry bushes are known as

   A. uredospores   B. teliospores
   C. basidiospores   D. aeciospores

25. Plants whose leaves are generally fleshy and waterproofed are known as

   A. hydrophytes   B. bryophytes
   C. mesophytes   D. xerophytes

26. Under anaerobic conditions yeast obtains energy through the process of

   A. oxidation   B. glycogenolysis
   C. fermentation   D. digestion

27. Antibodies that act on bacteria in such a way that phagocytes may more easily ingest them are known as

   A. opsonins   B. antitoxins   C. lysins   D. agglutinins

28. Commensalism is the type of association between organisms which may be

   A. helpful to both
   B. helpful to one and harmful to the other
   C. helpful to one and indifferent to the other
   D. harmful to both

29. Gill slits in the embryos of mammals are regarded as evidence of the fact that the

   A. embryo uses gills to breathe
   B. adult mammals use gills to breathe
   C. ancestors of mammals used gills to breathe
   D. mammals of the future will develop gills

30. Egestion is the process by which

   A. metabolic wastes are eliminated from an organism
   B. food substances pass from the digestive cavity into the body proper
   C. non-absorbable materials from the digestive cavity are eliminated from the body
   D. food substances are transported throughout the body of an organism

31. Brain waves may be detected through the use of a(n)

   A. sphygmomanometer B. electroencephalograph
   C. electrocardiograph D. oscillograph

32. The process by which protoplasm constructs new protoplasm, oxidizes food materials, and breaks down, is called

   A. anabolism B. catabolism C. metabolism D. diabolism

33. Of the following the smallest that can reduplicate itself is

   A. protozoan B. gene C. bacterium D. chromosome

34. A leaf from a plant kept in the dark for three days is boiled in alcohol to dissolve out the chlorophyll. When iodine is applied to the leaf, the leaf becomes

   A. brown B. violet
   C. orange-red D. blue-black

35. Control of hemophilia can be achieved now by

   A. supplementary doses of folic acid
   B. periodic injections of thromboplastinogen
   C. supplementary doses of vitamin B_{12}
   D. x-ray radiation of bone marrow

36. A person living at sea level who visits Pike's Peak for several weeks will most likely experience a

   A. fall in his white cell blood count
   B. fall in his red cell blood count
   C. rise in his white cell blood count
   D. rise in his red cell blood count

37. The thickest portion of the heart is the wall of the

   A. left auricle B. right auricle C. left ventricle D. right ventricle

38. The tricuspid valve lies between the

   A. left auricle and the left ventricle
   B. right auricle and the right ventricle
   C. right ventricle and the pulmonary artery
   D. left auricle and the right auricle

39. Of the molecules listed, the one with the highest potential-energy content may be represented as

    A. ADP B. ACTH C. ATP D. LH

40. The heart is in a state of contraction during

    A. diastole B. metastasis C. systole D. syncope

41. MOST of the stored food in a monocotyledonous seed is located in the

    A. endosperm B. cotyledon
    C. embryo sac D. hypocotyl

42. The process of invagination occurs during

    A. mitosis B. gastrulation
    C. maturation D. meiosis

43. Destruction of a group of cytons in the ventral horn of the grey matter of the spinal cord may result in

    A. loss of sensation B. paralysis
    C. loss of memory D. blindness

44. A vitamin involved in the "yellow" respiratory pigments found in cells is

    A. ascorbic acid B. carotene
    C. ergosterol D. riboflavin

45. The vitamin involved in formation of cocarboxylase which participates in oxidative decarboxylations is

    A. B_1 B. B_2 C. B_6 D. B_{12}

46. The vitamin MOST closely associated with intercellular material in tissues such as cartilage and bone is

    A. ascorbic acid B. inositol
    C. niacin D. riboflavin

47. Of the following hormones, the one NOT secreted by the pituitary gland is

    A. progesterone
    B. follicle stimulating hormone
    C. luteinizing hormone
    D. vasopressin

48. Myxedema is associated with atrophy of the

    A. thyroid B. pancreas C. pituitary D. adrenal

49. The hormone that serves primarily to sustain the corpus luteum during early pregnancy is

    A. estrogen
    B. progesterone
    C. luteotrophin
    D. oxytocin

50. A hormone derived from the ovary, uterus, and placenta which facilitates childbirth by its affect on the pubic symphysis is

    A. somatropin   B. relaxin   C. hypothalamin   D. progesterone

KEY (CORRECT ANSWERS)

1. B	11. C	21. A	31. B	41. A
2. A	12. D	22. C	32. C	42. B
3. D	13. B	23. A	33. B	43. B
4. A	14. C	24. C	34. A	44. D
5. C	15. D	25. D	35. B	45. A
6. D	16. D	26. C	36. D	46. B
7. A	17. B	27. A	37. C	47. A
8. B	18. C	28. C	38. B	48. A
9. B	19. A	29. C	39. C	49. C
10. A	20. B	30. C	40. C	50. B

TEST 5

DIRECTIONS: Each question or incomplete statement is followed by several suggested answers or completions. Select the one that BEST answers the question or completes the statement. PRINT THE LETTER OF THE CORRECT ANSWER IN THE SPACE AT THE RIGHT.

1. Students of science were not taught the Mendelian Laws before 1900 because   1.___

   A. the laws were not confirmed by research before the twentieth century
   B. the industrial revolution overshadowed the work of the obscure monk
   C. there was religious opposition to mechanistic explanations of life processes
   D. Mendel's scientific paper was neglected for nearly fifty years

2. Explosions of nuclear devices have increased the danger of damage to human bone tissue by substituting for one of the elements in normal bone a radioactive isotope of   2.___

   A. iodine   B. calcium   C. strontium   D. phosphorus

3. Smooth muscle cells are found in the   3.___

   A. muscles that cause the beating of the heart
   B. walls of the stomach
   C. muscles that cause movement of the legs
   D. striated muscle bundles

4. Composed of elongated cells with many nuclei BEST describes   4.___

   A. smooth muscle tissue   B. skeletal muscle tissue
   C. nerve tissue   D. vascular tissue

5. When an unknown food was tested, it yielded no color change when treated with iodine, or with nitric acid, or with Sudan III, but caused Benedict's solution to turn brick red upon heating. Of the following foods, the one MOST probably being tested was   5.___

   A. lean beef   B. white potato
   C. lemon juice   D. butter

6. In mammals, accommodation of the lens of the eye is a   6.___

   A. reflex   B. tropism   C. voluntary act   D. habit

7. In the fastest nerve fibers of mammals the nerve impulse travels at a rate, expressed in feet per second, of approximately   7.___

   A. 175   B. 350   C. 525   D. 700

8. In humans the sense of hearing is MOST closely associated with the   8.___

   A. anvil   B. organ of Corti
   C. semicircular canals   D. malleus

9. Fertilization in humans usually occurs in the   9.___

   A. vagina   B. uterus   C. oviduct   D. ovary

10. The great diversity of form and structure as seen in the bills and feet of birds can be described BEST by the biological principle of

    A. geographic isolation
    B. parallel evolution
    C. inbreeding
    D. adaptive radiation

11. The fact that many of the marsupials of Australia closely resemble different kinds of placental mammals in other parts of the world is an example of

    A. geographic isolation
    B. survival of the fittest
    C. parallel evolution
    D. divergent evolution

12. The internal connection of an embryonic gill slit with the pharynx is retained in adult humans as the

    A. endolymphatic duct
    B. uvula
    C. parotid gland
    D. Eustachian tube

13. The medulla of the human brain is associated with

    A. control of body equilibrium and muscular coordination
    B. sense perception: hearing, seeing, smelling
    C. control of limb movements and sense perception in the limbs
    D. control of swallowing, respiratory rhythm, blood pressure and heart beat

14. Muscular spasms – tetany – may result from the removal of the gland(s) called the

    A. pineal   B. thymus   C. thyroid   D. parathyroid

15. In diabetes insipidus the

    A. urine contains above normal concentrations of sugar
    B. anterior pituitary gland is damaged
    C. isles of Langerhans have degenerated
    D. urine is quite devoid of sugar

16. A reflex may become a conditioned reflex if it involves

    A. the original stimulus but no new stimulus
    B. the original stimulus and a different response
    C. a new stimulus and a new response
    D. a new stimulus and the same response

17. When a root of a plant is forced to lie horizontal on the ground, auxin will accumulate in the cell region near the ground and will bring about

    A. cell growth in this region thus causing the root to grow downward
    B. inhibition of cell growth in this region thus causing the root to grow downward
    C. development of root hairs in this region
    D. even elongation of the root along the horizontal axis

18. An acceptable explanation for the fact that the spores of ferns function in the distribution of the plant while the spores of flowering plants do not is

    A. the spores of ferns are produced in sporangia
    B. in ferns the sporophyte is the dominant generation

C. the gametophytes of ferns are independent plants whereas those of flowering plants are not
D. in flowering plants the zygote is formed by union of sperm and egg

19. The part of the seed that contains tissue which was part of the old sporophyte is the

    A. testa   B. hypocotyl   C. endosperm   D. cotyledon

20. Nucleoli found in cells

    A. arise at fixed points on specific chromosomes
    B. vary in number within the cells of a given species
    C. contain DNA
    D. are persistent structures

21. The foraminifera are characteristically

    A. naked protozoa
    B. all fresh water forms
    C. simple sponges
    D. animals with calcareous shells

22. Chlorophyll has a chemical structure which

    A. is identical with that of hemoglobin
    B. is like that of other enzymes
    C. resembles the hemo part of hemoglobin
    D. resembles the globin part of hemoglobin

23. Studies made with the electron microscope show that grana are the basic structural components of

    A. chromosomes   B. cytoplasm
    C. plasma membranes   D. chloroplasts

24. Experiments with radioactive carbon performed by M. Calvin on algae show that one of the first carbon compounds formed in photosynthesis is

    A. phosphoglyceric acid   B. fructose
    C. glucose   D. carbonic acid

25. In certain insects the sex formula is XX-XO. In both males and females there are 22 autosomes. The chromosome number found in sperm cells is

    A. 11   B. 12   C. 11 and 12   D. 23

26. In drosophila the sex of a fly of the genotype XY is determined primarily by genes located on the

    A. autosomes and Y-chromosomes   B. Y-chromosome
    C. autosomes   D. autosomes and X-chromosome

27. A corn grain dropped near a barnyard grew into a large corn plant which, after maturing, had ears with few kernels. The MOST probable explanation for the paucity of kernels is that the

A. barnyard fertilizer in high concentration affected kernel development
B. plant did not receive the same attention given to plants grown in the field
C. corn grain was probably not of selected seed variety
D. cross-fertilization did not occur

28. Two black guinea pigs, when mated, may produce a white offspring. This is probably a result of

    A. mutation
    B. heterozygosity
    C. independent assortment
    D. incomplete dominance

29. Accommodation of the eye for near vision results when the

    A. tension on the suspensory ligament increases
    B. ciliary muscle contracts
    C. ciliary muscle relaxes
    D. lens becomes flatter and broader as a result of stretching

30. An awareness by a person of the position or location of muscles and bones is attributed to the action of

    A. chemoreceptors
    B. proprioreceptors
    C. enteroreceptors
    D. tactoreceptors

31. Organs are grouped into systems on the basis of

    A. common structure
    B. related functions
    C. proximity to each other
    D. the order of their appearance in the embryo

32. The embryonic organ which meets the absorptive, respiratory and excretory needs of developing embryos of higher vertebrates is the

    A. allantois   B. amnion   C. gill   D. pronephros

33. The Krebs oxidative cycle appears to be determined largely, if not completely, by organized groups of enzymes derived from the

    A. Golgi bodies
    B. nuclear membrane
    C. nuclear sap
    D. mitochondria

34. The Feulgen reaction is a chemical aid to the identification of

    A. sex of unborn children
    B. growth hormones in plants
    C. pregnancy hormones in urine
    D. nucleic acid

35. If there are 16 chromosomes in each cell of a fern sporophyte, the number of chromosomes in each cell of the prothallus of this fern would be

    A. 4   B. 8   C. 16   D. 32

Questions 36-50

In each of the following 15 questions, 36-50, there are two statements, 1 and 2. You are to decide whether A. 1 and 2 are correct; or B. 1 and 2 are incorrect; or C. 1 is correct and 2 is incorrect; or D. 1 is incorrect and 2 is correct.

36. 1. The gene for color blindness in man is located on the X chromosome.
    2. The gene for hemophilia in man is located on the Y chromosome.

    A. 1 is correct and 2 is correct
    B. 1 is incorrect and 2 is incorrect
    C. 1 is correct and 2 is incorrect
    D. 1 is incorrect and 2 is correct

37. 1. Angiosperms are more primitive than gymnosperms.
    2. Bryophytes are more primitive than pteridophytes.

    A. 1 is correct and 2 is correct
    B. 1 is incorrect and 2 is incorrect
    C. 1 is correct and 2 is incorrect
    D. 1 is incorrect and 2 is correct

38. 1. A cell plate is formed in dividing animal cells.
    2. Centrosomes have never been found in plant cells.

    A. 1 is correct and 2 is correct
    B. 1 is incorrect and 2 is incorrect
    C. 1 is correct and 2 is incorrect
    D. 1 is incorrect and 2 is correct

39. 1. The endosperm cells of a ripe corn seed have the diploid number of chromosomes.
    2. The embryo cells of a ripe corn seed have the diploid number of chromosomes.

    A. 1 is correct and 2 is correct
    B. 1 is incorrect and 2 is incorrect
    C. 1 is correct and 2 is incorrect
    D. 1 is incorrect and 2 is correct

40. 1. Drone bees develop parthenogenetically.
    2. Worker bees are sterile females.

    A. 1 is correct and 2 is correct
    B. 1 is incorrect and 2 is incorrect
    C. 1 is correct and 2 is incorrect
    D. 1 is incorrect and 2 is correct

41. 1. The excretory system of man develops from the ectoderm.
    2. The nervous system of man develops from the mesoderm.

    A. 1 is correct and 2 is correct
    B. 1 is incorrect and 2 is incorrect
    C. 1 is correct and 2 is incorrect
    D. 1 is incorrect and 2 is correct

42. 1. Red corpuscles will burst when placed in a hypotonic solution.
    2. Red corpuscles will shrink when placed in an isotonic solution.

    A. 1 is correct and 2 is correct
    B. 1 is incorrect and 2 is incorrect
    C. 1 is correct and 2 is incorrect
    D. 1 is incorrect and 2 is correct

43. 1. Auricles have thinner walls than ventricles.
    2. The right ventricle has thinner walls than the left ventricle.

    A. 1 is correct and 2 is correct
    B. 1 is incorrect and 2 is incorrect
    C. 1 is correct and 2 is incorrect
    D. 1 is incorrect and 2 is correct

44. 1. The union of isogametes is a type of asexual reproduction.
    2. The union of heterogametes is a type of sexual reproduction.

    A. 1 is correct and 2 is correct
    B. 1 is incorrect and 2 is incorrect
    C. 1 is correct and 2 is incorrect
    D. 1 is incorrect and 2 is correct

45. 1. The part of a microscope on which the slide is placed for observation is called the base.
    2. The lenses in the eyepiece usually have greater magnifying power than the lenses in the objectives.

    A. 1 is correct and 2 is correct
    B. 1 is incorrect and 2 is incorrect
    C. 1 is correct and 2 is incorrect
    D. 1 is incorrect and 2 is correct

46. 1. The life process by which the protoplasm of a cell increases is called absorption.
    2. The sum total of the chemical and physical processes going on in a cell is called anabolism.

    A. 1 is correct and 2 is correct
    B. 1 is incorrect and 2 is incorrect
    C. 1 is correct and 2 is incorrect
    D. 1 is incorrect and 2 is correct

47. 1. The lichen is a parasite.
    2. Nitrogen-fixing bacteria are saprophytes.

    A. 1 is correct and 2 is correct
    B. 1 is incorrect and 2 is incorrect
    C. 1 is correct and 2 is incorrect
    D. 1 is incorrect and 2 is correct

48. 1. The drooping of the leaves of the mimosa plant is effected by auxins.
    2. The upward growth of a stem is an example of negative geotropism.

    A. 1 is correct and 2 is correct
    B. 1 is incorrect and 2 is incorrect
    C. 1 is correct and 2 is incorrect
    D. 1 is incorrect and 2 is correct

49. 1. It is more difficult to obtain a pure breed of animals with a dominant mutation than one with a recessive mutation.
    2. In most instances a mutation is beneficial to the organism in which it occurs.

    A. 1 is correct and 2 is correct
    B. 1 is incorrect and 2 is incorrect
    C. 1 is correct and 2 is incorrect
    D. 1 is incorrect and 2 is correct

50. 1. Bone is a type of connective tissue.
    2. Glands are composed of epithelial tissue.

    A. 1 is correct and 2 is correct
    B. 1 is incorrect and 2 is incorrect
    C. 1 is correct and 2 is incorrect
    D. 1 is incorrect and 2 is correct

KEY (CORRECT ANSWERS)

1. D	11. C	21. D	31. B	41. B
2. C	12. D	22. C	32. A	42. C
3. B	13. D	23. D	33. D	43. C
4. B	14. D	24. A	34. D	44. D
5. C	15. D	25. C	35. B	45. B
6. C	16. D	26. D	36. C	46. B
7. A	17. B	27. D	37. B	47. B
8. B	18. C	28. B	38. B	48. D
9. C	19. A	29. B	39. D	49. C
10. D	20. A	30. B	40. A	50. A

EXAMINATION SECTION
TEST 1

DIRECTIONS: Each question or incomplete statement is followed by several suggested answers or completions. Select the one that BEST answers the question or completes the statement. *PRINT THE LETTER OF THE CORRECT ANSWER IN THE SPACE AT THE RIGHT.*

1. A certain bacterium has the ability to make Substance D from Substance A through a series of steps:

    A → B → C → D

    Each step is dependent on the presence of an enzyme:
    Enzyme 1 Enzyme 2 Enzyme 3

    A → B → C → D

    A mutant form of the bacterium can make D ONLY if B is provided by the experimenter even though the mutant bacterium is found to contain adequate amounts of A. This result is explained by the fact that the mutant bacterium lacks

    A. Enzyme 1 *only*
    B. Enzyme 2 *only*
    C. Enzyme 3
    D. both Enzymes 1 and 2
    E. Enzyme 1, 2 and 3

2. _____ act as the PRINCIPAL site of protein synthesis in cells.

    A. Vacuoles
    B. Spindle fibers
    C. Centrosomes
    D. Ribosomes
    E. Mitochondria

3. For every human birth, the chance that the child will be a girl is one in two or 50 percent. The basic fact supporting this prediction is that

    A. the child's mother has two X chromosomes
    B. during meiosis, the chromosome number is reduced by half
    C. the child's father has one X chromosome and one Y chromosome
    D. during fertilization, the chromosome number is restored to the full value of 46
    E. None of the above

4. A student does an experiment to determine the effects of different concentrations of fertilizer on plant growth. She starts with five groups of plants all of the same species and of nearly equal size.
    The experimental treatment is as follows
    Group I: 50 ml/day of a 5% fertilizer solution
    Group II: 50 ml/day of a 10% fertilizer solution
    Group III: 50 ml/day of a 15% fertilizer solution
    Group IV: 50 ml/day of a 20% fertilizer solution
    Group V serves as a control
    What treatment should Group V receive?

    A. 50 ml of full-strength fertilizer not diluted in solution
    B. 50 ml of fertilizer solution, the concentration the average of that of the other four solutions

C. 50 ml of water and no fertilizer
D. Neither water nor fertilizer
E. 50 ml of water and 50 ml of fertilizer

5. In human beings, energy is used for all of the following EXCEPT the

   A. contraction of muscles
   B. maintenance of breathing
   C. maintenance of body temperature on cold days
   D. manufacture of food from CO_2 and H_2O
   E. exchange of blood gases

6. Insects introduced into a new environment may become serious pests PRINCIPALLY because

   A. the insects can make efficient use of the food in the new environment
   B. the insects and birds that usually prey on them are missing
   C. change leads to adaptations and survival of the fittest
   D. waste products of the insects have not yet reached a significant level of concentration in the new environment
   E. None of the above

7. The two hosts necessary for the completion of the life cycle of the sheep liver fluke are the sheep and a

   A. human being   B. pig
   C. rabbit   D. mosquito
   E. fresh-water snail

8. _____ in insects are physiologically comparable to the kidneys in man.

   A. Trachese   B. Malpighian tubules
   C. Nephridia   D. Ovipositors
   E. Green glands

9. The MOST practical control of wheat rust (Puccinia graminis) so far discovered is

   A. the destruction of one of its hosts
   B. the introduction and propagation of its natural enemies
   C. chemical treatment of the seed before planting
   D. control of insects that might spread spores of the fungus
   E. the spraying of infected fields

10. _____ is an event in the formation and discharge of the human egg which precedes the other four.

    A. Discharge of the egg from the ovary
    B. Rupture of the Graafian follicle
    C. Formation of the corpus luteum
    D. Formation of the follicular hormone (estrone)
    E. Formation of progestin (progesterone)

11. The FALSE statement about both aerobic and anaerobic respiration is that they 11.____

    A. produce ATP
    B. can use glucose as a substrate
    C. produce CO_2
    D. require oxygen
    E. All of the above

Questions 12-26.

DIRECTIONS: In Questions 12 through 26, each letter refers to the structure labeled with the same letter in the diagram below. For each item, select one of the five lettered words or phrases that appears above each set of questions which applies to the structure, and put the letter of your choice in the space at the right.

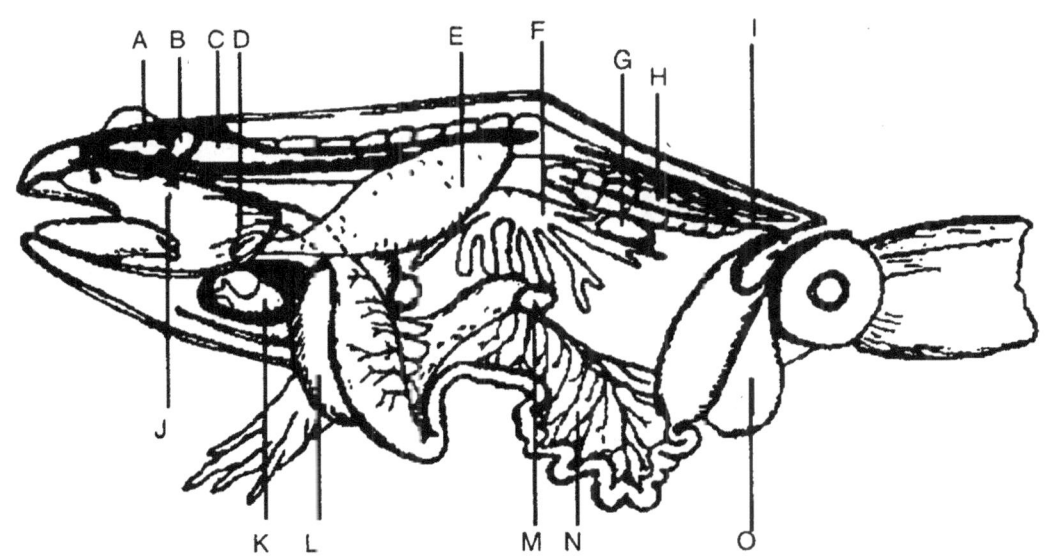

DISSECTION OF MALE FROG

Questions 12-14.

   A. Cerebrum
   B. Cerebellum
   C. Medulla
   D. Optic lobe
   E. Olfactory lobe

12. The structure at A is the 12.____

13. The structure at B is the 13.____

14. The structure at C is the 14.____

Questions 15-17.

    A. Spleen
    B. Testis
    C. Gall bladder
    D. Cloaca
    E. Kidney

15. The structure at G is the   15.____

16. The structure at H is the   16.____

17. The structure at M is the   17.____

Questions 18-20.

    A. Admits air to the mouth from the nostrils
    B. Admits food to the esophagus
    C. Admits air to the lungs
    D. Equalizes pressure on the two sides of the tympanum
    E. Aerates the blood

18. The structure at D   18.____

19. The structure at E   19.____

20. The structure at J   20.____

Questions 21-23.

    A. Produces spermatozoa
    B. Carries blood to the intestine
    C. Stores food in the form of fats
    D. Stores carbohydrates as glycogen
    E. Carries urine and sperm

21. The structure at F   21.____

22. The structure at L   22.____

23. The structure at I   23.____

Questions 24-26.

    A. Forces blood through the arteries
    B. Supports the digestive system
    C. Furnishes oxygen to the blood
    D. Stores liquid wastes
    E. Extracts digested food by osmosis

24. The structure at K   24.____

25. The structure at N   25.____

26. The structure at O   26.____

Questions 27-32.

DIRECTIONS: Questions 27 through 32 are to be answered on the basis of the following diagram. For each question, select one of the five lettered words or phrases that appears above each set of questions which applies to the question, and put the letter of your choice in the space at the right.

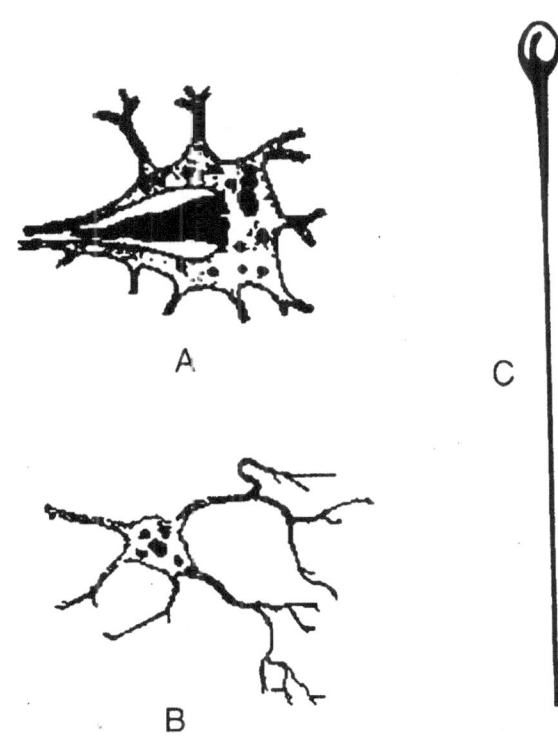

Questions 27-29.

    A. A flame cell
    B. An interstitial cell
    C. A nerve cell
    D. A sperm cell
    E. A phagocyte

27. Diagram A represents   27.____

28. Diagram B represents   28.____

29. Diagram C represents   29.____

Questions 30-32.

    A. Transmits paternal factors
    B. Paralyzes enemies of the hydra
    C. Transmits nerve impulses
    D. Digests foreign organisms in blood
    E. Excretes wastes in flatworms

30. The structure in Diagram A   30.____

31. The structure in Diagram B   31.____

32. The structure in Diagram C   32.____

Questions 33-35.

DIRECTIONS: Questions 33 through 35 are to be answered on the basis of the following diagrams. For each question, select one of the five lettered words or phrases that appears above the questions which applies to the question, and put the letter of your choice in the space at the right.

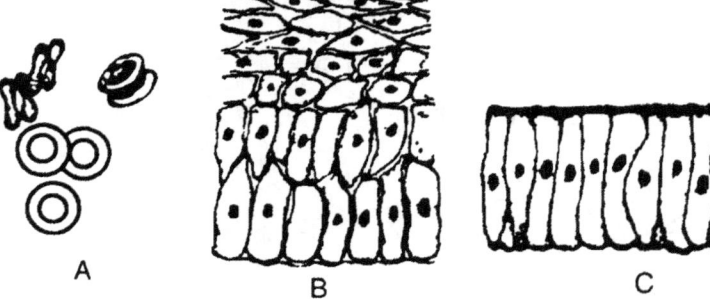

    A. Mammalian erythrocytes
    B. Amphibian erythrocytes
    C. Squamous epithelium
    D. Columnar epithelium
    E. Stratified epithelium

33. Diagram A represents   33.____

34. Diagram B represents   34.____

35. Diagram C represents   35.____

Questions 36-41.

DIRECTIONS: Questions 36 through 41 are to be answered on the basis of the following diagrams. For each question, select one of the five lettered words or phrases that appears above each set of the questions which applies to the question, and put the letter of your choice in the space at the right.

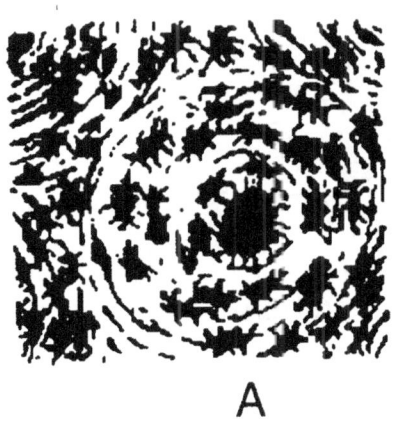
A

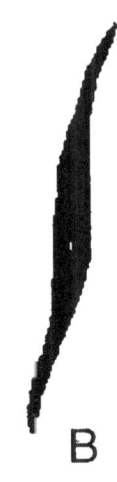
B

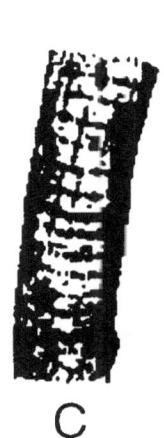
C

Questions 36-38.

    A. Striated muscle
    B. A smooth muscle cell
    C. Cartilage
    D. Bone
    E. Fibrous connective tissue

36. Diagram A represents   36._____

37. Diagram B represents   37._____

38. Diagram C represents   38._____

Questions 39-41.

    A. Absorbs shocks by its resiliency
    B. Produces movement of the limbs
    C. Produces peristaltic movement
    D. Connects striated muscle with bone
    E. Gives rigidity to the vertebrate

39. The structure in Diagram A   39._____

40. The structure in Diagram B   40._____

41. The structure in Diagram C   41._____

Questions 42-50.

DIRECTIONS: In Questions 42 through 50, each letter refers to the structure labeled with the same letter in the diagram below. For each item, select one of the five lettered words or phrases that appears above each set of questions which applies to the structure, and put the letter of your choice in the space at the right.

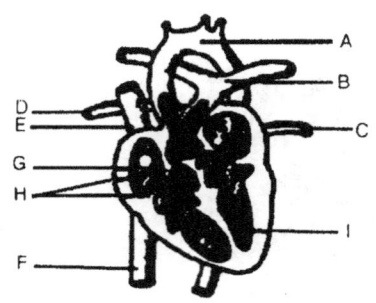

MAMMALIAN HEART

Questions 42-44.

42. A represents
43. B represents
44. C represents

A. Superior vena cava
B. Sinus venosus
C. Aorta
D. Pulmonary vein
E. Pulmonary artery

42.____
43.____
44.____

Questions 45-47.

45. The structure at D
46. The structure at E
47. The structure at F

A. Carries venous blood from the upper part of the body
B. Carries venous blood from the lower part of the body
C. Carries blood under the highest pressure in the body
D. Carries oxygenated blood from the right lung
E. Carries oxygenated blood to the right side of the body

45.____
46.____
47.____

Questions 48-50.

48. The structure at G
49. The structure at H
50. The structure at I

A. Receives oxygenated blood from the lungs
B. Prevents flow of blood from ventricle to auricle
C. Changes pulsating to smoothly flowing blood
D. Receives blood with high carbon dioxide content
E. Pumps arterial blood

48.____
49.____
50.____

KEY (CORRECT ANSWERS)

1. A	11. D	21. C	31. C	41. B
2. D	12. A	22. D	32. A	42. C
3. C	13. D	23. E	33. A	43. E
4. C	14. C	24. A	34. E	44. D
5. D	15. B	25. B	35. D	45. D
6. B	16. E	26. D	36. D	46. A
7. E	17. A	27. A	37. B	47. B
8. B	18. C	28. C	38. A	48. D
9. A	19. E	29. D	39. E	49. B
10. D	20. D	30. E	40. C	50. E

TEST 2

DIRECTIONS: Each question or incomplete statement is followed by several suggested answers or completions. Select the one that BEST answers the question or completes the statement. *PRINT THE LETTER OF THE CORRECT ANSWER IN THE SPACE AT THE RIGHT.*

1. A characteristic of the close of the Mesozoic Era was the

    A. formation of coal deposits
    B. dominance of cycads
    C. extinction of dinosaurs
    D. origin of primates
    E. origin of man

    1.____

2. Starvation in animals leads to the consumption of the reserves of the organic materials in the organs and organic materials in the organs and body cells.
The LIKELY order for consuming these substances is

    A. fats, proteins, and carbohydrates
    B. fats, carbohydrates, and proteins
    C. carbohydrates, proteins, and fats
    D. carbohydrates, fats, and proteins
    E. proteins, fats, and carbohydrates

    2.____

3. The effectiveness of a septic tank made for the disposal of sewage depends PRINCIPALLY on the action of

    A. filtrable viruses   B. bacteriophage
    C. aerobic bacteria   D. anaerobic bacteria
    E. nitrifying bacteria

    3.____

4. In man, lymph is returned to the bloodstream in the

    A. skin capillaries   B. glomeruli
    C. alveoli   D. inferior vena cava
    E. subclavian vein

    4.____

5. A HIGHLY branched digestive tract that transports digested food directly to the tissues, and the virtual absence of a circulatory system are characteristic of

    A. earthworms   B. flatworms   C. mollusks
    D. crustaceans   E. spiders

    5.____

6. In a growing root tip, root hairs FIRST appear

    A. at the root cap
    B. in the mature region
    C. in the region of differentiation
    D. in the region of elongation
    E. at the growing point

    6.____

7. The _____ develops from the embryonic endoderm in man.

    A. nervous system
    B. inner epithelium of the lungs

    7.____

C. muscles
D. bones
E. circulatory system

8. The Y-chromosome in man USUALLY differs from the X-chromosome in that the Y-chromosome

   A. contains fewer genes
   B. contains more genes
   C. is present only in germ cells
   D. is produced by reduction division
   E. is present in all gametes produced in the male body

9. The MOST reliable method of estimating the age of the oldest rocks in the earth is by determination of

   A. their chemical composition
   B. the number and kind of fossils they contain
   C. the rates of disintegration of radioactive substances
   D. their proximity to the surface of the earth
   E. the rates of evolutionary change

10. One characteristic of MOST dicotyledonous plants is the presence of

    A. flowers with parts in multiples of three
    B. vascular bundles scattered irregularly throughout the stem
    C. a continuous ring of cambium layer in the stem
    D. leaves with parallel veining
    E. seeds with several seed leaves

11. The _____ in the human ear transforms physical vibration into nerve impulses.

    A. tympanic membrane
    B. auditory nerve
    C. vestibulum
    D. organ of Corti
    E. utriculus

12. Bending of a young plant toward light is indirectly related to the presence in its growing parts of an unequal distribution of

    A. auxins
    B. diastase
    C. catalase
    D. chromatin
    E. plastids

13. The life cycle of the moss DIFFERS from that in flowering plants in that the sporophyte

    A. produces spores
    B. is in the form of a protonema
    C. is independent of the gametophyte
    D. is dependent on the gametophyte
    E. bears archegonia and antheridia

14. The structures in the human eye upon which the perception of color is MOST dependent are the

    A. peripheral cone cells
    B. peripheral rod cells

C. cone cells in the region of the fovea centralis
D. rod cells in the region of the fovea centralis
E. rods and cones at the point where the optic nerve passes through the retina

15. The existence today of a(n) _____ would be MOST improbable. 15.____

   A. parasitic plant containing chlorophyll
   B. living seed containing no embryo
   C. cell without a cell wall
   D. egg-laying mammal
   E. flowering fern

Questions 16-40.

DIRECTIONS: In answering Questions 16 through 40, select the word or phrase from the list appearing above each set of questions which applies to each question.

Questions 16-18.

   A. Lipase
   B. Trypsin
   C. Zymase
   D. Ptyalin
   E. Maltase

16. Accelerates the hydrolysis of starch to maltose 16.____

17. Accelerates the hydrolysis of proteoses and peptones to amino acids in an alkaline medium 17.____

18. Accelerates the hydrolysis of fats to fatty acids and glycerol 18.____

Questions 19-21.

   A. Maltase
   B. Rennin
   C. Lipase
   D. Erepsin
   E. Pepsin

19. Catalyzes the hydrolysis of proteins in an acid medium 19.____

20. Aids in changing maltose sugar to glucose by its action in the small intestine 20.____

21. In association with trypsin in the small intestine, completes the digestion of proteins 21.____

Questions 22-24.

   A. Sucrose
   B. Fat
   C. Glucose

D. Cellulose
E. Starch

22. Is a carbohydrate insoluble in cold water and unaffected by man's digestive juices   22.____

23. Is a carbohydrate that can be used directly by the human body without digestion   23.____

24. Is NOT a carbohydrate, although it contains the same chemical elements   24.____

Questions 25-27.

    A. Tendon
    B. Ligament
    C. Smooth muscle
    D. Striated muscle
    E. Cardiac muscle

25. Fibrous tissue connecting the ends of bones   25.____

26. Contractile tissue producing alimentary peristalsis   26.____

27. Connective tissue connecting muscles with the skeleton   27.____

Questions 28-30.

    A. Paramecium
    B. Spirogyra
    C. Field mushroom
    D. Corn smut
    E. Frog

28. Autophytic   28.____

29. Saprophytic   29.____

30. Parasitic   30.____

Questions 31-33.

    A. Trapezius
    B. Ciliary
    C. Gastrocnemius
    D. Biceps
    E. Triceps

31. Extends the foot at the ankle joint   31.____

32. Straightens the arm at the elbow   32.____

33. Varies the curvature of the lens in the eye   33.____

Questions 34-40.

    A. True of crayfishes only
    B. True of grasshoppers only
    C. True of spiders only
    D. True of two of the above, but not all three
    E. True of all three of the above

34. The adults have compound eyes only   34.____

35. The adults have no antennae   35.____

36. The adults have head and thorax fused into one   36.____

37. The food of the adult consists principally of plant materials   37.____

38. The main part of the nervous system is a ventral nerve chain of ganglia   38.____

39. The adults breathe by means of book lungs   39.____

40. Lost legs and eyes of adults may regenerate   40.____

Questions 41-43.

DIRECTIONS: Questions 41 through 43 are to be answered on the basis of the following concepts.
    A. Life came from simple molecules.
    B. The acquired traits of an individual can be transmitted to her offspring.
    C. The fitness of an organism will determine its survival.
    D. Living organisms are necessary to produce other living organisms.

For each question, select the concept that is appropriate. A concept may be the answer to one question, more than one question, or no question.

41. Maggots emerge when meat is exposed to flies; they do NOT emerge if the flies are prevented from laying eggs on the meat.   41.____

42. This principle would be illustrated if a cow were to lose one leg and her calves were then born with three legs each.   42.____

43. Amino acids have been prepared from methane, water, ammonia, and hydrogen after an electric spark was passed through them.   43.____

44. If a freshwater fish is placed in salt water, which of the following BEST summarizes the result?   44.____

    A. The fish loses water from its tissues.
    B. The fish swells and becomes turgid.
    C. Salt diffuses out of the cells into the surrounding salt water.
    D. The fish absorbs salt until the salt concentration in its tissues equals that of the salt water.
    E. None of these

45. Large numbers of certain species of ladybird beetles are liberated in the orange groves of California PRIMARILY because the ladybird beetles

    A. attract birds
    B. are the best pollinating insects known
    C. controls rusts and smuts
    D. secrete a substance beneficial to the trees
    E. feed upon scale insects

45.____

46. The number of bacteria present in a tube of liquid medium can be measured indirectly by the amount of light that passes through the tube. The greater the number of bacteria, the less the light that is transmitted through the tube.
Which graph BEST represents this relationship?

46.____

A.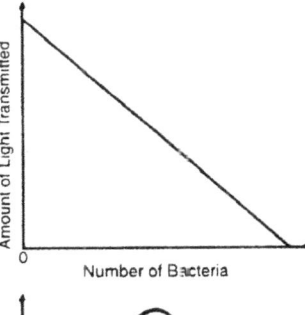

B.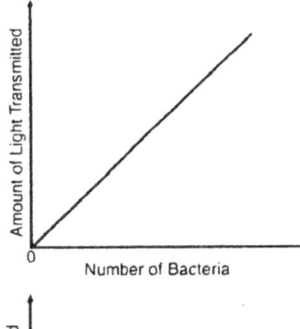

C.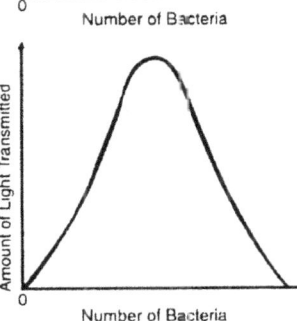

D.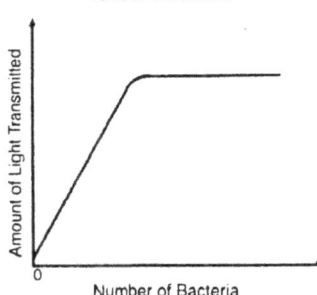

E. None of these

47. During the fifteenth century, a few European rabbits were introduced into the Madeira Islands off the west coast of Africa. Today, the island rabbits are smaller and darker than their ancestors and can no longer be mated with present day European rabbits.
These observations BEST illustrate which point?

    A. A species change resulting from geographic isolation
    B. Separation of alleles that act as independent units
    C. The appearance of recessive traits that were formerly concealed by dominant traits
    D. Environmental changes resulting in phenotypic changes only
    E. None of these

47.____

Questions 48-49.

DIRECTIONS: Questions 48 and 49 are to be answered on the basis of the following table.

	Gestation Period (in days)	Earliest Breeding Age of Females
White Rat	21-22	4 months
Mouse	20-22	60 days
Guinea Pig	62-64	9 months
Golden Hamster	16-19	70 days
Rabbit	30-32	10 months

48. According to the above table, the _____ has the LONGEST period of development before birth.

   A. Mouse
   B. Guinea Pig
   C. Golden hamster
   D. Rabbit
   E. White Rat

49. According to the above table, which animal is the OLDEST when it is FIRST able to breed?

   A. White Rat
   B. Guinea Pig
   C. Golden hamster
   D. Rabbit
   E. Mouse

50. Each of these is a procedure for determining the effectiveness of a bird disease vaccine. Which would be considered MOST satisfactory from a scientific viewpoint?
   Vaccinate

   A. 100 birds and expose all 100 to the disease
   B. 100 birds and expose *only* 50 of them to the disease
   C. 50 birds, do NOT vaccinate 50 other birds, and expose all 100 to the disease
   D. 50 birds, do NOT vaccinate 50 other birds, and expose *only* the vaccinated birds to the disease
   E. All of the above

KEY (CORRECT ANSWERS)

1. C	11. D	21. D	31. C	41. D
2. D	12. A	22. D	32. E	42. B
3. D	13. D	23. C	33. B	43. A
4. E	14. C	24. B	34. A	44. A
5. B	15. E	25. B	35. C	45. E
6. C	16. D	26. C	36. D	46. A
7. B	17. B	27. A	37. B	47. A
8. A	18. A	28. B	38. E	48. B
9. C	19. E	29. C	39. C	49. D
10. C	20. A	30. D	40. A	50. C

TEST 3

DIRECTIONS: Each question or incomplete statement is followed by several suggested answers or completions. Select the one that BEST answers the question or completes the statement. *PRINT THE LETTER OF THE CORRECT ANSWER IN THE SPACE AT THE RIGHT.*

1. Below are four possible body shapes for one-celled animals. 1.____
   If all have the same volume, which form can exchange materials with its surroundings MOST quickly?

   A. (elongated rounded rectangle)   B. (wavy elongated shape)

   C. (circle)   D. (curved elongated shape)

   E. One cannot determine from the information given

2. A certain nontoxic chemical compound in solution is red at a pH of 7 and blue at a pH of 2.____
   5; that is, the compound changes to blue as the solution becomes acid. The red solution may be used to impart a red color to yeast cells. After paramecia ingest red yeast cells, the cells can be seen concentrated within food vacuoles.
   If in time the cells turn blue, a logical interpretation of the color change would be that

   A. the cytoplasm of the paramecium has a pH below 7
   B. paramecia prefer foods that have an acid reaction
   C. within food vacuoles, a chemical reaction such as digestion is taking place
   D. if yeast cells are ingested quickly by paramecia, the cells change color
   E. None of these

3. Complications associated with antibody formation sometimes affect newborn babies if 3.____
   the mother is _____ and the father is _____.

   A. AB; A   B. A; O   C. Rh⁻; Rh⁻
   D. Rh⁻; Rh⁺   E. O; A

4. _____ is NOT a function of blood. 4.____

   A. Protection of the body against disease
   B. Transport of oxygen to cells
   C. Transport of digestive enzymes to cells
   D. Transport of metabolic wastes from cells
   E. None of these

5. Photosynthesis and respiration are ALIKE in that both 5.____

   A. are energy-releasing processes
   B. are performed by all plants and animals
   C. convert stored chemical energy to useful heat energy
   D. involve energy conversions
   E. require oxygen

6. A student believes that male roaches are attracted to female roaches by certain chemical gases released by the females and that it is NOT necessary for the males to see the females. The best way to test this hypothesis is to have male roaches that are free and to place the females in a cage.
   This experimental cage should have which of these qualities?
   I. One-way entrances
   II. Porous walls
   III. Transparent walls
   The CORRECT answer is:

   A. I and II
   B. I and III
   C. II and III
   D. I, II, III
   E.

Questions 7-8

DIRECTIONS: Questions 7 and 8 are to be answered on the basis of the table below, which lists a few enzymes, the substance that each digests (substrate), and the acidity at which each functions most effectively (optimal pH). The acidity is reported by use of the pH scale; a pH of 1 is highly acid, a pH of 7 is neutral, and a pH of 14 is highly alkaline.

Enzyme	Substrate	Optimal pH
Amylase (pancreas)	Starch	6.7-7.0
Lactase	Lacrose	5.7
Pepsin	Protein	1.5-1.6
Lipase (pancreas)	Fat	8.0
Trypsin	Protein	7.8-8.7
Maltase	Maltose	6.1-6.8

7. Which series CORRECTLY lists the enzymes according to optimal pH, from most acid to least acid?

   A. Pepsin, lactase, maltase, lipase
   B. Pepsin, amylase, trypsin, maltase
   C. Trypsin, lipase, amylase, pepsin
   D. Lipase, amylase, lactase, pepsin
   E. Lipase, lactose, pepsin, amylase

8. From the data in the table, identify the CORRECT conclusion concerning the enzymes which digest proteins.

   A. Enzymes that digest proteins function best in acid media.
   B. Enzymes that digest proteins function best in alkaline media.
   C. Enzymes that digest proteins function best in neutral media.
   D. Pepsin functions best in acid media; trypsin functions best in alkaline media.
   E. None of these

Questions 9-16.

DIRECTIONS: Questions 9 through 16 are to be answered on the basis of the following data on the inheritance of dominant and recessive traits.

In summer squashes, the gene for white is dominant over the gene for yellow, and the gene for disc shape is dominant over the gene for sphere shape.

Two white disc squash plants were crossed and produced offspring as follows:

9 white disc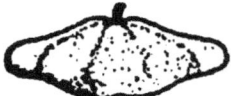

3 yellow disc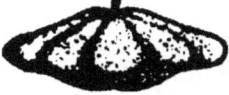

3 white sphere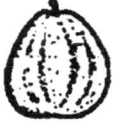

1 yellow sphere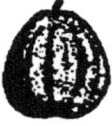

Let: W represent the gene for white color

w represent the gene for yellow color

D represent the gene for disc shape

d represent the gene for sphere shape

The KEY below lists five possible crosses involving the traits: white (W), yellow (w), disc (D), and sphere (d). For each question, determine which cross given in the KEY applies. Mark the letter of the CORRECT answer in the space at the right.

KEY–Crosses
A. WwDd x WwDd
B. WWDD x WWDD
C. WWdd x wwDD
D. wwdd x wwdd
E. WwDd x wwdd

9. Which cross would yield ONLY pure dominant offspring for both traits? 9.____

10. Which cross should a truck gardener use if he wanted to raise only pure yellow sphere squashes? 10.____

11. If a truck gardener desired to raise white disc squashes ONLY, season after season, which cross should he select as the source of seed? 11.____

12. Which cross would produce squashes all of which would breed true for the recessive traits? 12.____

13. The two squashes that were crossed to produce the four kinds of offspring given above are represented by which one of the crosses? 13.____

14. Which cross represents a mating between the yellow sphere offspring and a squash like one of its parents? 14.____

15. The parents of the two squashes that were crossed are represented by which one of the crosses? 15.____

16. Which cross would yield only hybrid offspring? 16.____

Questions 17-20.

DIRECTIONS: Questions 17 through 20 are concerned with the functions of certain endocrine glands. For each question, select from the sketch below the gland whose secretion is involved.

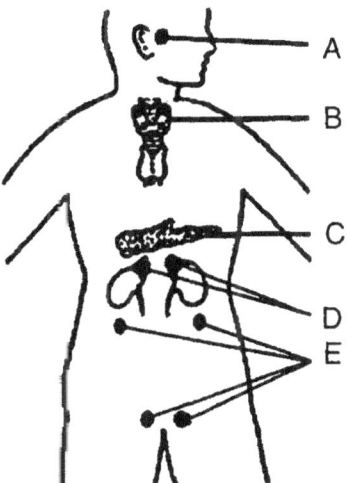

17. A hormone from this(these) gland(s) is associated with the changes of the *awkward age* through which many young people pass in their transition from childhood to young adulthood 17.____

18. This hormone regulates the body's utilization of carbohydrate foods. The gland(s) whose islets secrete it also discharge(s) enzymes capable of digesting proteins, starches, and fats. 18.____

19. The life of a patient lying on the operating table seems to be ebbing away. The doctor administers a substance which causes the heart to beat faster, the arteries to contract, the hair to bristle, and the breathing rate to increase.
Such a substance is manufactured by which gland(s)?

19._____

20. A basal metabolism test reveals that a young lady is consuming more than the normal amount of oxygen for her height, weight, and age. She is the author of several novels which have been bestsellers. She seems to thrive on long hours of work and little sleep.

20._____

Questions 21-35.

DIRECTIONS: Match the statements or words in Questions 21 through 35 with the items listed above each set of questions. Write the CORRECT letter for each question in the space at the right.

Questions 21-23.

    A. Riboflavin
    B. Ethylene
    C. Thiamin
    D. Carotene
    E. Colchicine

21. Used as a means of increasing the number of chromosomes in cells of plants.   21._____

22. Used to hasten the ripening of fruits.   22._____

23. Is a precursor of vitamin A in the animal body.   23._____

Questions 24-26.

    A. Thallophytes
    B. Bryophytes
    C. Pteridophytes
    D. Gymnosperms
    E. Angiosperms

24. Leafy sporphyte, both generations USUALLY independent, no seeds develop.   24._____

25. Seed plants, ovule NOT surrounded by ovary wall.   25._____

26. Relatively little cell differentiation, may be single-celled, colonial, or multicellular.   26._____

Questions 27-29.

    A. Coelenterata
    B. Annelida
    C. Nemathelminthes
    D. Platyhelminthes
    E. Echinodermata

27. Bilaterally symmetrical, triploblastic, contain a single gastrovascular cavity, no anus, flame cells.   27.____

28. Radially symmetrical, triploblastic, contain a well-developed coelom, anus usually present.   28.____

29. Radially symmetrical, diploblastic, contain a single gastrovascular cavity, no anus.   29.____

Questions 30-32.

    A. Chaetopoda
    B. Nematoda
    C. Mastigophora
    D. Reptilia
    E. Arachnida

30. The class to which the earthworm belongs.   30.____

31. The class to which the scorpion belongs.   31.____

32. The class to which Euglena belongs.   32.____

Questions 33-35.

    A. Mushrooms
    B. Yeasts
    C. Ferns
    D. Mosses
    E. Flowering plants

33. Gills   33.____

34. Prothallium   34.____

35. Embryo sac   35.____

Questions 36-44.

DIRECTIONS: Questions 36 through 44 are to be answered on the basis of the following diagram. Match the statements or words in these questions with the items listed above each set of questions. Write the CORRECT letter for each question in the space at the right.

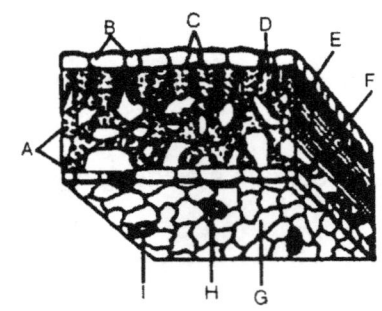

CROSS-SECTION OF LEAF

Questions 36-38.

    A. Transpiration is most actively taking place from these cells
    B. Photosynthesis is most active here
    C. Conducts sap to the root
    D. Protects the leaf, transmits light
    E. No respiration takes place in these cells

36. The structure at A

37. The structure at B

38. The structure at C

Questions 39-41.

    A. Regulates leaf temperature
    B. Utilizes solar energy in the synthesis of glucose
    C. Conducts water coming from the root
    D. Protects the leaf from mechanical injury
    E. Conducts organic food from the leaf

39. The structure at D

40. The structure at E

41. The structure at F

Questions 42-44.

    A. Sieve cell
    B. Guard cell
    C. Mesophyll
    D. Lower epidermis
    E. Stoma

42. G represents   42._____

43. H represents   43._____

44. I represents   44._____

Questions 45-47.

DIRECTIONS: Questions 45 through 47 are to be answered on the basis of the following chart.

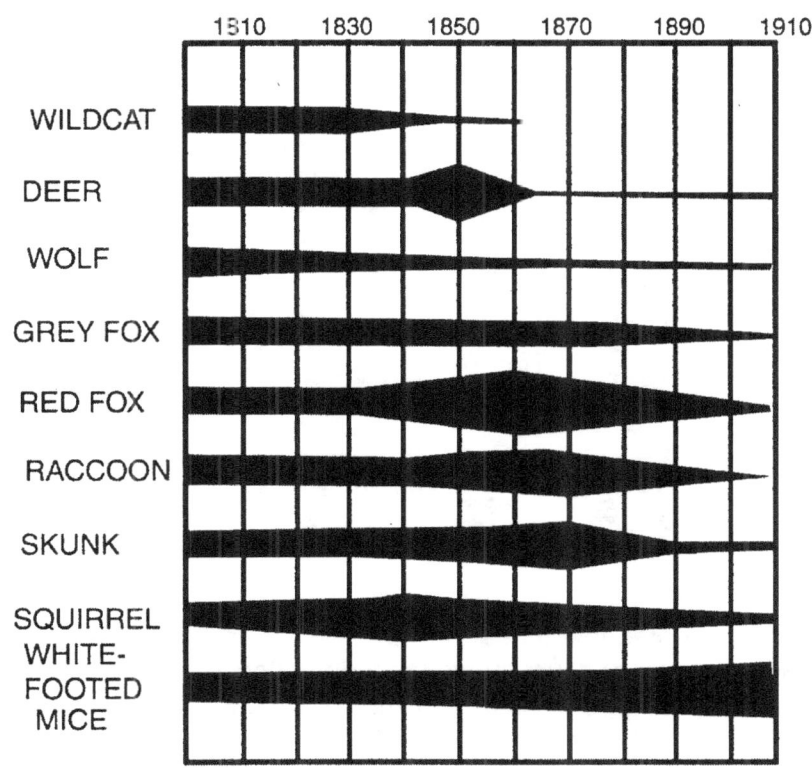

45. The cheapest and most practical way in which the population of white-footed mice could be decreased is to   45._____

    A. raise more cats
    B. spread poisoned bran in the fields
    C. put much of the crop land back in pasture
    D. set traps and hire boys to tend them
    E. encourage hawks and owls to increase by enacting protective hunting laws

46. On the basis of other data in this graph, the 1850 peak of the deer population was VERY likely   46._____

    A. due to an increase in available food
    B. due largely to increased breeding activity
    C. due in part to the decline of the wildcat-wolf population in that period
    D. unrelated to the trend of the wildcat-wolf population in 1850
    E. related directly to the increase in white-footed mice

47. The MOST probable explanation of the increase in white-footed mice in 110 years is that   47._____

    A. man considers white-footed mice harmless
    B. man is more friendly to carnivorous animals than to herbivorous animals
    C. white-footed mice have no natural enemies
    D. white-footed mice are protected by law
    E. man has greatly reduced the carnivore link of the food chain

Questions 48-50.

DIRECTIONS: Questions 48 through 50 are to be answered on the basis of the following experiment.

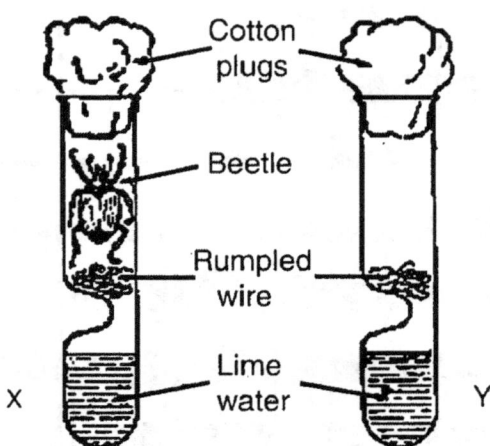

Two specially indented test tubes, X and Y, were one-third filled with limewater. A piece of rumpled wire was then lodged just above the indentation in each tube. A live beetle was placed over the rumpled wire in Tube X, but not in Tube Y. A cotton plug was inserted as a stopper in each tube, after which both tubes were allowed to stand for 20 minutes. At the end of that time, the limewater in Tube X had become cloudy, while the limewater in Tube Y remained clear.

48. This experiment provided evidence that   48._____

    A. carbon dioxide was being set free in Tube X
    B. a beetle cannot live in the presence of limewater
    C. oxygen was being used up in Tube X
    D. oxygen was being set free in Tube X
    E. carbon dioxide was being used up in Tube X

49. How would the experiment have been affected if the beetle had been placed in a cyanide jar before being put in Tube X?   49._____

    A. The beetle would have withstood the limewater much better.
    B. The limewater would have become more cloudy.
    C. The limewater would have turned yellow in color.
    D. The limewater would have remained clear.
    E. There would have been no appreciable change in the results.

50. A scientist would call that part of the experiment which involved test tube Y and its contents the 50._____

    A. follow-up   B. verification   C. reserve
    D. duplicate   E. control

KEY (CORRECT ANSWERS)

1. B	11. B	21. E	31. E	41. E
2. C	12. D	22. B	32. C	42. D
3. D	13. A	23. D	33. A	43. E
4. C	14. E	24. C	34. C	44. B
5. D	15. C	25. D	35. E	45. E
6. A	16. C	26. A	36. A	46. C
7. A	17. E	27. D	37. D	47. E
8. D	18. C	28. E	38. B	48. A
9. B	19. D	29. A	39. B	49. D
10. D	20. B	30. A	40. C	50. E

EXAMINATION SECTION
TEST 1

DIRECTIONS: Each question or incomplete statement is followed by several suggested answers or completions. Select the one that BEST answers the question or completes the statement. *PRINT THE LETTER OF THE CORRECT ANSWER IN THE SPACE AT THE RIGHT.*

1. What is the volume occupied by 73g of a solution with a specific gravity of 1.23? _____ ml.

    A. 89.79   B. 59.35   C. 23.0   D. 1.23

    1._____

2. Of the following, an example of a pair of isotopes is

    A. H and D
    B. C and N
    C. Li and Na
    D. cis and trans HClC = CClH

    2._____

3. What is the weight of 3.2 moles of NaCl?

    A. 3.2 g
    B. 18.26 g
    C. 19.26×10^{23} g
    D. 187 g

    3._____

4. The chemical formula for sodium phosphate is

    A. $NaPO_4$ B. Na_3PO_4 C. $NaHPO_4$ D. Na_3P

    4._____

5. The name of the MnO_4^- ion is

    A. manganese (II)
    B. manganate
    C. permanganate
    D. ammonium

    5._____

6. Which one of the following is an example of a hydrocarbon?

    A. Hexane   B. Ethanol   C. Acetone   D. Graphite

    6._____

7. How many moles of ethane are contained in a pure sample weighing 95 g?

    A. 2850   B. 95   C. 30   D. 3.17

    7._____

8. Calculate the percentage by weight of Mg in $Mg(NO_3)_2$.
   The CORRECT answer is:

    A. 4.11   B. 16.39   C. 24.31   D. 48.3

    8._____

9. How many oxygen atoms are contained in one mole of O_2 gas?

    A. 32×10^{-23}
    B. 12.04×10^{-23}
    C. 12.04×10^{23}
    D. 6.02×10^{23}

    9._____

10. A compound was found to contain 72.0% (by weight) Mn and the remainder was oxygen. The empirical formula of this compound is

    A. MnO_2 B. MnO C. Mn_3O_4 D. Mn_4O_3

    10._____

11. Calculate the number of grams of CO_2 produced per one gram of sucrose consumed for the following reaction of sucrose with excess oxygen: $C_{12}H_{22}O_{11} + 12O_2 \rightarrow 12CO_2 + H_2O$
The CORRECT answer is:

    A. .128 g   B. 1.54 g   C. 12 g   D. 44 g

12. How many moles of Li_2O can be produced from 1.0 g of Li and 1.5 g of O_2 according to the reaction: $4Li + O_2 \rightarrow 2Li_2O$

    A. .0144   B. .0720   C. .0938   D. 2.0

13. The number 0.00532 is written in scientific notation as

    A. 532   B. 5.32   C. 5.32×10^3 D. 5.32×10^{-3}

14. The product of 1.3×10^{-4} times $2.1 \times 10^{+2}$ is

    A. .273
    B. 2.73×10^{-2}
    C. $2.73 \times 10^{+2}$
    D. 27.3

15. One micron is one millionth of a meter ($1\mu = 10^{-6}$ m) and there are one hundred million angstroms in one centimeter ($1 \overset{\circ}{A} = 10^{-8}$ cm).
How many angstroms equal one micron?

    A. $10^{-2} \overset{\circ}{A}$ B. $10^{-4} \overset{\circ}{A}$ C. $10^2 \overset{\circ}{A}$ D. $10^4 \overset{\circ}{A}$

16. Calculate the concentration of (Na^+) in moles/liter i a solution prepared by adding 100 g of NaCl to sufficient water to make 0.50 liters of solution.
The CORRECT answer is:

    A. .855   B. 1.71   C. 3.42   D. 8.69

17. How many moles of chloride ion, Cl^-, are present in 50 ml of 0.20 M $BaCl_2$?

    A. 0.020   B. 0.20   C. 0.010   D. 0.05

18. If 40.0 ml of an HCl solution requires 32.0 ml of 0.10 M NaOH for neutralization during a titration, the molarity of the HCl solution should be _____ M.

    A. .4   B. 3.2   C. 0.10   D. 0.080

19. A sample of gas is contained in a fixed volume at 20° C and heated until the pressure doubles.
What is the FINAL temperature of the gas?

    A. 313.2° C   B. 313.2° K   C. 273.2° K   D. 40° C

20. At 27° C and 750 mm of Hg pressure, 0.60 g of a pure gas occupies 0.50 liters. The molecular weight of the pure gas is _____ g/mole.

    A. 60   B. 2.66   C. 30   D. 26.6

21. $H^+ + I^- + SO_4^{2-} \rightarrow I_2 + H_2S + H_2O$

    Balance the above equation and determine the number of moles of I^- consumed for each mole of H_2S produced. The number of moles should be

    A. 2 B. 4 C. 6 D. 8

22. What will be the effect of doubling the total pressure on an equilibrium mixture for the reaction:

    $H_2(g) + I_2(g) \rightleftharpoons 2HI(g)$? (g = gas)

    A. More HI will be consumed.
    B. More HI will be produced.
    C. Ha will be consumed and I_2 produced.
    D. There is no change in the number of moles of $H_2(g)$, $I_2(g)$, and $HI(g)$.

23. Ten grams of AgCl are shaken in one liter of water until equilibrium is established. If K_{sp} for AgCl is 10^{-1}, the weight of AgCl dissolved per liter of solution should be _____ g.

    A. 10
    B. 1.43×10^{-3}
    C. 10^{-9}
    D. 143×10^{-10}

24. The temperature, in degrees Fahrenheit, that is equivalent to 40° C (degrees Centigrade) is _____ F.

    A. -40 B. 54.2 C. 72 D. 104

25. If eleven (11.0) g of $NaNO_3$ are dissolved in 100 g of H_2O, then the NaNOs concentration is expressed as the percent solution of

    A. 12.9% B. 11.0% C. 9.9% D. 1.29%

KEY (CORRECT ANSWERS)

1.	B	11.	B
2.	A	12.	B
3.	D	13.	D
4.	B	14.	B
5.	C	15.	D
6.	A	16.	C
7.	D	17.	A
8.	B	18.	D
9.	C	19.	A
10.	C	20.	C

21. D
22. D
23. B
24. D
25. C

TEST 2

DIRECTIONS: Each question or incomplete statement is followed by several suggested answers or completions. Select the one that BEST answers the question or completes the statement. *PRINT THE LETTER OF THE CORRECT ANSWER IN THE SPACE AT THE RIGHT.*

1. A label on a bottle of nitric acid reads 60% by weight HNO_3 and specific gravity equals 1.2.
   Then, the molar concentration of HNO_3 is

   A. 0.95   B. 11.4   C. 60   D. 720

   1.____

2. How many grams of NaOH are contained in 250 ml of a 0.2M (molar) solution?
   _____ g.

   A. 10.0   B. 8.0   C. 6.2   D. 2.0

   2.____

3. How many milliliters (ml) of 18 M (molar) H_2SO_4 should be diluted to 200 ml to prepare a 3.3 N (normal) solution of acid?
   _____ ml.

   A. 36.6   B. 18.3   C. 9.15   D. 5.45

   3.____

4. Which one of the following indicates the HIGHEST purity of a chemical when it appears on a commercial label?

   A. C.P.
   B. Tech.
   C. Anal. Reagent
   D. Pract.

   4.____

5. An example of a triprotic acid is

   A. HCl   B. H_2SO_4 C. H_3PO_4 D. $La(OH)_3$

   5.____

6. Calculate the pH for a solution with $(H^+) = 2 \times 10^{-3}$ M (molar).
   The CORRECT answer is

   A. 3.2   B. 2.7   C. 2   D. 2×10^{-3}

   6.____

7. Calculate the molar concentration of (H^+) in a solution of pOH = 7.3.
   The CORRECT answer is _____ M.

   A. 2.0×10^{-7} B. 5×10^{-8} C. 7.8   D. 6.7

   7.____

8. What is the pH of buffer prepared by mixing 200 ml of 2M CH_3COOH with 200 ml of 1M CH_3COONa if $Ka\ (CH_3COOH) = 1.8 \times 10^{-5}$?

   A. 2.22
   B. 3.6×10^{-5}
   C. 4.44
   D. 4.75

   8.____

9. Which one of the following compounds is used as an oxidizing agent in redox titrations?

   A. HCl
   B. $KMnO_4$
   C. Oxalic acid
   D. Sodium dithonite

   9.____

10. Which instrument is used to measure the optical density of a solution?

    A. refractometer
    B. spectrophotometer
    C. pyknometer
    D. pH meter

11. Which one of the following compounds is NOT aromatic?

    A. Benzene
    B. Xylene
    C. Butyne
    D. Aniline

12. Oxidation of a primary alcohol produces a(n)

    A. olefin
    B. aldehyde
    C. ketone
    D. secondary alcohol

13. The formula for diethyl ether is

    A. $CH_3C(O)CH_3$
    B. $C_2H_5OC_2H_5$
    C. CH_3OCH_3
    D. $C_2H_5COO\,C_2H_5$

14. An ester is produced by a reaction between an

    A. organic acid and an alcohol
    B. organic acid and a base such as NaOH
    C. acid anhydride and water
    D. alcohol and a mineral acid

15. Proteins are composed of chains of

    A. nucleic acids
    B. amino acids
    C. carbohydrates
    D. alkaloids

16. Which one of the following atomic species is NOT radioactive?

    A. ^{14}C
    B. ^{3}H
    C. ^{32}P
    D. ^{14}N

17. For which one of the following tasks is an infrared spectrophotometer useful? The

    A. identification of organic compounds
    B. determination of the concentration of sodium in water
    C. measurement of radioactivity
    D. observation of fluorescence

18. Which one of the following procedures should be used when preparing a solution of sulfuric acid from concentrated acid?

    A. Pouring acid into water
    B. Pouring water into acid
    C. Pouring acid and water into the same beaker rapidly
    D. Distilling the acid into water

19. Which one of the following solutions has the LOWEST freezing point?

    A. Pure H_2O
    B. 2 molal $CaCl_2$
    C. 2 molal NaCl
    D. 1 molal Na_2SO_4

20. At the end point of a titration of acetic acid with sodium hydroxide, the pH of the solution is

   A. 0   B. below 7.0   C. 7.0   D. above

21. What is the pressure, in mm, of Hg which corresponds to 1.31 atm?

   A. 17.8   B. 1.31   C. 19.2   D. 995.6

22. In the process of weighing samples, the tare weight refers to the

   A. weight of the sample
   B. weight of the container
   C. total weight of the sample plus container
   D. error in the measurement

23. The electronic configuration of sodium metal is

   A. $1s^1, 2s^1, 2p^1, 3s^1$
   B. $1s^2, 2s^2, 2p^6, 3s^1$
   C. $1s^2, 2s^2, 2p^6$
   D. $1s^{11}$

24. Which atom is MOST easily ionized to the +1 state?

   A. H   B. Li   C. Na   D. K

25. Which one of the following colored light rays contains photons of the HIGHEST energy? _____ light.

   A. Red   B. Infrared   C. Green   D. Blue

KEY (CORRECT ANSWERS)

1. B		11. C	
2. D		12. B	
3. B		13. B	
4. C		14. A	
5. C		15. B	
6. B		16. D	
7. A		17. A	
8. C		18. A	
9. B		19. B	
10. B		20. D	

21. D
22. B
23. B
24. D
25. D

EXAMINATION SECTION
TEST 1

DIRECTIONS: Each question or incomplete statement is followed by several suggested answers or completions. Select the one that BEST answers the question or completes the statement. *PRINT THE LETTER OF THE CORRECT ANSWER IN THE SPACE AT THE RIGHT.*

1. The formula for nitrogen (IV) oxide is 1.____
   A. N_2O B. NO_2 C. NO_4 D. N_4O

2. Which compound has the GREATEST degree of ionic character? 2.____
   A. Na_2O B. H_2O C. CO_2 D. NO_2

3. Hydrogen bonds are formed between molecules in which hydrogen is covalently bonded to an element having 3.____
   A. low electronegativity
   C. low ionization energy
   B. high electronegativity
   D. high atomic mass

4. Using electronegative values as a guide, which formula is CORRECTLY written? 4.____
   A. F_6S B. Cl_2O C. Br_4C D. I_3P

5. Which atom has the GREATEST affinity for an electron? 5.____
   A. Li   B. Br   C. Na   D. Cl

6. The group in the Periodic Table which contains the MOST active metals is Group 6.____
   A. IA   B. IB   C. VIIA   D. VIIB

7. Which ion has the SMALLEST radius? 7.____
   A. Mg^{+2} B. Na^+ C. K^+ D. Ca^{+2}

8. Which group in the Periodic Table contains solid, liquid, and gaseous elements at room temperature? 8.____
   A. 0   B. IIA   C. VIA   D. VIIA

9. Which metallic ion would MOST likely produce a colored solution? 9.____
   A. K^+ B. Ca^{+2} C. Cr^{+3} D. Al^{+3}

10. Which element in Group VA of the Periodic Table is BEST described as a metalloid? 10.____
    A. N   B. P   C. As   D. Bi

11. If the gram-molecular mass of a gas is 44.0 at STP, the number of liters occupied by 11.0 g of the gas is 11.____
    A. 5.60   B. 11.2   C. 22.4   D. 44.8

12. What is the TOTAL number of moles of $CaCl_2$ needed to make 500 ml of 4 M $CaCl_2$? 12.____
    A. 1   B. 2   C. 8   D. 4

13. The mass of one mole of nitrogen gas molecules at STP is _____ grams.

    A. 7 B. 14 C. 16 D. 28

14. Which expression represents the molarity (M) of a solution?

    A. $\dfrac{\text{moles of solvent}}{1,000 \text{ gm of solution}}$

    B. $\dfrac{\text{moles of solute}}{1,000 \text{ gm of solution}}$

    C. $\dfrac{\text{moles of solvent}}{1,000 \text{ ml of solution}}$

    D. $\dfrac{\text{moles of solute}}{1,000 \text{ ml of solution}}$

15. The percentage by mass of oxygen in CuO is _____ percent.

    A. 16 B. 20 C. 25 D. 50

16. In the reaction A(s) + B(s) → C(g) + D(g) + heat, the entropy of the system _____ and the reaction is _____

    A. increases; exothermic
    B. increases; endothermic
    C. decreases; exothermic
    D. decreases; endothermic

17. Given the reaction A + B ⇌ AB + 50 kcal.
    If an activation energy of 5 kcal is required, the activation energy of the reverse reaction is _____ kcal.

    A. 5 B. 45 C. 50 D. 55

Questions 18-20.

DIRECTIONS: For each of Questions 18 through 20, select the letter of the expression, chosen from the list below, that BEST answers that question.

EXPRESSIONS

A. $[A^+][B^-]$

B. $\dfrac{[A^+]}{[B^+]}$

C. $\dfrac{[A^+][B^-]}{[AB]}$

D. $\dfrac{[A^+]}{[B^-]}$

18. Given the ionization equation of a weak acid:
    AB(aq) ⇌ A^+(aq) + B^-(aq). Which expression is equal to its equilibrium constant, K_a?

19. The equation for the reaction of a metal replacing a metallic ion B^+ from aqueous solution is
    A(s) + B^+(aq) ⇌ A^+(aq) + B(s). Which expression is equal to its equilibrium constant, K?

20. Given the dissociation equation of a saturated solution of a slightly soluble salt: AB(s) ⇌ A^+(aq) + B^-(aq). Which expression is equal to its solubility product constant, K_{sp}?

Questions 21-22.

DIRECTIONS: Questions 21 and 22 are to be answered on the basis of the information below.

An aqueous solution has a H_3O^+ concentration of 1×10^{-9} mole per liter. [Kw = $[H_3O^+][OH^-] = 1 \times 10^{-14}$]

21. The OH⁻ concentration of this solution is 1 x _____ M.

    A. 10^{-5} B. 10^{-7} C. 10^{-9} D. 10^{-14}

22. This solution is _____ and will turn litmus paper _____.

    A. acidic; blue
    B. acidic; red
    C. basic; blue
    D. basic; red

23. In the neutralization reaction between hydrochloric acid and sodium hydroxide, the spectator ions are

    A. H⁺ and OH⁻
    B. Cl⁻ and OH⁻
    C. Na⁺ and H⁺
    D. Na⁺ and Cl⁻

24. In the reaction $CH_3COOH + H_2O \rightleftharpoons H_3O^+ + CH_3COO^-$, a conjugate acid-base pair is

    A. CH_3COOH and H_3O^+
    B. CH_3COOH and CH_3COO^-
    C. CH_3COOH and H_2O
    D. CH_3COO^- and H_2O

25. What volume of 0.1 M KOH is needed to EXACTLY neutralize 10 ml of 0.01 M HNO_3? _____ ml.

    A. 1   B. 0.1   C. 10   D. 100

26. In the reaction $Cl_2 + 2KI \rightarrow 2KCl + I_2$, which species is reduced?

    A. K₊   B. Cl_2 C. I_2 D. I⁻

27. In the reaction $Zn + CuSO_4 \rightarrow ZnSO_4 + Cu \downarrow$, one mole of zinc will _____ mole(s) of electrons.

    A. lose 1   B. gain 1   C. lose 2   D. gain 2

28. A chemical cell DIFFERS from an electrolytic cell in that a chemical cell

    A. produces an electric current by means of a chemical reaction
    B. produces a chemical reaction by means of an electric current
    C. has oxidation and reduction occurring at the electrodes
    D. has ions migrating between the electrodes

29. In the reaction 2KClO₃ → 2KCl + 3O₂, the oxidation number of chlorine

    A. decreases
    B. increases
    C. remains the same
    D. cannot be determined from the information given

30. When a neutral atom undergoes reduction, its oxidation number

    A. decreases   B. increases
    C. remains the same   D. decreases, then increases

31. An unsaturated hydrocarbon may be represented by the formula

    A. C_2H_6 B. C_3H_6 C. C_4H_{10} D. C_5H_{12}

32. Which is the CORRECT structural formula for methanol?

    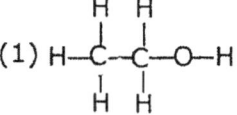

33. What is the CORRECT I.U.C. name of the compound represented by the structural formula shown at the right?
    A. n-pentane
    B. Isobutane
    C. 2-methylbutane
    D. n-butane

    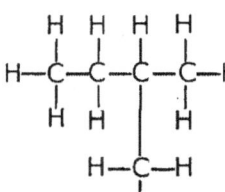

34. An isomer of 2, 2,dimethylpropane is

    A. ethane   B. propane   C. n-pentane   D. n-butane

35. In a homologous series, the second member has the formula C_3H_6. What is the formula for the fourth member of the series?

    A. C_4H_6 B. C_4H_{10} C. C_5H_{10} D. C_5H_{12}

KEY (CORRECT ANSWERS)

1.	B	16.	A
2.	A	17.	D
3.	B	18.	C
4.	B	19.	B
5.	D	20.	A
6.	A	21.	A
7.	A	22.	C
8.	D	23.	D
9.	C	24.	B
10.	C	25.	A
11.	A	26.	B
12.	B	27.	C
13.	D	28.	A
14.	D	29.	A
15.	B	30.	A

31. B
32. D
33. C
34. C
35. C

TEST 2

DIRECTIONS: Each question or incomplete statement is followed by several suggested answers or completions. Select the one that BEST answers the question or completes the statement. *PRINT THE LETTER OF THE CORRECT ANSWER IN THE SPACE AT THE RIGHT.*

1. Which salt is LEAST soluble in water at 25° C?

    A. Lithium carbonate ($K_{sp} = 1.7 \times 10^{-3}$)
    B. Calcium carbonate ($K_{sp} = 0.87 \times 10^{-8}$)
    C. Silver carbonate ($K_{sp} = 6.2 \times 10^{-12}$)
    D. Barium carbonate ($K_{sp} = 8.1 \times 10^{-9}$)

    1.____

2. When formed from its elements at 25° C, the compound _____ would be produced by an exothermic reaction.

    A. dinitrogen monoxide(g) B. ethyne (acetylene)(g)
    C. nitrogen monoxide (g)   D. carbon dioxide (g)

    2.____

3. Which chemical species could be classified as both a Bronsted acid and a base?

    A. H_2O B. OH^- C. NH_4^+ D. H_2SO_4

    3.____

4. An acidic solution DIFFERS from a basic solution in that an acidic solution

    A. turns litmus blue
    B. contains hydronium ions
    C. has a pH less than 7
    D. is a conductor of electricity

    4.____

5. The conjugate base of the acid HBr is

    A. H^+ B. Br^- C. H_3O^+ D. OH^-

    5.____

6. How many moles of H_3O^+ ions will be required to exactly neutralize 34 grams of OH^- ions?

    A. 1.0   B. 2.0   C. 0.5   D. 4.0

    6.____

7. Which is the WEAKEST acid? (K_A values are taken at 25° C.)

    A. Acetic acid ($K_A = 1.8 \times 10^{-5}$)
    B. Hydrofluoric acid ($K_A = 7.2 \times 10^{-4}$)
    C. Hypobromous ($K_A = 2.0 \times 10^{-9}$)
    D. Nitrous acid ($K_A = 4.5 \times 10^{-4}$)

    7.____

8. A gas whose water solution is basic is

    A. CO_2 B. SO_2 C. HCl D. NH_3

    8.____

9. The hydronium ion concentration of a solution is 1 x 10⁻⁶ mole per liter. This solution is

   A. slightly acidic
   B. strongly acidic
   C. slightly basic
   D. strongly basic

10. Nitrogen has an oxidation number of +2 in the compound

    A. NH_3
    B. HNO_2
    C. N_2
    D. NO

11. Which atom-ion pair will react spontaneously?
    Ag +

    A. Au^{+3}
    B. H^+
    C. Fe^{+2}
    D. Fe^{+3}

12. Which pair of half cells would produce a cell with the HIGHEST potential ($E°$)?
    _____ and H_2, H^+ (1 M)

    A. Zn, Zn^{+2}(1 M)
    B. Mg, Mg^{+2} (1 M)
    C. Fe, Fe^{+2}(1 M)
    D. Al, Al^{+3} (1 M)

13. The electronic equation $Mg^{+2} + 2e^- \rightarrow Mg^0$ indicates that the magnesium

    A. ion is being oxidized
    B. ion is being reduced
    C. atom is being oxidized
    D. atom is being reduced

14. When Cu^0 replaces Ag^+ from a water solution, the Cu^0 is _____ and its oxidation number _____.

    A. reduced; increases
    B. reduced; decreases
    C. oxidized; increases
    D. oxidized; decreases

15. What is the MAXIMUM $E°$ voltage for the cell with the net equation $Zn + Cu^{+2} \rightarrow Zn^{+2} + Cu$?

    A. -0.42
    B. +0.42
    C. -1.10
    D. 1.10

16. The first two members of the benzene family are benzene (C_6H_6) and toluene (C_7H_8). The general formula of this series is

    A. C_nH_n
    B. C_nH_{-+1}
    C. C_nH_{2n-6}
    D. C_nH_{2n}

17. Which class of compounds has the general formula R-OH?

    A. Alkanes
    B. Alkenes
    C. Alcohols
    D. Acids

18. One of the products produced by the reaction between CH_3COOH and CH_3OH is

    A. HOH
    B. H_2SO_4
    C. HCOOH
    D. CH_3CH_2OH

19. Which molecule contains four carbon atoms?

    A. Ethane
    B. Butane
    C. Methane
    D. Propane

20. As the average kinetic energy of the molecules of a sample increases, the temperature of the sample

    A. decreases
    B. increases
    C. remains the same
    D. decreases, then increases

21. As the elements in Period 3 are considered in order of increasing atomic number, the number of principal energy levels in each successive element

    A. decreases
    B. increases
    C. remains the same
    D. decreases, then increases

22. If the concentration of one of the reactants in a chemical reaction is increased, the rate of the reaction

    A. decreases
    B. increases
    C. remains the same
    D. cannot be determined from the information given

23. As the molecular mass of the compounds of the alkane series increases, their boiling point

    A. decreases
    B. increases
    C. remains the same
    D. cannot be determined from the information given

24. When a radioactive element forms a chemical bond with another element, its half-life

    A. decreases
    B. increases
    C. remains the same
    D. increases, then decreases

25. When two chlorine atoms combine to form a molecule of chlorine, the oxidation number of the chlorine

    A. decreases
    B. increases
    C. remains the same
    D. cannot be determined from the information given

Questions 26-27.

DIRECTIONS: Questions 26 and 27 are to be answered on the basis of the diagram below, which represents a movable piston and a cylinder. The cylinder contains 1,000 ml. of gas G at STP.

26. If the temperature remains constant and the pressure on gas G is increased to 4 atmospheres, the new volume of the gas will be _____ ml.

    A. 250   B. 500   C. 2,000   D. 4,000

27. If the pressure remains constant and the temperature of gas G is raised to 273° C, the piston will move until the new volume of gas G is _____ ml.

    A. 273   B. 500   C. 2,000   D. 273,000

28. How many calories are required to change 100. grams of ice at 0° C to water at 0° C? (Heat of fusion of H_2O = 80. cal/gram.)

    A. .80   B. 80.   C. 8.0×10^2 D. 8.0×10^3

29. Deviations from ideal gas behavior become MOST significant at _____ pressure and _____ temperature.

    A. high; high
    B. high; low
    C. low; low
    D. low; high

30. What will be the temperature of water when its vapor pressure is 760 mm. of Hg? _____ ° C.

    A. 0   B. 100   C. 273   D. 760

31. The number of orbitals in a p sublevel is

    A. one   B. six   C. three   D. seven

32. A sample contains 100 milligrams of iodine-131. At the end of 32 days, the number of milligrams of iodine-131 that will remain will be

    A. 25.00   B. 12.50   C. 6.250   D. 3.125

33. Which is the electron configuration of the fluoride ion (F^-)?

    A. $1s^2 2s^8$ B. $1s^2 2s^2 2p^4$ C. $1s^2 2s^2 2p^6$ D. $1s^2 2s^2 2p^8$

34. The TOTAL number of s-electrons for a chlorine atom in the ground state is

    A. 1   B. 2   C. 6   D. 4

35. Energy is emitted when an electron moves from sublevel

    A. 2s to 2p   B. 2p to 3d   C. 3p to 3d   D. 3d to 3s

KEY (CORRECT ANSWERS)

1. C
2. D
3. A
4. C
5. B

6. B
7. C
8. D
9. A
10. D

11. A
12. B
13. B
14. C
15. D

16. C
17. C
18. A
19. B
20. B

21. C
22. B
23. B
24. C
25. C

26. A
27. C
28. D
29. B
30. B

31. C
32. C
33. C
34. C
35. D

TEST 3

DIRECTIONS: Each question or incomplete statement is followed by several suggested answers or completions. Select the one that BEST answers the question or completes the statement. *PRINT THE LETTER OF THE CORRECT ANSWER IN THE SPACE AT THE RIGHT.*

1. If 15 calories of heat energy are added to 1 gram of water at 20° C, the resulting temperature of the water will be _____ °C.

    A. -10   B. 5   C. 35   D. 50

2. Sublimation is a change directly from the _____ phase to the _____ phase.

    A. solid; gaseous B. solid; liquid
    C. liquid; gaseous D. gaseous; liquid

3. At a pressure of one atmosphere, the temperature of a mixture of ice and water at equilibrium would be _____ °K.

    A. 25   B. 32   C. 273   D. 298

4. A 1.00-liter sample of a gas at a pressure of 1.00 atmosphere is compressed to 0.25 liter at constant temperature.
    What is the new pressure of the gas?
    _____ atm.

    A. 0.50   B. 2.0   C. 0.25   D. 4.0

5. One mole of any gas at STP will occupy a volume of _____ liters.

    A. 2.24×10^1 B. 2.73×10^2
    C. 3.73×10^2 D. 6.02×10^{23}

6. A liter of chlorine at STP has a mass of APPROXIMATELY

    A. 1   B. 1.5   C. 3   D. .3

7. How many neutrons are in the nucleus of an atom that has an atomic number of 17 and a mass number of 35?

    A. 17   B. 18   C. 35   D. 52

8. Which atom has the LARGEST radius?

    A. Li   B. Be   C. C   D. F

9. Which element has the HIGHEST first ionization energy?

    A. Barium   B. Bismuth   C. Beryllium   D. Bromine

10. Isotopes are atoms which have different

    A. atomic masses B. atomic numbers
    C. atomic radii D. electron configurations

11. When the aluminum atom is in the ground state, how many orbitals contain ONLY one electron?

   A. 1 B. 2 C. 3 D. 13

12. Which is the electron dot structure for the atom whose electronic structure is $1s^2 2s^2 2p^6 3s^2 3p^5$?

   A. $\dot{X}\cdot$ B. $\cdot\ddot{X}\cdot$ C. $\dot{X}\cdot$ D. $\cdot\ddot{X}:$

13. The empirical formula of the compound N_2O_4 is

   A. NO B. NO_2 C. N_2O D. N_2O_3

14. Van der Waals forces will increase when there is a DECREASE in the _____ molecules.

   A. number of B. size of
   C. distance between D. mass of

15. When the equation $N_2 + H_2 \rightarrow NH_3$ is balanced, the sum of the coefficients is

   A. 6 B. 2 C. 8 D. 4

16. The abnormally high boiling point of water is PRIMARILY due to _____ bonding.

   A. covalent B. ionic
   C. coordinate covalent D. hydrogen

17. Which type of bond would MOST likely be formed between phosphorous and chlorine?

   A. Nonpolar covalent B. Polar covalent
   C. Electrovalent D. Network

18. Which represents a molecule at STP?

   A. H B. O C. Ne D. Cl

19. A certain solid, when it is in the liquid state or dissolved in water, will conduct electricity. In the solid state, it will not conduct electricity.
   This solid MUST contain _____ bonds.

   A. ionic B. metallic C. covalent D. coordinate

20. The element with an atomic number of 34 is MOST similar in its chemical behavior to the element with an atomic number of

   A. 19 B. 31 C. 36 D. 52

21. A Ba^{+2} ion DIFFERS from a Ba atom in that the ion has

   A. more electrons B. more protons
   C. fewer electrons D. fewer proton

22. Which period contains elements in which electrons from more than one principal energy level may be involved in bond formation?

   A. 1 B. 2 C. 3 D. 4

23. In the ground state, Al and Mg atoms both have the same number of electrons in the   23._____
    A. 3p subshell
    B. 3s subshell
    C. 3rd principal energy level
    D. outermost principal energy level

24. Which group of elements in the ground state would have electrons with an S^2P^3 configuration in the outermost shell?   24._____
    A. VA   B. IIA   C. IIIA   D. IVA

25. Which element in Group VIIA forms the MOST stable compounds?   25._____
    A. Fluorine   B. Chlorine   C. Bromine   D. Iodine

26. Which represents a mole of calcium at STP?   26._____
    A. 23 liters
    B. 22.4 grams
    C. 6.02×10^{23} atoms
    D. 3.01×10^{23} molecules

27. Consider the following reaction: 27._____
    $Na(s) + H_2O(\ell) \rightarrow Na^+(aq) + OH^-(aq) + 1/2 H_2(g)$.
    How many moles of $Na^+(aq)$ are produced when 46 grams of Na(s) react with an excess of $H_2O(\ell)$?
    A. 1.0   B. 2.0   C. 0.50   D. 4.0

28. Which gas has a density of 1.34 grams per liter at STP?   28._____
    A. NO_2 B. NO   C. N_2 D. H_2

29. As the temperature increases from 30° to 40° C, the solubility of potassium nitrate in 100 ml of water increases by APPROXIMATELY _____ grams.   29._____
    A. 5   B. 10   C. 15   D. 20

30. The number of moles in 2.16 grams of silver is   30._____
    A. 2.00×10^{-2}
    B. 4.59×10^{-2}
    C. 2.00×10^{2}
    D. 2.33×10^{2}

31. The solution with the LOWEST freezing point would be produced when 1.0 gram of $C_6H_{12}O_6$ is dissolved in _____ grams of H_2O.   31._____
    A. 18   B. 100   C. 180   D. 1,000

32. The difference between the heat content of the products and the heat content of the reactants is   32._____
    A. entropy of reaction
    B. heat of reaction
    C. free energy
    D. activation energy

33. Which change results in an increase in entropy?

    A. $Br_2(\ell) \rightarrow Br_2(s)$
    B. $Cl_2(g) \rightarrow Cl_2(\ell)$
    C. $F_2(\ell) \rightarrow F_2(g)$
    D. $I_2(g) \rightarrow I_2(s)$

34. The purpose of a catalyst in a reaction is to

    A. change the activation energy required of the reaction
    B. provide the energy necessary to start the reaction
    C. increase the amount of product formed
    D. decrease the amount of reactants used

35. Which is the CORRECT equilibrium expression for the reaction A(g) + B(g) = C(g) + D(g)?
    K =

    A. $\dfrac{[A][C]}{[B][D]}$
    B. $\dfrac{[B][D]}{[A][C]}$
    C. $\dfrac{[A][B]}{[C][D]}$
    D. $\dfrac{[C][D]}{[A][B]}$

KEY (CORRECT ANSWERS)

1.	C	16.	D
2.	A	17.	B
3.	C	18.	C
4.	D	19.	A
5.	A	20.	D
6.	C	21.	C
7.	B	22.	D
8.	A	23.	B
9.	D	24.	A
10.	A	25.	A
11.	A	26.	C
12.	D	27.	B
13.	B	28.	B
14.	C	29.	C
15.	A	30.	A

31. A
32. B
33. C
34. A
35. D

EXAMINATION SECTION
TEST 1

DIRECTIONS: Each question or incomplete statement is followed by several suggested answers or completions. Select the one that BEST answers the question or completes the statement. *PRINT THE LETTER OF THE CORRECT ANSWER IN THE SPACE AT THE RIGHT.*

1. The equivalent weight of $CaCl_2$ (M.W. = 110) is

    A. 37   B. 55.5   C. 110   D. 220

2. 40.8 gm of mercury is used for the calibration of a pipette (Density = 13.6). What is the volume?

    A. 1   B. 2   C. 3   D. 4

3. In gas-liquid chromatography, it is necessary for the sample to be

    A. precipitated   B. pulverized
    C. soluble in water   D. volatilized

4. In flame photometry, the color of sodium in the flame is

    A. green   B. purple   C. red   D. yellow

5. Thin layer chromatography has a distinct ADVANTAGE over paper chromatography in that it

    A. can be used with aqueous solutions
    B. is cheaper
    C. is faster
    D. uses less sample

6. Of the following, the one that the halogen ions do NOT include is

    A. chloride   B. fluoride   C. iodide   D. sulfide

7. Beer's Law relates to

    A. calorimetry   B. colorimetry
    C. gas volumes   D. oxidation-reduction

8. The sulfides of lead and mercury are

    A. colloidal   B. insoluble
    C. red in color   D. soluble

9. The inert gases include all EXCEPT

    A. argon   B. krypton   C. methane   D. neon

10. Of the following metals, the one which is in a different group from the others in the periodic table is

    A. lithium   B. sodium   C. magnesium   D. cesium

11. The reaction of equimolar concentrations of NaOH and HCl is

    A. amphoteric titration
    B. coulemetric titration
    C. neutralization
    D. oxidation-reduction

12. 10.0 ml of a 0.1 normal solution contains

    A. 1 equivalent
    B. 1 microequivalent
    C. 1 milliequivalent
    D. 1 milligram

13. The assay of a compound that has maximum absorbency at 300 mu requires a spectrophotometer sensitive in which one of the following spectral regions?

    A. Infra-red
    B. Red
    C. Ultraviolet
    D. Visible

14. Which of the following is NOT an oxidizing agent?

    A. Ceric sulfate
    B. Citrate
    C. Ferricyanide
    D. Permanganate

15. A buffer solution contains

    A. a strong acid
    B. a weak acid or base
    C. an oxidizing agent
    D. sodium chloride

16. When a procedure calls for the d- or l-isomer of a substance, it may be possible to

    A. substitute the d- or l-isomer of a related substance
    B. use 1/2 the weight of a racemic mixture of the substance
    C. use twice the weight of the racemic mixture of the substance
    D. use the meso form of the substance

17. Hercuric ion will combine with which one of the following to form an undissociated salt?

    A. Carbonate   B. Chloride   C. Fluoride   D. Sulfate

18. pH is defined as

    A. $[H^+]$
    B. $[H^+]+[OH^+]$
    C. $-\log[H^+]$
    D. $2 - \log[H^+]$

19. Which of the following can be used to prepare a pH standard?

    A. Acetate
    B. Phosphate
    C. Potassium acid phthalate
    D. Veronal

20. The PREFERRED indicator to observe a pH change at 9.0 is

    A. bromthymol blue
    B. methyl orange
    C. methyl red
    D. phenolphthalein

21. The MOST effective buffer at pH of 6.8 is

    A. acetate
    B. barbiturate
    C. borate
    D. phosphate

22. The reaction involved in the titration of sodium oxalate by potassium permanganate is   22.____

   A. amphoteric titration   B. coulemetric titration
   C. neutralization   D. oxidation-reduction

23. Density is expressed BEST as   23.____

   A. mass/unit volume
   B. solubility per 100 ml
   C. specific gravity/unit volume
   D. volume/unit mass

24. 60° C converted to Fahrenheit is   24.____

   A. 110° F   B. 120° F   C. 130° F   D. 140° F

25. A substance with a melting point of +28° C at room temperature (25° C) will be a   25.____

   A. gas   B. liquid   C. mixture   D. solid

26. Which of the following has the HIGHEST boiling point?   26.____

   A. Acetic acid   B. Ethyl alcohol
   C. Methyl alcohol   D. Water

27. At constant pressure, which of the following will have the LOWEST freezing point?   27.____

   A. 0.1M NaCl   B. 0.2M NaCl
      0.1M Na_2HPO_4 C. 0.2M NaH_2PO_4

28. In one liter, a 5% solution contains _____ gm.   28.____

   A. 5   B. 25   C. 50   D. 100

29. Which one of the following compounds, in aqueous solution, absorbs ultraviolet light?   29.____

   A. Fumaric acid   B. Glutamic acid
   C. Malic acid   D. Succinic acid

30. Which of the following statements is LEAST likely to be correct?   30.____
    Automated procedures

   A. are less costly than manual ones
   B. speed the rate of performance
   C. conserve laboratory space
   D. can be performed by less skilled personnel

31. The principle of the AutoAnalyzer is based on _____ analysis.   31.____

   A. sequential   B. discrete
   C. single   D. multiple

32. Atomic absorption is used to determine   32.____

   A. anions   B. atomic numbers
   C. cations   D. methyl groups

33. A nanogram of material is

    A. 1×10^{-3} g
    B. 1×10^{-6} g
    C. 1×10^{-9} g
    D. 1×10^{12} g

34. The Henderson-Hasselbalch equation is pH =

    A. $-\log[H]$
    B. $\log[H]$
    C. $pK_a + \log \frac{[Acid]}{[Salt]}$
    D. $pK_a + \log \frac{[Salt]}{[Acid]}$

35. In gas chromatography, the sample must be

    A. liquid
    B. inorganic
    C. solid
    D. volatilized

36. Atomic absorption spectroscopy requires

    A. an extremely hot flame
    B. a hollow cathode lamp
    C. nuclear energy
    D. vigorous mixing

37. Absolute temperature is _____ °C.

    A. -100
    B. -273
    C. +100
    D. +273

38. Gravimetric analysis PRIMARILY involves

    A. amperometric voltages
    B. colorimetry
    C. titration
    D. weighing

39. A gram molecular weight of a gas at standard conditions of temperature and pressure occupies _____ ml.

    A. 1,000
    B. 10,000
    C. 22,400
    D. 44,800

40. Infra-red analysis is MOST often used in

    A. analytical chemistry
    B. electrochemistry
    C. organic chemistry
    D. physical chemistry

41. Enzymes are

    A. complex collagens
    B. complex lipids
    C. polysaccharides
    D. protein catalysts

42. Vitamin A is

    A. a nitrogenous compound
    B. a protein catalyst
    C. water insoluble
    D. water soluble

43. Which of the following is destroyed in pasteurization?

    A. Alkaline phosphatase
    B. Calcium
    C. Iron binding protein
    D. Lactose

44. In the human cell, energy is stored as

    A. adenosine monophosphate
    B. adenosine triphosphate
    C. creatine phosphokinase
    D. nicotine adenine dinucleotide

45. The acid found in normal gastric juice is

    A. citric   B. HCl   C. H_2SO_4 D. lactic

46. Albumin can be precipitated by addition of

    A. blood serum   B. sodium chloride
    C. sodium sulfate   D. water

47. Which of the following is NOT a reducing carbohydrate?

    A. Fructose   B. Galactose   C. Glucose   D. Sucrose

48. The kinetic theory of matter explains that

    A. the space between molecules of a gas is greater than the space occupied by the molecule itself
    B. molecules of matter do not move unless agitated
    C. molecules of matter are the ultimate particles of individual elements
    D. molecules of matter are always in motion

49. Of the following, the PRIMARY purpose of standards and controls is to obtain

    A. accuracy   B. priorities
    C. replicates   D. reproducibility

50. Of the following, the BEST definition for accuracy in laboratory practice is

    A. nearness to truth
    B. reproducibility of replicates
    C. within biological variation
    D. within 2 standard deviations of the mean

KEY (CORRECT ANSWERS)

1. B	11. C	21. D	31. A	41. D
2. C	12. C	22. D	32. C	42. C
3. D	13. C	23. A	33. C	43. A
4. D	14. B	24. D	34. D	44. B
5. C	15. B	25. D	35. D	45. B
6. D	16. C	26. A	36. B	46. C
7. B	17. B	27. D	37. B	47. D
8. B	18. C	28. C	38. D	48. D
9. C	19. C	29. A	39. C	49. A
10. C	20. D	30. D	40. C	50. A

TEST 2

DIRECTIONS: Each question or incomplete statement is followed by several suggested answers or completions. Select the one that BEST answers the question or completes the statement. *PRINT THE LETTER OF THE CORRECT ANSWER IN THE SPACE AT THE RIGHT.*

1. Which of the following formulas does NOT correspond to a known substance?   1.____
   A. $NaClO_2$ B. $NaPO_3$ C. $NaSO_2$ D. $Na_2S_2O_3$

2. In the reaction between zinc and concentrated nitric acid, shown UNBALANCED as   2.____
   ____Zn + ____HNO_3 = ____$Zn(NO_3)_2$ + ____NO + ____H_2O,
   the number which should appear in front of the formula for nitric acid after the equation has been balanced is
   A. 3   B. 4   C. 6   D. 8

3. The element whose valence electrons have the quantum designation $4s^2$, $4p^5$ is No.   3.____
   A. 7   B. 25   C. 28   D. 35

4. In the case of the following equilibrium reaction, heat, which of the following actions will result in a CHANGE in the numerical value of the equilibrium constant?   4.____
   A. Addition of NO_2
   B. Increase in the temperature
   C. Increase in the total pressure
   D. Introduction of a catalyst

5. Of the following, the STRONGEST oxidizing agent is   5.____
   A. Br_2 B. F_2 C. Na D. O_2

6. The ionization constant of acetic acid is 1.8×10^{-5}. What is the pH of a liter of a solution containing 0.5 moles of acetic acid and 0.25 moles of sodium acetate?   6.____
   A. 1.8   B. 3.2   C. 4.44   D. 5.05

7. The volume of 0.42 M H_2SO_4 solution which will be EXACTLY neutralized by 230 ml of 0.70 M NaOH is   7.____
   A. 138   B. 192   C. 276   D. 384

8. Of the following, the substance which will NOT react with 1 M NaOH is   8.____
   A. Al   B. $Al(OH)_3$ C. Fe   D. SO_2

9. Of the following precipitates, the one which will NOT dissolve in 0.3 M HCl is   9.____
   A. As_2S_3 B. CuS   C. $MnNH_4PO_4$ D. ZnS

10. The ionization constant, K_B, of ammonium hydroxide is 1.8×10^{-5}. What is the USEFUL range of pH's of the buffer solutions that can be made up from various mixtures of ammonium hydroxide and ammonium chloride?   10.____
    A. 8.5 to 10.5   B. 7 to 13   C. 5.5 to 7.5   D. 2 to 6

11. The atomic number of an element is equal to the

    A. number of neutrons in the nucleus
    B. number of protons in the nucleus
    C. sum of the protons and the electrons
    D. sum of the protons and the neutrons

12. What will be the APPROXIMATE increase in the reaction rate for every 10° C rise in temperature?
    _____ fold.

    A. 1.5   B. 2.0   C. 2.5   D. 3.0

13. At standard temperature and pressure, one liter of hydrogen gas contains APPROXIMATELY the same number of molecules as

    A. 0.5 liter of oxygen
    B. 1.0 liter of sulfur dioxide
    C. 1.5 liters of ozone
    D. 2.0 liters of helium

14. The amount of $CuSO_4 \cdot 5H_2O$ that must be dissolved in 100 ml of water to produce a solution containing 1 mg Cu^{++} per ml is _____ g.

    A. 0.100   B. 0.252   C. 0.393   D. 0.635

15. Of the following techniques, the one which would be the BEST to use in order to obtain absolute ethanol from the standard commercial product (95% ethanol, 5% water) is

    A. fractional distillation
    B. reaction with sodium, followed by distillation
    C. reaction with zinc, followed by filtration
    D. solvent extraction

16. Based upon mutual solubility considerations, which of the following would you expect to be the BEST solvent for a heavy machine oil?

    A. Acetone   B. Benzene   C. Dioxane   D. Ethanol

17. The specific gravity of concentrated hydrochloric acid reagent is 1.19. The solution contains 37% HCl.
    The molarity of the reagent is

    A. 2   B. 6   C. 8   D. 12

18. The purpose of a magnetic damper is to

    A. activate balance pans
    B. eliminate counting of swings
    C. keep the humidity down
    D. remove static electricity

19. Quantities of waste flammable organic liquids should be destroyed by

   A. burning under controlled conditions
   B. dumping in a secluded area
   C. evaporating on a water bath in a hood
   D. flushing down the sink

20. Of the following determinations, which would be BEST for routine use in the quality control (i.e., testing of purity) of a solid benzene derivative?

   A. Diffusion coefficient
   B. Melting range
   C. Solubility in toluene
   D. Vapor pressure

21. The MEDIAN value in a column of figures is the _____ value.

   A. highest   B. lowest   C. mean   D. middle

22. The R_F in paper chromatography designates the

   A. distance between two solutes
   B. rate at which the fastest component migrates
   C. rate at which the slowest component migrates
   D. rate of solute migration compared to the solvent

23. An internal standard is used in flame photometry because it

   A. corrects for gas fluctuations
   B. forms a binary mixture
   C. increases the excitation
   D. simplifies calculations

24. In calcium analysis by atomic absorption, lanthanum is added to

   A. intensify the absorption
   B. intensify the emission
   C. prevent PO_4 interference
   D. reduce iron

25. The pressure of a mixture of three gases will be

   A. the product of the individual partial pressures
   B. the average of the partial pressures
   C. the sum of the partial pressures
   D. the partial pressure of the most volatile gas

26. Which of the following guides to the chemical literature deals EXCLUSIVELY with organic compounds?

   A. Abegg   B. Gmelin   C. Beilstein   D. Mellor

27. Of the following, the reagent which is employed in the separation and purification of ketones is

   A. Na_2CO_3 B. $NaHSO_3$ C. Cu_2Cl_2 D. $Ag(NH_3)_2OH$

28. Of the following, the compound which exists as two geometrical isomers is

   A. HOOCCH=CH$_2$
   B. HOOCCH$_2$CH$_2$COOH
   C. HOOCCH=CHCOOH
   D. HOOCC≡CH

29. The monomer from which Teflon plastic is produced is

   A. CF$_2$=CF$_2$
   B. CF$_3$COOH
   C. CH$_2$=CH$_2$
   D. CHF=CHF

30. Of the following, the substance to start with in order to obtain the BEST yield of m-phenylenediamine is

   A. aniline
   B. benzenediazonium chloride
   C. m-dichlorophenol
   D. m-dinitrobenzene

31. What is the MOST likely reason for a blood glucose to be exceedingly high (above 1000 mg per 100 ml)?
   The

   A. patient ingested large amounts of carbohydrates
   B. patient ingested reducing substances
   C. patient was not fasting
   D. specimen was contaminated from an infusion

32. If the pH of blood plasma is 7.1 and the dissolved CO$_2$ is 2.0 mmoles, then the HCO$_3$ is _____ mmoles.

   A. 10
   B. 20
   C. 30
   D. 40

33. A triglyceride is a compound of three

   A. fatty acids
   B. fatty acids and one glycerol
   C. glycerols and one fatty acid
   D. glycerol molecules

34. Starch can be determined by measuring the intensity of the blue color when it reacts with

   A. alkaline copper
   B. amylase
   C. iodine
   D. silver

35. After the complete hydrolysis of lecithin, which of the following is NOT present?

   A. Choline
   B. Ethanolamine
   C. Glycerol
   D. Phosphoric acid

36. Fehling's Solution is used in the analysis of

   A. fat
   B. protein
   C. reducing sugar
   D. starch

37. An antimetabolite that inhibits an enzyme reaction is

   A. a heayy metal
   B. a substance that chelates with the substrate
   C. structurally related to the enzyme
   D. structurally related to the substrate

38. Of the following enzymes, the one that is NOT present in the carbohydrate citric acid cycle is

    A. fumarase
    B. isocitric dehydrogenase
    C. succinic dehydrogenase
    D. triose phosphate isomerase

39. The xylose test, as performed in the clinical laboratory, is a test for

    A. glomerular filtration
    B. kidney function
    C. liver function
    D. malabsorption

40. Serum acid phosphatase will be FALSELY elevated when the

    A. patient has urinary retention
    B. patient was not fasting
    C. serum alkaline phosphatase is elevated
    D. serum is hemolyzed

41. The *diurnal* variation of a blood substance infers that it varies with the

    A. age of the patient
    B. procedure used
    C. sex of the patient
    D. time of day

42. A single peak in the Tiselius electrophoresis indicates that the

    A. substance is a pure protein
    B. substance is not a protein
    C. solution contains mucopolysaccharides
    D. solution is a mixture of proteins

43. 68 ml. of gastric juice were titrated to pH 7.0 and found to contain 138 mmoles per liter of acid.
    What is the acidity in mmoles of the total volume of gastric juice?

    A. 20.3 B. 14.4 C. 9.4 D. 4.9

44. The glucose oxidase method for blood glucose is PREFERRED over any other blood glucose test because

    A. it is the fastest procedure
    B. it requires the least expensive reagents
    C. the reagents are readily stable
    D. there is no interference from other reducing substances

45. Fluoride is used as a blood anticoagulant for glucose determinations because it

    A. inhibits bacterial growth
    B. inhibits glycolytic enzymes
    C. precipitates calcium
    D. prevents hemolysis

46. Deoxyribonucleoproteins form viscous solutions because they

    A. are elongated
    B. are spherical
    C. contain protein
    D. have a high molecular weight

47. Bromsulphonphthalein (BSP) is used as a liver function test because the dye is

    A. excreted by the kidney
    B. excreted by the liver
    C. not adsorbed to proteins
    D. stored in the liver

48. Proteins will NOT migrate in an electric field at _____ pH.

    A. a neutral
    B. an acid
    C. an alkaline
    D. an isoelectric

49. A pooled serum may be used as a

    A. daily control
    B. gas analysis control
    C. primary standard
    D. secondary standard

50. Which of the following is NOT a hormone?

    A. Carotene
    B. Estriol
    C. Epinephrine
    D. Secretin

KEY (CORRECT ANSWERS)

1. C	11. B	21. D	31. B	41. D
2. D	12. B	22. D	32. D	42. A
3. D	13. B	23. A	33. A	43. C
4. B	14. C	24. C	34. A	44. D
5. B	15. B	25. C	35. C	45. C
6. C	16. B	26. C	36. C	46. D
7. B	17. D	27. B	37. C	47. C
8. C	18. B	28. C	38. B	48. D
9. B	19. C	29. A	39. B	49. B
10. A	20. B	30. D	40. C	50. A

TEST 3

DIRECTIONS: Each question or incomplete statement is followed by several suggested answers or completions. Select the one that BEST answers the question or completes the statement. *PRINT THE LETTER OF THE CORRECT ANSWER IN THE SPACE AT THE RIGHT.*

1. One liter is APPROXIMATELY one

   A. pint
   B. quart
   C. half-gallon
   D. gallon

   1._____

2. The temperature on the Kelvin (absolute) scale which corresponds to -60° C is

   A. -333   B. +213   C. +273   D. +333

   2._____

3. How many liters of H_2 at STP would be displaced from 500 ml of 4M HCl by excess zinc?

   A. 11.2   B. 22.4   C. 44.8   D. 89.6

   3._____

4. Metallic sodium should be stored in

   A. alcohol   B. kerosene   C. sawdust   D. water

   4._____

5. The reaction,
   $MnO_2 + H^+ + H_2C_2O_4 \rightarrow CO_2 + H_2O + MN^{++}$, is not balanced.
   After balancing it, select, of the following, the CORRECT number of moles of $H_2C_2O_4$ required to react with one mole of MnO_2.

   A. 1/2   B. 1   C. 2   D. 4

   5._____

6. The pH of .01M HCl is

   A. 10^{-2} B. 1   C. 2   D. 3

   6._____

7. The ionization constant of acetic acid is 1.8×10^{-5}. The hydrogen ion concentration in a solution of 0.5M acetic acid and 0.5M sodium acetate is

   A. $.9 \times 10^{-5}M$
   B. $1.8 \times 10^{-5}M$
   C. $3 \times 10^{-3}M$
   D. $3.3 \times 10^{-12}M$

   7._____

8. A 50.0 ml sample of NaOH solution requires exactly 27.8 ml of 0.100M acid in titration. What is the normality of the NaOH?

   A. 0.0278   B. 0.0556   C. 0.112   D. 0.556

   8._____

9. The solubility of $Pb(IO_3)_2$ in water is 4.0×10^{-5} moles/liter. What is the K_{sp} (solubility product) for $Pb(IO_3)_2$?

   A. 1.6×10^{-9}
   B. 2.4×10^{-13}
   C. 4.0×10^{-5}
   D. 12×10^{-5}

   9._____

10. Light of 5000 Å wave length

    A. is in the ultraviolet region
    B. is in the visible region
    C. contains twice as much energy as light of 2500 Å wave length
    D. is in the infra-red region

11. The compound Na_2S contains what percentage S?

    A. 33%   B. 41%   C. 59%   D. 69%

12. A compound that has the power to neutralize an acid and form a salt is called a(n)

    A. buffer   B. hetone   C. anhydride   D. alkali

13. Which of the following isotopes is NOT radioactive?

    A. C^{12} B. C^{14} C. Co^{60} D. H^3

14. The organic compound C_4H_{10}

    A. is a unique compound with no isomers
    B. exists in two isomeric forms
    C. exists in three isomeric forms
    D. exists in many (more than three) isomeric forms

15. Of the following, the STRONGEST reducing agent is _____ acid.

    A. acetic   B. nitric   C. oxalic   D. phosphoric

16. Which of the following solutions has the LOWEST freezing point? 1M

    A. calcium sulfate   B. calcium chloride
    C. sodium chloride   D. sugar

17. The general formula for an organic aldehyde is

    A. RCHO   B. RCOOH   C. RCOR   D. ROR

Questions 18-19.

DIRECTIONS: Questions 18 and 19 are to be answered on the basis of the following reversible reaction.

$$N_2O_4 \text{ (gas)} \rightleftarrows 2NO_2 \text{ (gas)}$$

18. Which expression CORRECTLY describes the equilibrium constant? (P stands for pressure)

    A. $P_{N_2O_4} / P^2_{NO_2}$ B. $P^2_{NO_2} / P_{N_2O_4}$
    C. $P_{NO_2} / P_{N_2O_4}$ D. $2(P_{NO_2}) / P_{N_2O_4}$

19. If the total pressure on the reaction at equilibrium is suddenly increased at constant temperature,

    A. nothing would happen
    B. the equilibrium constant would change
    C. the reaction would shift toward NO_2 (gas)
    D. the reaction would shift toward N_2O_4 (gas)

20. A reaction requires 1 hour to run to completion at 30° C. The same reaction will run to completion in 15 minutes at APPROXIMATELY _____ ° C.

    A. 20 B. 40 C. 50 D. 120

21. A quality control chart is used to

    A. check day-to-day variability
    B. define the laboratory accuracy
    C. define the laboratory workload
    D. find normal values

22. A primary standard is prepared by

    A. dilution of a solution
    B. always using oxidizing agents
    C. weighing on a gross balance
    D. weighing on an analytical balance

23. What part of a population will be included within 2 standard deviation in a normal distribution curve?
    _____ percent.

    A. 65 B. 75 C. 85 D. 95

24. When a frozen control material is thawing and a portion is taken before complete melting and mixing, the obtained values are LIKELY to be

    A. high B. low C. unchanged D. variable

25. The PROPER use of a volumetric pipette requires

    A. allowing it to drain
    B. blowing it out
    C. washing it out
    D. weighing the contents

26. When the skin is splashed with acid, it should

    A. immediately be covered with oil
    B. immediately be flushed with water
    C. immediately be flushed with weak acid
    D. not be touched

27. Fume hoods are used in laboratories to

    A. allow the use of a flame
    B. exhaust noxious fumes
    C. provide a well-lit work area
    D. provide storage space

28. How many milligrams of nitrogen are there in 40 milligrams of urea?

    A. 16.8   B. 18.5   C. 21.6   D. 24.6

29. The presence of barbiturates in a blood sample can BEST be determined by

    A. cellulose acetate electrophoresis
    B. fractional distillation
    C. paper electrophoresis
    D. thin layer chromatography

30. Urease is a(n)

    A. major constituent of urine
    B. nucleic acid metabolite
    C. protein metabolite
    D. enzyme

31. The MAJOR urinary excretory product of steroid metabolism is

    A. cholesterol   B. estrogen
    C. 17-ketosteroids   D. lanosteroid

32. The MAJOR polysaccharide involved in human metabolism is

    A. a-amylopectin   B. amylose
    C. glycogen   D. starch

33. The chemical identification of glucose can be made by the formation of a

    A. boron bead
    B. complex with bathophenanthrolene
    C. phenylhydrazine
    D. polymer

34. Which of the following has an asymmetric carbon atom? _____ acid.

    A. Acetic   B. Lactic   C. Oleic   D. Succinic

35. Nitrogen is NOT present in

    A. glucuronic acid   B. glutathione
    C. glycolic acid   D. glycine

36. The MAJOR intracellular ion is

    A. calcium   B. carbonate   C. potassium   D. sodium

37. The blood volume in a normal adult approximates _____ ml.

    A. 1000   B. 3000   C. 5000   D. 8000

38. The pH of normal blood is

    A. 6.40   B. 6.90   C. 7.40   D. 7.90

39. The serum protein involved in the clotting of blood is

   A. fibrinogen
   B. 1-globulin
   C. 2-globulin
   D. haptoglobin

40. Which one of the following tests can NOT be done on oxalated blood plasma?

   A. Calcium   B. Creatinine   C. Glucose   D. Urine

41. The nitrogen content of proteins is MOST NEARLY _____ percent.

   A. 16.5   B. 18.5   C. 20.5   D. 22.5

42. Protein-bound iodine is a measure of _____ function.

   A. adrenal   B. cardiac   C. liver   D. thyroid

43. Which of the following is NOT a liver function test?

   A. Cephalin flocculation
   B. Glucose tolerance
   C. Serum bilirubin
   D. Thymol turbidity

44. Heparin is often used as a(n)

   A. anticoagulant
   B. chelating agent in Ca^{++} analysis
   C. colored complex
   D. primary standard

45. Amino acids are bound together to form a protein through

   A. alcohol acid esters
   B. glycosidic linkages
   C. peptide bonds
   D. 3'5' phosphate bonds

46. Inulin is a polysaccharide of

   A. fructose   B. galactose   C. glucose   D. lactose

47. A characteristic of isoenzymes is that

   A. the enzymes have identical activities at a given pH
   B. the protein moieties have the same charge densities
   C. the protein moieties have the same molecular weight
   D. a substrate is common to all the enzymes

48. The MOST likely journal to contain articles about elemental analysis is

   A. Analytical Chemistry
   B. Clinical Chemistry
   C. Journal of Chromatography
   D. Journal of Organic Chemistry

49. The Index Medicus contains

   A. abstracts of journal articles
   B. information about disease
   C. information about drugs
   D. references to journal articles by subject and author

50. When it is necessary to refer to published articles in the field of chemistry when only the subject is known, the BEST source of reference is 50.____

   A. CHEMICAL ABSTRACTS
   B. INDEX OF AMERICAN CHEMICAL SOCIETY
   C. INDEX OF CLINICAL CHEMISTRY
   D. INDEX MEDICUS

KEY (CORRECT ANSWERS)

1. B	11. B	21. A	31. B	41. D
2. B	12. D	22. D	32. B	42. C
3. B	13. A	23. D	33. B	43. A
4. B	14. B	24. D	34. C	44. A
5. B	15. C	25. A	35. B	45. C
6. C	16. B	26. B	36. C	46. D
7. B	17. A	27. B	37. D	47. C
8. B	18. B	28. C	38. C	48. A
9. B	19. D	29. A	39. A	49. D
10. B	20. C	30. D	40. B	50. A

EXAMINATION SECTION
TEST 1

DIRECTIONS: Each question or incomplete statement is followed by several suggested answers or completions. Select the one that BEST answers the question or completes the statement. *PRINT THE LETTER OF THE CORRECT ANSWER IN THE SPACE AT THE RIGHT.*

1. John is 1/6 of his father's age. In 20 years, he will be 1/2 of his father's age at that time. How old is the father?

    A. 24   B. 30   C. 36   D. 42   E. 48

2. $(.7/.07)(49/100) = 4 + x$ $x =$

    A. 4.9   B. .09   C. .9   D. 3.1   E. 3.95

3. Which is the largest?

    A. 23/25   B. 27/30   C. 15/16   D. 14/15   E. 7/8

4. Clyde received a 10% raise in each of the last two years. His present salary is $43,560. What was his starting salary?

    A. $36,000   B. $38,000   C. $40,000   D. $42,700   E. $52,708

5. At a convention of dentists, 1,000 dentists are from the east coast. One hundred dentists are women; 60 of the women are not from the east coast. How many male dentists are from the east coast?

    A. 900   B. 850   C. 800   D. 960   E. 940

6. 1/3 of 1/4 is what percent of 5/12?

    A. .2   B. 5   C. 12   D. 20   E. 500

7. Which line is parallel to the y axis?

    A. $x = 4y$ B. $x = 2y^0$
    C. $x = y + 6$ D. $xy = 2$
    E. $xy = 2 + 4y^{-1}$

8. The five tires that come with Mary's new car were rotated frequently so that each tire was used for exactly the same amount of time as the others. They were replaced when the odometer read 24,000 miles. How many miles had each been driven?

    A. 18,000 miles   B. 30,000 miles
    C. 20,000 miles   D. 24,000 miles
    E. 19,200 miles

9. $\dfrac{-\binom{7646}{x}}{4---}$ What is the smallest number x could be?

    A. 2647   B. 4000   C. 3000   D. 646   E. 3646

10. A bug sits at the edge of a 12 inch (diameter) phonograph record playing at 33 1/3 r.p.m. Approximately how fast (in feet/minute) is the bug moving?

   A. 3   B. 33   C. 50   D. 100   E. 396

11. An object floats if it weighs less than an equal volume of water. One cc of water weighs 1 gram. Each of the following objects weighs 2 kilograms.
Which ones float? (All dimensions in cm.)

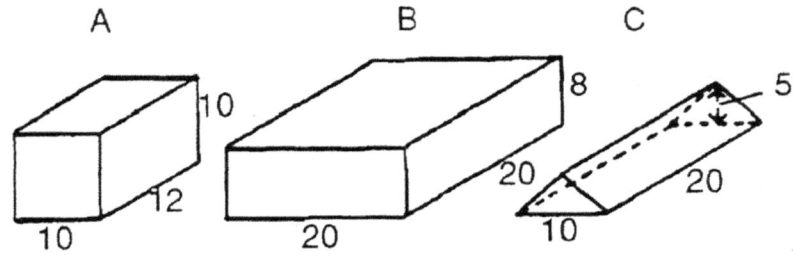

   A. A only   B. B only   C. C only   D. B & C   E. A & B

12. .04 is 25% of

   A. 0.01   B. 0.16   C. 0.1   D. 1.0   E. 1.6

13. $x^2 + 3x + 2 = 2$, $x < 0$.
   x =

   A. $\dfrac{3-\sqrt{8}}{2}$ B. -1   C. -2   D. -3   E. -4

14. if $3x/4y = 1/8$, then $4x/3y =$

   A. 1/6   B. 1/3   C. 2/3   D. 24   E. 2/9

15. .3% of 25% equals

   A. 7.5   B. .75   C. .075   D. .0075   E. .00075

16. Arrange from least to greatest:

   I. .07   II. $\sqrt{.49}$ III. .075   IV. $(.835)^2$

   The CORRECT answer is:

   A. I, III, IV, II B. III, I, IV, II
   C. IV, I, II, III D. I, III, II, IV
   E. IV, II, III, I

17. A television set is priced at $490.00. The installment payment contract requires 20% of the price as a down-payment, plus installments of $47.75 per month over a period of 10 months to pay for the set, including interest charges.
What is the total amount of interest charged?

   A. $83.00   B. $83.50   C. $85.50   D. $85.75   E. $125.50

18. A florist bought some plants for $150. He sold enough at 75 cents to meet the cost and had 100 plants left. How many were originally purchased by the florist?

    A. 150   B. 250   C. 300   D. 350   E. 400

19. If $3x + y = 5$ and $5x + y = 6$, then $y =$

    A. 2/7   B. .5   C. 1   D. 2   E. 3.5

20. A purse contains $3.20 in dimes and quarters. There are 3 less dimes than quarters. How many dimes are there?

    A. 7   B. 10   C. 13   D. 16   E. 20

21. A lawn fertilizer is most effective if 25 pounds is spread over 10,000 square feet. A weed killer must be mixed with the fertilizer but only 3 pounds should be used on every 15,000 square feet. What should the ratio be between the fertilizer and the weed killer when mixed?

    A. 12.5 to 1   B. 3 to 2
    C. 8.33 to 1   D. 5.5 to 1
    E. 25 to 3

22. If 1 yard = .9 meters, then 1.5 meters = how many yards?

    A. 1.65   B. 1.80   C. 1.60   D. 1.67   E. 1.35

23. ( ) is to 40 as x/5 is to ( ).

    A. 4; x/50   B. 10; 40x   C. 8; x   D. 10; 8x   E. 5; x/40

24. What is the approximate value of $\sqrt{360}$?

    A. 60   B. 18   C. 6   D. 16   E. 19

25. An auto travels at an average of 45 mi/hr for 1 hour and then an average of 60 mi/hr for the next half hour. What is the average speed for the entire time period in miles/hr.?

    A. 47.5   B. 50   C. 52.5   D. 55   E. 62.5

KEY (CORRECT ANSWERS)

1.	B		11.	B
2.	C		12.	B
3.	C		13.	D
4.	A		14.	E
5.	D		15.	E
6.	D		16.	A
7.	B		17.	C
8.	E		18.	C
9.	A		19.	E
10.	D		20.	A

21. A
22. D
23. C
24. E
25. B

5 (#1)

SOLUTIONS TO PROBLEMS

1. Let the father's current age = x and John's current age = 1/6 x. In 20 years, their ages will be x + 20 and 1/6 x + 20. Then, 1/6 x + 20 = 1/2(x+20), which becomes 1/6 x + 20 = 1/2 x + 10. Solving, x = 30.

2. The left side of this equation becomes (10)(.49) = 4.9 Now, 4.9 = 4 + x. Solving, x = .9

3. Converting each fraction into a decimal equivalent, we get: .92, .9, .9375, .93, and .875, respectively. The largest is .9375 corresponding to 15/16.

4. Let x = initial salary. With the first 10% raise, his salary is 1.10x. The second 10% raise will bring his salary to (1.10x)(1.10) = 1.21x. Now, 1.21x = $43,560. Solving, x = $36,000

5. The number of female dentists from the east coast is 100 - 60 = 40. Thus, the number of male dentists from the east coast must be 1000 - 40 = 960.

6. 1/3 of 1/4 means (1/3)(1/4) = 1/12. Then, $\frac{1}{12} \div \frac{5}{12} = \frac{1}{5}$, and $\frac{1}{5}$ = 20%

7. Any line parallel to the y-axis has no slope, and so must be of the form x = c (c is a constant). x = 2/y° can be written as x = 2/1 or x = 2.

8. Since only 4 tires are used at the same time, each of the 5 tires will be used 4/5 or 80% of the elapsed time before replacement. (24,000)(.80) = 19,200.

9. To find the minimum x, we need to find the maximum for the answer (since this is a subtraction). The maximum answer upon subtracting is 4999. Solving, 7646 - x = 4999, we get x = 2647.

10. The circumference = (π)(1 foot) = 3.14 feet (approximately) 33 1/3 revolutions = (33 1/3)(3.14) = 104 2/3 feet, which is the rate per minute.

11. 2 kilograms = 2000 grams. The only object(s) which float must correspond to more than 2000 cc. Object A has a volume of only 1200 cc. Object B has a volume of 3200 cc. Object C has a volume of only (1/2)(10)(5)(20) = 500 cc. Object B will float since 3200 cc. of water weighs 3200 grams and 2000 < 3200. Objects A and C will not float.

12. Solve .04 = .25x to get x = .16.

13. Rewrite the equation as x^2 + 3x = 0. Then, x(x+3) = 0. The two answers are x = 0 and x = -3. With the restriction x < 0, we have x = -3.

14. 3x/4y = 1/8. Dividing both sides by 3/4, we get x/y =1/6. Now, multiply the entire equation x/y = 1/6 by 4/3 to get 4x/3y = (1/6)(4/3) = 2/9

15. .3% of 25% becomes (.003)(.25) = .00075

16. The equivalent decimals are .07, .7, .075, and .697225. Arranging from least to greatest: .07, .075, .697225, and .7, which correspond to I, III, IV, and II.

17. The actual payments are (.20)($490) + (10)($47.75) = $575.50 Interest amount = $575.50 - $490 = $85.50

18. The number of plants he sold = $150 ÷ $0.75 = 200.
    Since he had 100 plants left, he originally purchased 200 + 100 = 300 plants.

19. Subtract the first equation from the second to get $2x = 1$. So, $x = .5$. Substitute this x value in either equation. Choosing the first equation, $(3)(.5) + y = 5$. Then, $y = 3.5$

20. Let x = number of dimes, x + 3 = number of quarters.
    Then, $.10x + .25(x+3) = 3.20$. Simplifying, $.35x + .75 = 3.20$. Finally, $x = 7$

21. For the weed killer, since 3 pounds should be used on 15,000 square feet, this translates into 2 pounds per 10,000 square feet. The ratio on the 10,000 square feet of lawn for fertilizer to weed killer is 25 to 2. This reduces to 12.5 to 1.

22. 1.5 meters = 1.5 ÷ .9 = 1.67 yards

23. Substituting choice C, 8 to 40 = 1/5 and x/5 to x = 1/5

24. $18^2 = 324$ and $19^2 = 361$. Thus, $\sqrt{360} \approx 19$

25. Total miles = 45 + (1/2)(60) = 75. Total time = 1 + 1/2 = 1 1/2 hours
    Average speed = 75 ÷ 1 1/2 = 50 mi/hr.

TEST 2

DIRECTIONS: Each question or incomplete statement is followed by several suggested answers or completions. Select the one that BEST answers the question or completes the statement. *PRINT THE LETTER OF THE CORRECT ANSWER IN THE SPACE AT THE RIGHT.*

1. 1/3 of 15 = 15% of

   A. 3/4   B. 45   C. 75   D. 5   E. 33 1/3

2. A tree in an apartment building courtyard died, and the cost of cutting down the tree is $350.00. The city will share the cost with the landlord on a 2 to 3 ratio, the landlord paying the larger part. How much will the landlord have to pay?

   A. $233.00 B. $175.00
   C. $117.00 D. $150.00
   E. $210.00

3. $\dfrac{1}{2} + \dfrac{4}{2x-1} = 6$. x =

   A. -1/2   B. 13/22   C. 19/22   D. -1/4   E. -15/22

4. The capacity of a car's cooling system if 17 quarts. 1 3/4 gallons of antifreeze plus 1 pint of rust inhibitor are required to drop the freezing point to -18°. How much water is required to fill the system to capacity?

   A. 21 pints   B. 9 pints
   C. 19 pints   D. 10 quarts
   E. 18 pints

5. If 1 inch = 2.54 cm., 3/4 cm. = how many inches?

   A. 1.9   B. 3.39   C. .75   D. .19   E. .3

6. A box has the shape of a rectangular solid, with a base measuring 16 inches by 10 inches and a height of 8 inches. What is the approximate length of the sides of a cubic container having the same volume?

   A. 9.75 inches   B. 10.00 inches
   C. 10.85 inches D. 12.65 inches
   E. 13.15 inches

7. What is a valid formula for the line plotted on the graph?
   A. x = y
   B. x = 10/y
   C. x = 10 - y
   D. x = y/10
   E. x = y + 10

8. In the fraction x/y, when 1 is added to the numerator, the fraction equals 1/3. When 3 is added to the denominator of x/y, the fraction equals 1/6. What is x/y?

   A. 2/6   B. 2/3   C. 2/9   D. 6/17   E. 2/12

9. What is the *approximate* value of $\frac{(.03)^2(\sqrt{.25} + 3.5)}{.12}$?

   A. .03   B. .36   C. .003   D. 3.0   E. .0036

10. A woman is now three times as old as her son. In four years, the son will be one-half as old as the woman is now. How old is the woman now?

    A. 24   B. 28   C. 30   D. 21   E. 33

11. 1/5 of 27 = 25% of

    A. 21 3/5   B. 5.4   C. 1.35   D. 105/5   E. 21.5

12. A rancher had 70 head of cattle. A buyer made four purchases of cattle from the rancher. The rancher now has eighteen cattle remaining. On the average, how many cattle exchanged hands at EACH purchase?

    A. 10.5   B. 13   C. 15   D. 20   E. 52

13. $\sqrt{16 + x} = 4 + 2$ x =

    A. 36   B. 4   C. -10   D. 20   E. 2

14. If 10 cc of 20% acid is mixed with 20 cc of 40% acid, the percentage of acid in the resulting solution is

    A. 50   B. 30   C. 33 1/3   D. 35   E. 60

15. 5/6 + 5/9 - 2/3 + x = a whole number. Then x = ?

    A. 5/18   B. 13/16   C. 17/18   D. 18/13   E. 2/9

16. A piece of lumber is 63 inches long. It is to be cut in three pieces. Two pieces are to be of equal length, while the third piece is to be 9 inches longer than each of the other two pieces. How long will the longer piece of lumber be?

    A. 54 inches   B. 36 inches
    C. 30 inches   D. 27 inches
    E. 18 inches

17. The sun shining on a tree casts a shadow 45 feet long. A boy five feet tall standing near the tree has a 2 foot 10 inch shadow. How tall is the tree?

    A. 54 feet   B. 22.5 feet
    C. 37.5 feet   D. 79.4 feet
    E. 18 feet

18. x/95 = 7.5% x =

    A. 12.7   B. 7.1   C. 8.0   D. 1.26   E. 713

19. A street light shining on a signpost casts a shadow 6 feet long. A child 5 feet tall standing near the signpost casts a shadow 2 feet 3 inches long. How tall is the signpost?

    A. 13.3 feet   B. 6.6 feet
    C. 12 feet   D. 20 feet
    E. 15.3 feet

20. $\dfrac{(-2)^{15}}{(-2)^{12}} = ?$

    A. -4   B. +4   C. -8   D. +8   E. -16

21. Five consecutive whole numbers have a sum of 50. What is the second of the five numbers?

    A. 5   B. 7   C. 9   D. 10   E. 11

22. If z = 35% of w, and y = 15% of z, then y = _____ % of w.

    A. 2.33   B. 42.9   C. 5.25   D. 2.25   E. 4.3

23. If (y + 2)x = 1/4, y =

    A. 1/4 - 2x   B. 1/4x - 2
    C. 1/4x + 8   D. x/4 - 2
    E. 1 - 8x/4

24. A set of drill bits are being sold for $200.00. The bits cost the dealer $160.00, plus a $20.00 shipping fee. What percent of the selling price will be profit for the dealer?

    A. 7%   B. 10%   C. 11%   D. 21%   E. 30%

25. Let A be the area of a circle whose diameter is 8. Which of the following numbers is closest to A?

    A. 50   B. 70   C. 100   D. 120   E. 200

KEY (CORRECT ANSWERS)

1.	E	11.	A
2.	E	12.	B
3.	C	13.	D
4.	C	14.	C
5.	E	15.	A
6.	C	16.	D
7.	C	17.	D
8.	C	18.	B
9.	A	19.	A
10.	A	20.	C

21. C
22. C
23. B
24. B
25. A

SOLUTIONS TO PROBLEMS

1. 1/3 of 15 = 5. Then, 5 ÷ .15 = 33 1/3

2. Let 2x = city's cost and 3x = landlord's cost. 2x + 3x = $350 Solving, x = $70. Then, landlord's cost is (3)($70) = $210

3. Multiplying the equation by (2)(2x-1), we get (1)(2x-1) + (4)(2) = (6)(2)(2x-1). Simplifying, 2x - 1 + 8 = 24x - 12.
This reduces further to 19 = 22x. So, x = 19/22

4. 1 3/4 gallons = (1 3/4)(4) = 7 quarts = 14 pints of antifreeze.
The capacity of the cooling system = 17 quarts = 34 pints. Since 1 pint of rust inhibitor is needed, the amount of water required is 34 - 14 - 1 = 19 pints.

5. 3/4 cm = 3/4 ÷ 2.54 = .295 or about .3 inches

6. The volume of the box = (16)(10)(8) = 1280 cubic inches. If a cubic container has a volume of 1280 cubic inches, each side must be $\sqrt[3]{1280}$ ≈ 10.85 inches.
(Actually, the answer is slightly closer to 10.86)

7. Since the coordinates of the two given points are (10,0) and (0,10), the slope of the line is (10-0) ÷ (0-10) = -1. Y = -1x + B, where B is the y-intercept. Now, B = 10 since (0,10) lies on this line. Y = -1x + 10 is the equation and this can be written as x = 10 - y.

8. From the given information, (x+1)/y = 1/3 and x/(y+3) = 1/6 Rewriting, we have y = 3x + 3 and y = 6x - 3. Adding these equations, 2y = 9x. Thus, x/y = 2/9.

9. $(.03)^2$ = .0009. ($\sqrt{.25}$ + 3.5) = 4.0. The answer becomes (.0009)(4)/.12 = .03. (Change the word *approximate* to *exact*.)

10. Let x = woman's age, 1/3x = son's age. Then, 1/3 x + 4 = 1/2 x.
This reduces to 1/6 x = 4, so x = 24.

11. 1/5 of 27 = (.2)(27) = 5.4. Then, 5.4 ÷ .25 = 21.6 = 21 3/5

12. 70 - 18 = 52. Then, 52 ÷ 4 = 13.

13. $\sqrt{16+x}$ = 6. Square both sides to get 16 + x = 36. Then, x = 20

14. The amount of acid in the resulting solution is (.20)(10) + (.40)(20) = 10 cc. The solution is 10 + 20 = 30 cc. Percentage of acid is (10/30)(100) = 33 1/3

15. 5/6 + 5/9 -2/3 = (15 + 10 - 12)/18 = 13/18. Since choice A is 5/18, 13/18 + 5/18 = 18/18 = 1, which is a whole number.

16. Let x = length of each shorter piece and x + 9 = length of the longer piece. x + x + x + 9 = 63. Solving, x = 18. So, the longer piece must be 27 inches.

17. The ratio of the boy's height to his shadow is 60 inches to 34 inches = 30 to 17 (reduced). Let x = height of the tree. Then, x/45 = 30/17. Solving, x ≈ 79.4 feet

18. $x/95 = .075$. $x = (.075)(95) = 7.125$ or about 7.1

19. The ratio of the child's height to his shadow is 60 inches to 27 inches = 20 to 9 (reduced). Let x = height of the signpost. Then, $x/6 = 20/9$. Solving, x - 13.33 or about 13.3 feet.

20. In division, we subtract exponents to get $(-2)^3 = -8$. Of course, the base must remain the same.

21. Let x, x+1, x+2, x+3, x+4 represent the numbers. Then, $x + x+1 + x+2 + x+3 + x+4 = 50$. Solving, x = 8. The second number must be 9.

22. $y = .15z = (.15)(.35)w = .0525w$. Thus, y is 5.25% of w.

23. $(y+2)(x) = 1/4$. Dividing both sides by x, we get $y + 2 = 1/4x$. Finally, $y = 1/4x - 2$

24. The dealer's total cost is $180 and his profit is $20. The percent profit on the selling price is $(20/200)(100) = 10\%$.

25. $A = (\pi)(4)^2 = 16\pi = 50.265$ or about 50. Note that the formula is Area = (π) (radius)^2.

EXAMINATION SECTION
TEST 1

DIRECTIONS: Each question or incomplete statement is followed by several suggested answers or completions. Select the one that BEST answers the question or completes the statement. *PRINT THE LETTER OF THE CORRECT ANSWER IN THE SPACE AT THE RIGHT.*

1. At 7:00 A.M., a student leaves his home in his automobile to drive to school 28 miles away. He averages 50 mph until 7:30 A.M., when his car breaks down. The student has to walk and run the rest of the way.
   If he wants to arrive at school at 8:00 A.M., how fast, in mph, must he travel on foot?
   A. 3   B. 4   C. 5   D. 6   E. 7

   1.____

2. Express $1 + \dfrac{\frac{1}{2+1}}{1+\frac{1}{4}}$ in simplest terms.
   A. 27/28   B. 30/43   C. 1 1/9   D. 1 1/27   E. 1 13/30

   2.____

3. A theater charges $5.00 admission for adults and $2.50 for children. At one showing, 240 admissions brought in a total of $800.
   How many adults attended the showing?
   A. 40   B. 80   C. 120   D. 160   E. 266

   3.____

4. $\sqrt{25+?} = 5 + 8$
   A. 8   B. 12   C. 64   D. 144   E. 169

   4.____

5. The perimeter of a square is 20.
   Which of the following represents the area?
   A. 5   B. 10   C. 20   D. 25   E. 100

   5.____

6. Evaluate the expression $\dfrac{1}{4} + \dfrac{3}{8} - \dfrac{6}{15} - \dfrac{8}{32}$
   A. 7/16   B. 1/32   C. 1/8   D. 1/4   E. 0

   6.____

7. Bill spent 20% of the money he initially had in his wallet on groceries and 25% on gas. He had $66.00 left.
   How much money did he have before he shopped?
   A. $85   B. $100   C. $110   D. $111   E. $120

   7.____

8. Express the product $(2x+5y)^2$ in simplest form.
   A. $4x^2 + 25y^2$ B. $4x^2 + 20xy + 25y^2$ C. $4x^2 + 10y + 25y^2$
   D. $4x^2 - 20xy + 25y^2$ E. $4x + 25y$

   8.____

9. A student received test grades of 83, 90, and 88.
   What was her grade on a fourth test if the average for the four tests is 84?
   A. 85   B. 80   C. 75   D. 70   E. 65

   9.____

10. A rectangular room is 3 meters wide, 4 meters long, and 2 meters high. How far is it from the northeast corner at the floor to the southwest corner at the ceiling?
 _____ meters.
 A. $\sqrt{29}$ B. $\sqrt{11}$ C. $\sqrt{9}$ D. 9   E. 5

11. If an electron has a mass of 9.109×10^{-31} kg and a proton has a mass of 1.672×10^{-27} kg, approximately how many electrons are required to have the same mass as one proton?
 A. 150,000
 B. 1,800
 C. 5.4×10^4
 D. 5.4×10^{-4}
 E. 15×10^{-58}

12. The introduction of a new manufacturing process will affect a saving of $1,450 per week over the initial 8-week production period. New equipment, however, will cost 1/4 of the total savings.
 How much did the equipment cost?
 A. $11.600.00
 B. $2,900.00
 C. $725.00
 D. $362.50
 E. $181.25

13. If P dollars is invested at r percent compounded annually, at the end of n years it will have grown to $A = P(1+r)^n$. An investment made at 16% compounded annually. It grows to $1,740 at the end of one year.
 How much was originally invested?
 A. $150
 B. $278.40
 C. $1,461.60
 D. $1,500
 E. $1,700

14. What is 1/4% of 200?
 A. 0.05   B. 0.5   C. 5   D. 12.5   E. 50

15. Which of the following is .5% of .95?
 A. .000475   B. .00475   C. .0475   D. .475   E. 4.75

16. What is the value of (5 lbs. 1 oz.)/(3 lbs. 6 oz.) in ounces?
 A. 22   B. 1.66   C. 1.5   D. 0.66   E. 0.28

17. If 1 inch = 2.56 centimeters, 3/8 centimeter equals which of the following in inches?
 A. 6.77   B. .95   C. .39   D. .38   E. .15

18. If $2x + y = 7$ and $x - 4y = 4$, then x equals which of the following?
 A. -15/9   B. -1/9   C. 7/15   D. 11/9   E. 32/9

19. What part of an hour is 6 seconds?
 A. 1/600   B. 1/10   C. 1/360   D. 1/60   E. 1/5

20. If $1/3 + 5(x-1) = 8$, then which of the following is the value of x?
 A. 8/13   B. 8/5   C. 38/25   D. 38/15   E. 38

21. Which line is perpendicular to the x-axis?
    A. x = 3   B. y = 3   C. x = y   D. x = y/3   E. y = x/3

22. If a dental hygienist at a certain office is paid H dollars a week, the dental assistant works 36 hours a week at A dollars per hour, and the receptionist works 40 hours a week and receives R dollars every other week, which of the following represents the weekly payroll for these three employees?
    A. H/3 + 36A + 40R/3
    B. H + 36A + R/2
    C. H/3 + 12A + R/6
    D. 5H + 36 + 20R
    E. H/3 + 12A + 40R

23. Company A ordered five units of anesthetic at $12.00 per unit. Company B ordered 10 units at $13.00 per unit, and Company C ordered 4 at $10.00 per unit. Since all these companies were at one address, the three orders were put on one bill.
    Approximately what percent of the total bill did Company A have to pay?
    A. 5   B. 18   C. 26   D. 36   E. 55

24. Which of the following is the value of A, if 50(A/100) = 2A²?
    A. 25   B. 1   C. 5/2   D. 1/4   E. 1/2

25. Five-eighths of the employees in the company are single males. What percentage of the employees in the company are single males?
    A. 12.5   B. 20.0   C. 25.0   D. 32.0   E. 62.5

26. If x = 20% of y, and z = 35% of x then z = _____ % of y.
    A. 70   B. 57   C. 7   D. 1.75   E. .07

27. Which of the following is the value of the expression $\frac{|14-3|-|7-16|}{3|(-2)+1}$?
    A. -20/3   B. -2/3   C. 0   D. 23   E. 20/3

28. A tank can be filled by a pipe in 30 minutes and emptied by another pipe in 50 minutes.
    How many minutes will it take to fill the tank if both pipes are open?
    A. 45   B. 60   C. 75   D. 80   E. 100

29. If (4/5)x = (2/5)y, then which of the following is equal to y/x?
    A. 1/2   B. 2/5   C. 25/8   D. 2   E. 3

30. Which of the following would NOT result in a straight line? x =
    A. 1/y   B. 2y + 5   C. (y+6)/(2)   D. 5 − y   E. 4(x+3y)

31. $\frac{5}{4} + \frac{4}{5} + \frac{3}{2}$ − _____ = a positive integer.
    A. 10/20   B. 11/20   C. 71/20   D. 3/20   E. 4/20

32. If $\frac{2}{x} + \frac{3}{5} = \frac{4}{3}$, then which of the following is the value of x?
    A. 30/11 B. 30/29 C. 11/30 D. -11/6 E. -5/2

33. Optometry school applicants decreased by 25% during a 4-year period. During the same time, the number of first-year openings in optometry school increased by 12%.
    If the ratio of applicants to first-year student openings had been 3 to 1, then which of the following would be the APPROXIMATE ratio at the end of the 4-year period?
    A. 1.5 to 1 B. 2 to 1 C. 3 to 2 D. 4 to 3 E. 6 to 5

34. If then which of the following is the value of x?
    A. 4 B. 27 C. 29 D. 40 E. 729

35. Two cars start at the same point and travel north and west at the rate of 24 and 32 mph, respectively.
    How far apart are they at the end of 2 hours?
    A. 63 B. 80 C. 112 D. 116 E. 100

36. Right triangle ABC with right angle C and AB = 6, BC = 3, find AC.
    A. 3 B. 6 C. 27 D. 33 E. $3\sqrt{3}$

37. When each of the sides of a square is increased by 1 yard, the area of the new square is 53 square yards more than that of the original square. What is the length of the sides of the original square?
    A. 25 B. 26 C. 27 D. 52 E. 54

38. Evaluate: $3(2)^2 + \sqrt{25} - (-2)^3$.
    A. 9 B. 24 C. 25 D. 33 E. 76

39. Which of the following is the length of the line segment BC if AB = 14, AD = 5, and angle BAD = 30°?
    A. $\sqrt{221}$
    B. $\sqrt{171}$
    C. $7\sqrt{3}$
    D. 7
    E. 9

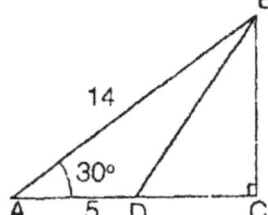

40. A bowl contains 7 green and 3 red marbles.
    What is the probability that two marbles selected at random from this bowl without replacement are both red?
    A. 1/15 B. 9/100 C. 21/100 D. 47/90 E. 6/10

41. If x pens cost 75 cents and y pencils cost 57 cents, then which equation below can be used to find the cost of 2 pens and 3 pencils?
    A. 2(75/x) + 3(57/y) B. 3x/75 + 2y/57 C. 75/2x + 57/3y
    D. 2(x/75) + 3(y/57) E. 3(75/x) + 2(57/y)

42. Maria has a number of dimes and quarters whose total value is less than $9.00. There are twice as many dimes as quarters.
    At most, how many quarters could she have?
    A. 14 B. 15 C. 19 D. 20 E. 35

43. The number (1, 2, 3, 6) have an average (arithmetic mean) of 3 and a variance of 3.5.
    What is the average (arithmetic mean) and variance of the set of numbers (3, 6, 9, 18)?
    A. 9, 31.5 B. 3, 10.5 C. 3, 31.5 D. 6, 7.5 E. 9, 27.5

44. A fence encloses a triangular-shaped region whose sides are 20 feet, 20 feet, and 10 feet in length.
    If the number of inches between fence posts (centers) is 30 inches, how many posts will be needed?
    A. 17 B. 20 C. 21 D. 22 E. 23

45. A ceiling 6 feet by 7 feet can be painted for $52.
    Find the cost of painting a ceiling 18 feet by 21 feet, all things equal except the dimensions.
    A. $104 B. $126 C. $156 D. $378 E. $468

46. Three consecutive odd numbers have a sum of 51.
    What is the LARGEST of these numbers?
    A. 15 B. 17 C. 18 D. 19 E. 21

47. It takes 5 hours for a qualified typist to complete a report. Coffee break begins at 10:15 A.M. It is now 9:55 A.M.
    How much of the task can the typist be expected to complete by coffee break?
    A. 1/8 B. 1/25 C. 1/3 D. 1/6 E. 1/15

48. A container in the form of a rectangular solid is 10 feet long, 9 feet wide, and 2 feet deep. The container is filled with a liquid weighing 100 pounds per cubic foot.
    A. 90 B. 180 C. 1,800 D. 9,000 E. 18,000

49. The value of $\cos(\pi/3)$ equals the value of
    A. $-\cos(2\pi/3)$ B. $\cos(2\pi/3)$ C. $\cos(6\pi/3)$
    D. $-\cos(5\pi/3)$ E. $\cos(4\pi/3)$

50. If $5 \leq x \leq 12$ and $-2 \leq y \leq 9$, then is as large as possible when x = _____ and y = _____.
    A. 12; 9 B. 12; 0 C. 12; -2 D. 0; 0 E. 0; 0

KEY (CORRECT ANSWERS)

1. D	11. B	21. A	31. B	41. A
2. E	12. B	22. B	32. A	42. C
3. B	13. D	23. C	33. B	43. A
4. D	14. B	24. D	34. C	44. B
5. D	15. B	25. A	35. B	45. E
6. E	16. C	26. C	36. E	46. D
7. E	17. E	27. D	37. B	47. E
8. B	18. E	28. C	38. C	48. E
9. C	19. A	29. D	39. D	49. A
10. A	20. D	30. A	40. A	50. B

SOLUTIONS TO PROBLEMS

1. Let x = rate of walking/running. Then, (50)(1/2) + (x)(1/2) = 28. Simplifying, 1/2x = 3. Solving, x = 6.

2. $3 + \frac{1}{4} = 3\frac{1}{4}$, $1/3 \frac{1}{4} = \frac{4}{13}$, $2 + \frac{4}{13} = 2\frac{4}{13}$, $1/2 \frac{4}{13} = \frac{13}{30}$
   Finally, $1 + \frac{13}{30} = 1\frac{13}{30}$

3. Let x = number of adults, 240-x = number of children.
   Then, 5x + 2.50(240-x) = 800. Simplifying, we get 5x + 600 – 2.50x = 800. This reduces to 2.50x = 200. Solving, x = 800

4. $\sqrt{25 + x}$ = 13 squaring both sides, 25 + x = 169. So, x = 144.

5. If the perimeter of a square is 20, each side must be 5. The area is 5^2 = 25.

6. Changing to a denominator of 32, we get 8/32 + 12/32 + 12/32 – 12/32 – 8/32 = 0/32 = 0

7. Let x = original amount. 100% - 20% - 25% = 55%. Then, $66 = .55x. Solving, x = $120

8. $(2x+5y)^2 = 4x^2 + 10xy + 25y^2 = 4x^2 + 20xy + 25y^2$

9. Let x = grade on her 4th test. Then, (83+90+88+x)/4 = 84. This becomes (261+x)/4 = 84. Further reduction leads to 261 + x = 336, so x – 75.

10. The required distance is $\sqrt{3^2 + 4^2 + 2^2} = \sqrt{9 + 16 + 4} = \sqrt{29}$

11. $(1.672 \times 10^{-27}) \div (9.1109 \times 10^{-31})$. $1836 \times 10^4 \approx 1800$

12. Total savings is $1450)(8) = $11,600. Equipment costs (1/4)($11,600) = $2900.

13. $1740 = P(I+.16)'. Then, P = $1740 ÷ 1.16 = $1500.

14. 1/4% of 200 is (.0025)(200) = .5

15. .5% of .95 is (.005)(.95) = .00475

16. 5 lbs. 1 oz. = 81 oz. and 3 lbs. 6 oz. = 54 oz. Then, 81 oz. ÷ 54 oz. = 1.5

17. 3/8 cm = 3/8 ÷ 2.54 = .375 ÷ 2.54 ≈ .1476 ≈ .15 inch.

18. From equation 1, y = 7 – 2x. Substituting into equation 2, x – 4(7-2x) = 4.
    Simplifying, x – 28 + 8x = 4. This reduces to 9x = 32, so x = 32/9

19. Since there are 3600 seconds in 1 hour, 6 seconds would represent 6/3600 = 1/600 of an hour.

20. $1/3 + 5(x-1) = 8$. Simplify to $1/3 + 5x - 5 = 8$. This will reduce to $5x = 12\ 2/3$, so $x = 38/15$.

21. A line perpendicular to the x-axis must have an undefined slope. The equation must be x = constant. The only choice fitting this format is $x = 3$.

22. The receptionist works 40 hours at R/2 dollars per week. Thus, the weekly payroll for all three workers is $H + 36A + R/2$. (The 40 hours is not used in computing.)

23. The total bill was $(5)(\$12) + (10)(\$13) + (4)(\$20) = \$230$. Company A's bill was $60. Thus, $\$60/\$230 \approx 26.1\% \approx 26\%$.

24. $50(A/100) = 2A^2$ becomes $A/2 = 2A^2$. Simplifying further, we get $A = 4A^2$. Simplifying further, we get $A = 4A^2$ or $A(4A-1) = 0$. The two values of A are 0 and 1/4.

25. The number of single males is represented as $(5/8)(1/5)(100)\% = 12.5\%$

26. $z = .35x$ and $x = .20y$. Thus, $z = (.35)(.20)y = .07y$.

27. The numerator is $|11| - |-9| = 11 - 9 = 2$. The denominator is $3|-1| = 3$. Thus, the fraction = 2/3.

28. Let x = required number of minutes. Then, $1/30x - 1/50x = 1$. Multiplying by 150, $5x - 3x = 150$. Solving, $x = 75$.

29. $\frac{4}{5}x = \frac{2}{5}y$. Then, $\frac{y}{x} = \frac{4}{5} \div \frac{2}{5} = 2$

30. $x = \frac{1}{y}$ becomes $xy = 1$, which represents a hyperbola.

31. $\frac{5}{4} + \frac{4}{5} + \frac{3}{2} = (25+16+30)/20 = 71/20$. If $71/20 - x$ = a positive integer, then the only correct values of x are 11/20, 31/20, 51/20.

32. Multiplying the equation by 15x, we get $30 + 9x = 20x$. Then, $30 = 11x$, so $x = 30/11$.

33. Let 3x = number of applicants, x = 1st year student openings. Over the 4-year period, the number of applicants dropped to $.75(3x) = 2.25x$ and the number of openings rose to $1.12x$. Now, $2.25x \div 1.12x \approx 2$ to 1.

34. $\sqrt{x - 25} = 2$. Squaring both sides, $x - 25 = 4$, so $x = 29$.

35. At the end of 2 hours, their individual <u>distances</u> are 48 miles and 64 miles. Their distance apart is = 80 miles.

36. $AC^2 + 3^2 = 6^2$. This simplifies to $AC^2 = 27$. Thus, $AC = \sqrt{27} = 3\sqrt{3}$

37. Let x = original length of each side, so that x + 1 = new length of each side of the square. Then, $(x+1)^2 - x^2 + 53$. This simplifies to $x^2 + 2x + 1 = x^2 + 53$. Then, $2x + 1 = 53$, so $x = 26$.

38. $3(2)^2 + \sqrt{25} - (-2)^3 = 12 + 5 + 8 = 25$.

39. Sine 30° = BC/14 1/2 = BC/14, so BC = 7.

40. Probability of 2 red marbles being drawn without replacement is (3/10)(2/9) = 1/15.

41. Each pen costs 75/x cents and each pencil costs 57/y cents. Then, 2 pens and 3 pencils cost 2(75/x) + 3(57/y).

42. Let x = number of quarters, 2x = number of dimes. Then, .25x + .10(2x) < 9.00. Solving, x < 20, so x = 19.

43. The new set of numbers is 3 times as large as the original set. Therefore, the mean is 3 times as big, which is 9, and the variance is 3^2 or 9 times as big, which is (9)(3.5)= 31.5.

44. Using the diagram shown at the right, for the fence $\overline{BC}$, we'll need 5 posts whose distance from each other is 12 1/2'. (This includes a post at B and a post at C.) Now along $\overline{AB}$, since AB = 20' and $20 \div 2\frac{1}{2} = 8$, we'll need 8 posts (including a post at A). Finally, starting at A and ending at C, we need to place only 20 ÷ 2 1/2 – 1 = 7 posts since a post already exists at A and at C. Thus, the total number of posts is 5 + 8 + 7 = 20.

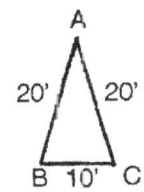

45. (6')(7') = 42 square feet costing $52, which means $52/$42 or $(26/21) per square foot. Now a ceiling 18 ft. by 21 ft. is 378 square feet and will cost (26/21)(378) = $468.

46. Let x, x+2, x+4 represent the three odd numbers. Then, x + x+2 + x+4 = 51. This reduces to 3x + 6 = 51, from which x = 15. The three numbers are 15,17, 19 and so the largest is 19.

47. From 9:55 A.M. to 10:15 A.M. represents 20 minutes. Then, 20 minutes/5 hours = 20 minutes/300 minutes, which reduces to 1/15.

48. Volume is (10)(9)(2) = 180 cu. ft. The weight of the liquid is (100)(180) = 18,000 lbs.

49. Cosine $\frac{\pi}{3}$ = .5, which is also the value of -Cosine $\frac{2\pi}{3}$.

50. To make $(3x-4)(4+5y^2)$ as large as possible, we maximize the numerator and minimize the denominator. Given the restriction $5 \le x \le 12$, use x = 12. Given the restriction use y = 0. (Note carefully that y = 0 yields a smaller value of $4 + 5y^2$ than y = -2)

MATHEMATICS PROBLEM SOLVING
EXAMINATION SECTION
TEST 1

DIRECTIONS: Each question or incomplete statement is followed by several suggested answers or completions. Select the one that BEST answers the question or completes the statement. *PRINT THE LETTER OF THE CORRECT ANSWER IN THE SPACE AT THE RIGHT.*

1. If a man travels r miles an hour for h hours and s miles an hour for t hours, what is his *average* rate in miles per hour for the ENTIRE distance traveled?   1.____

   A. $rh + st$ B. $\dfrac{r}{h} + \dfrac{s}{t}$ C. $\dfrac{rh+st}{2}$ D. $\dfrac{rh+st}{h+t}$
   E. *None of these answers*

2. A certain square 18 feet on a side has the same area as a rectangle. If *one* side of the rectangle is 9 feet, what is the number of feet in the *other* dimension?   2.____

   A. 9   B. 2   C. 27   D. 36
   E. *None of these answers*

3. A dealer paid 72 cents for a fountain pen listed at 90 cents. What was the *rate* of discount allowed him?   3.____

   A. 5%   B. 2%   C. 8%   D. 20%
   E. *None of these answers*

4. The tax rate in a certain district is 8 1/2 mills on the dollar. What would this be if expressed as *dollars per thousand?*   4.____

   A. $.085   B. $8.50   C. $85   D. $8500
   E. *None of these answers*

5. The wheel of the average bicycle is 28 inches in diameter. How many feet will be covered in 9 turns of the wheel? (Use $\pi = 22$)   5.____

   A. 21 ft   B. 66 ft   C. 462 ft.   D. 792 ft
   E. *None of these answers*

6. If light travels approximately 186,000 miles a second and the sun is 93 million miles away, how long does it take a ray of light to travel from the sun to the earth? (Find answer to the nearest minute.)   6.____

   A. 5 min.   B. 2 min.   C. 8 min.   D. 500 min.
   E. *None of these answers*

7. The Acme Company offers a gas range for $63 cash or for $5 down and 10 monthly payments of $6.50 each. The install-ment price is what percent GREATER than the cash price? (Find answer to the nearest whole percent.)   7.____

   A. 7%   B. 9%   C. 10%   D. 11
   E. *None of these answers*

2 (#1)

8. The earth revolves through 360 degrees of longitude in 24 hours. How many minutes does it take to revolve through 1 degree?   8.____

   A. .25   B. 6   C. 15   D. 25
   E. *None of these answers*

9. A small factory with 3 machines has a job of stamping out a number of pan covers. The newest machine can do the job in 3 days, another machine can do it in 4 days, and the third machine can do it in 6 days.   9.____
   How many days will it take the factory to do the job, using *all three* machines?

   A. 1 1/3   B. 4 1/3   C. 6   D. 13
   E. *None of these answers*

10. If 1 gallon of water is added to 6 quarts of a mixture of alcohol and water that is 50% alcohol, what percent alcohol is the resulting mixture?   10.____

    A. 25%   B. 30%   C. 33 1/3%   D. 50%
    E. *None of these answers*

SOLUTIONS TO PROBLEMS

1. Answer (D) $\dfrac{rh+st}{h+t}$ Formula: Distance = rate x time

   First distance traveled: rh = r x h
   Second distance traveled: st = s x t
   Total distance traveled: rh + st   Total time traveled: h + t

   Formula: Distance ÷ time = rate or $\dfrac{rh+st}{h+t}$ = average rate in miles per hour

2. Answer (D) 36

   18^2 = 324 sq. ft., area of square (area of square = (side)^2), which is also the area of the rectangle (given).
   Formula: Area of rectangle = length x width
   Let x = the number of feet in other dimension

   ∴ 9x = 324, x = 36 feet.

3. Answer (D) 20%

   Formula: Rate of discount = $\dfrac{\text{amount of discount}}{\text{list price}}$

   by substitution = $\dfrac{90-72}{90} = \dfrac{18}{90} = \dfrac{1}{5} = 20\%$

4. Answer (B) $8.50
   10 mills = 1 cent; 100 mills = 10 cents; 1000 mills = 1 dollar

   ∴ 8 1/2 mills per $1 = 8 1/2 x 1000 mills = 8500 mills per $1000 or
   $8.50 per $1000 (8500 mills / $1000).

5. Answer (B) 66 ft.
   Formula: Circumference = π x diameter

   $= \dfrac{22}{7} \times 28$ in.

   = 88 in.
   Formula: Distance covered = circumference x no. of turns
   = 88 x 9 (given)
   = 792 in.
   = 66 ft. (792 / 12).

6. Answer (C) 8 min. $\dfrac{93{,}000{,}000}{186{,}000} = 500$ sec

   ∴ 500 ÷ 60 (60 sec. = 1 min.) = 8 1/2 min. (to the nearest min.)

7. **Answer (D) 11%**

    Formula: Percent of increase = $\dfrac{\text{amount of increase}}{\text{cash price}} \times 100\%$

    cash price Since the installment price = $70 ($5 + 10 × $6.50) and
    the cash price = $63 (given),
    the installment price is $7 greater

    ∴ by substitution, percent increase of installment price =

    $\dfrac{\$70 - \$63}{\$63} \times 100 = \dfrac{7}{63} \times 100 = 11\dfrac{1}{9}$ (to the nearest whole percent)

8. **Answer (E) None of these answers**
    Change 24 hours to minutes = 1440 min. (24 × 60).

    ∴ $\dfrac{1440}{360}$ = 4 minutes (time it takes the earth to revolve through 1°)

9. **Answer (A) 1 1/3**

    Formula: $\dfrac{\text{time worked}}{\text{time required}}$ = part of the job completed

    Let x = time for all three machines
    Let x/3 = part of job done by newest machine
    Let x/4 = part of job done by second machine
    Let x/6 = part of job done by third machine

    ∴ $\dfrac{x}{3} + \dfrac{x}{4} + \dfrac{x}{6} = 1$ (complete job) or 9x = 12, x = 1 1/3 days.

10. **Answer (B) 30%**

    Formula: $\dfrac{\text{quantity of alcohol}}{\text{quantity of solution}} \times 100$ = percent of alcohol

    6 quarts × 50% alcohol = 3 quarts alcohol
    Second solution contains 6 quarts + 4 quarts (1 gal.) = 10 quarts

    ∴ $\dfrac{3 \text{ quarts}}{10 \text{ quarts}} \times 100 = 30\%$

TEST 2

DIRECTIONS: Each question or incomplete statement is followed by several suggested answers or completions. Select the one that BEST answers the question or completes the statement. *PRINT THE LETTER OF THE CORRECT ANSWER IN THE SPACE AT THE RIGHT.*

1. On a $9840 bill for equipment, what is the *difference* between a discount of 30% and a discount series of 20% and 10%?

    A. No difference B. $196.80 C. $787.20
    D. $2755.20 E. *None of these answers*

    1.____

2. If the fuel consumption of a 110-horsepower engine is 0.75 lb. per hp per hour, how many pounds of fuel will be used in 40 minutes?

    A. 0.50 B. 30 C. 50 D. 55
    E. *None of these answers*

    2.____

3. A clock that loses 4 minutes every 24 hours was set right at 6 a.m. on January 1. What was the time indicated by this clock when the right time was 12 o'clock noon on January 6?

    A. 11:36 B. 11:38 C. 11:39 D. 11:40
    E. *None of these answers*

    3.____

4. The sides of a church spire are four congruent triangles, each with an altitude of 40 feet and a base of 10 feet. Find the area of the spire.

    A. 200 sq. ft. B. 400 sq. ft. C. 600 sq. ft
    D. 1600 sq. ft. E. *None of these answers*

    4.____

5. If a man's salary is $b per month and if during a certain month he spends $c, what *fractional part* of his salary does he save?

    A. b-c B. c/d C. b-c/b D. b/c
    E. *None of these answers*

    5.____

6. A bowler has an average of 150 points a game for 12 games. If he bowls 6 more games, how high an average must he make in these games to raise his average for the 18 games to 160?

    A. 170 B. 180 C. 210 D. 225
    E. *None of these answers*

    6.____

7. A store offers for sale five packages of cereal, all of the same kind and quality but manufactured by different firms and containing different amounts. Determine which of the following is MOST economical?

    A. 6 oz. for 5¢ B. 1 lb. for 12 1/2¢ C. 11 oz. for 9¢
    D. 14 oz. for 11¢ E. 1 lb. 3 oz. for 16¢

    7.____

8. From the formula $K = 1/2h(b + b_1)$, find the value of b_1 in terms of K, h and b.

    A. 2K-b/h B. k/2h - b C. 2k-hb/h D. kh/2 - 2
    E. *None of these answers*

    8.____

213

2 (#2)

9. In measuring a distance of 1 mile, an error of 11 feet was made. Which of the following CORRECTLY represents the size of the error?

   A. 1 inch in 40 ft
   B. 1 ft. in 150 yd
   C. 0.2%
   D. 1:500
   E. None of these answers

10. A coffee shop blends two kinds of coffee, putting in 2 parts of the 33¢ a pound grade to 1 of the 24¢ grade. If the mixture is changed to 1 part of the 33¢ kind and 2 parts of the 24¢ kind, how much will the shop save in blending 100 lb.?

    A. $1
    B. $0.90
    C. $3
    D. $9
    E. None of these answers

SOLUTIONS TO PROBLEMS

1. Answer (B) $196.80
   30% of $9840 = $2952; $9840 - $2952 = $6888
   20% of $9840 = $1968; $9840 - $1968 = $7872
   10% of $7872 = $787.20; $7872 - $787.20 = $7084.80
   ∴ $7084.80 - $6888 = $196.80

2. Answer (D) 55
   Since 0.75 lb. produces one hp per hr., .75 x 110 = 82.5 lbs. (no. lbs. of fuel used to produce 110 hp in 1 hr.)
   40/60 = 82.5 or 2/3 x 82.5 = 55 lbs.

3. Answer (C) 11:39
   Total time between the two given dates = 5 days + 6 hrs. or 5 x 24 + 6 = 126 hrs.
   The object is to find the total number of minutes lost by the clock during the 126 hrs.
   Let us call this loss x.

   ∴ $\frac{4}{24} = \frac{x}{126}$ or $24x = 504$, $x = 21$ min. lost

   the time indicated by the clock at 12 o'clock noon on
   ∴ January 6 was 11:39 (12 o'clock - 21 min.).

4. Answer (E) None of these answers
   Formula: area of triangle = 1/2 base x altitude
   area of spire = 4 x 1/2 base x altitude
   by substitution = 4 x 1/2 x 10 x 40 = 800 sq. ft.

5. Answer (C) $\frac{b-c}{b}$

   If the man earns b and spends c, he saves b - c.

   Formula: $\frac{\text{amount saved}}{\text{amount earned}}$ = fractional part of salary saved

   by substitution, $\frac{b-c}{b}$ = fractional part of salary saved.

6. Answer (B) 180
   The bowler has achieved a total of 1800 points (150 x 12). His aim is to achieve 2880 points (160 x 18) in 6 more games; which means 1080 points more (2880 - 1800)
   ∴ 1080 / 6 = 180 points (the new average he must achieve).

7. Answer (B) 1 lb. for 12 1/2¢
   Method: find the cost per oz. in each of the five statements and compare.

   A. .05 / 6 = $.0083   B. .12 1/2 = $.00781 (most economical)
   C. .09 / 11 = $.0081   D. .11 / 14 = $.00785
   E. .16 / 19 = $.0084

8. Answer (C) $\dfrac{2K-hb}{h}$

   $K = 1/2\,h(b + b_1)$ or $2K = h(b + b_1)$ or $2K = hb + hb_1$ or $2K - hb = hb_1$; finally, $2K - hb/h = b_1$.

9. Answer (C) 0.2%

   $\dfrac{11\,\text{ft}}{5280\,\text{ft.}(1\,\text{mile})} = \dfrac{1}{480} = .002$ or .2%

10. Answer (C) $3
    Blend 1: 2 lbs. x .33 + 1 lb. x .24 = .90 per 3 lbs. = .30 per 1 lb. Blend 2: 1 lb. x .33 + 2 lbs. x .24 = .81 per 3 lbs. = .27 per 1 lb. Saving per lb., using blend 2 = .03 per 1 lb. (.30 - .27). Saving per 100 lbs., using blend 2 = $3 (100 x .03).

TEST 3

DIRECTIONS: Each question or incomplete statement is followed by several suggested answers or completions. Select the one that BEST answers the question or completes the statement. *PRINT THE LETTER OF THE CORRECT ANSWER IN THE SPACE AT THE RIGHT.*

1. What is the largest integer that is a factor of *all three* of the following numbers: 2160, 1344, 1440?

    A. 6   B. 8   C. 12   D. 16
    E. *None of these answers*

2. Divide 49 by .035.

    A. 1.4   B. 14   C. 140   D. 1400
    E. *None of these answers*

3. Find the value of (4 5/8 - 2 3/4) / 5/4.

    A. 1   B. 2   C. 1 7/10   D. 2 3/10
    E. *None of these answers*

4. Express .3% as a common fraction.

    A. 1/3   B. 3/10   C. 3/100   D. 3/1000
    E. *None of these answers*

5. The annual income of a family is budgeted as follows: 1/10 for clothing, 1/3 for food, and 1/5 for rent. This leaves $1320 for other expenses and savings. Find the annual income.

    A. $2156   B. $3600   C. $23,760   D. $39,600
    E. *None of these answers*

6. Mr. Smith's tax on his house for a certain year was $283.79. If the tax rate for that year was $3.835 per $100 of assessed valuation, for what amount was Mr. Smith's house assessed?

    A. $10.88   B. $74   C. $1038.33   D. $7400
    E. *None of these answers*

7. A furniture dealer has put a chair on sale with discounts of 25% and 10% from $60, the marked price. How much will it cost to buy the chair?

    A. $13.50   B. $21   C. $39   D. $40.50
    E. *None of these answers*

8. The distance between Chicago and Cleveland is 354 miles. If a person leaves Chicago at 9:50 a.m. Central Time and arrives in Cleveland at 5:30 p.m. the same day Eastern Time, at what *average* speed does he travel, correct to the nearest mile?

    A. 46 mph   B. 50 mph   C. 53 mph   D. 55 mph
    E. *None of these answers*

9. The oil burner in a certain house is used to heat the house and to heat the hot water. During the seven cold months when the house is heated, an average of 200 gallons of oil a month is used. In the remaining five months, when the house is not heated, a total of 200 gallons of oil is used. What percentage of the year's oil supply is required to heat water during these five months?

    A. 1/8%   B. 7%   C. 12 1/2%   D. 14%
    E. *None of these answers*

9._____

10. The distance s in feet that a body falls in t seconds is given by the formula $s = 16t^2$. If a body has been falling for 5 seconds, how far will it fall during the 6th second?

    A. 16 ft   B. 80 ft   C. 176 ft   D. 576 ft
    E. *None of these answers*

10._____

SOLUTIONS TO PROBLEMS

1. Answer (E) None of these answers
   2160: the factors are 2, 2, 2, 2, 3, 3, 3, 5
   1344: the factors are 2, 2, 2, 2, 2, 2, 3, 7
   1440: the factors are 2, 2, 2, 2, 2, 3, 3, 5
   By inspection, we see that the factors are 2 x 2 x 2 x 2 x 3 = 48

2. Answer (D) 1400
   49 ÷ .035 = 49000 ÷ 35 (moving decimals 3 places to the right). Then solve by using the algorism 35) 49000

3. Answer (E) None of these answers
   The problem may be solved as follows:

   $$(4\frac{5}{8} - 2\frac{3}{4}) + \frac{5}{4} = (\frac{37}{8} - \frac{11}{4}) + \frac{5}{4} = (\frac{37}{8} - \frac{22}{8}) + \frac{5}{4} = \frac{15}{8} + \frac{5}{4}$$

   $$= \frac{15}{8} \times \frac{4}{5} = \frac{3}{2} = 1\frac{1}{2}$$

4. Answer (D) $\frac{3}{1000}$ .3% = $\frac{.3}{100} = \frac{3}{1000}$

5. Answer (B) $3600
   If x represents the annual income, then x/10 = amount spent for clothing, x/3 = amount spent for food, and x/5 = amount spent for rent.

   $$\therefore \frac{x}{10} + \frac{x}{3} + \frac{x}{5} + \$1320 = x.$$ We find x = $3600.

6. Answer (D) $7400
   Let x = assessment of Mr. Smith's house.
   Since the tax rate was $3.835 per $100., this was = .03835.
   Formula: assessment x tax rate = tax paid.
   By substitution, .03835x = $283.79. Solving, we find that x=$7400.

7. Answer (D) $40.50
   Formula: marked price minus discounts = cost.
   $60 minus $15 (25% x $60) = $45 (price after first discount)
   $45 minus $4.50 (10% x $45, the second discount) = $40.50 (cost).

8. Answer (C) 53 mph
   Time interval = 6 hours 40 min. or 6 2/3 hrs. (Note: In converting Central Time to Eastern Time, add 1 hour.)

   Formula: Rate = $\frac{\text{Distance}}{\text{Time}} = \frac{354}{6\frac{2}{3}} = 354 \times \frac{3}{20} = \frac{1062}{20} = 53.1$ mph or

   53 mph (to the nearest mile).

9. Answer (C) 12 1/2%
   Year's oil supply = 1600 gallons (200 x 7 = 1400 gallons + 200 for the remaining 5 months)

   $\therefore \dfrac{200}{1600} = \dfrac{1}{8} = \dfrac{1}{2}\%$ (percentage of the year's oil supply required to heat water during the 5 months when the house is not heated)

10. Answer (C) 176 ft.   Formula: $s = 16t^2$
    By substitution, $s = 16 \times 5^2 = 16 \times 25 = 400$ ft. (distance covered in 5 seconds). By substitution: $s = 16 \times 6^2 = 16 \times 36 = 576$ ft. (distance covered in 6 seconds).

    $\therefore$ 576 - 400 = 176 ft. (distance body will fall during 6th sec.)

TEST 4

DIRECTIONS: Each question or incomplete statement is followed by several sug-gested answers or completions. Select the one that BEST answers the question or completes the statement. *PRINT THE LETTER OF THE CORRECT ANSWER IN THE SPACE AT THE RIGHT.*

1. A can do a piece of work in r days and B, who works faster, can do the same work in s days. Which of the following expressions, if any, represents the number of days it would take the *two of them* to do the work if they worked together?   1.____

   A. r + s/2   B. r - s   C. 1/r + 1/s   D. rs/r + s
   E. *None of these answers*

2. If y represents the tens digit and x the units digit of a two-digit number, then the number is represented by   2.____

   A. y + x   B. yx   C. 10x + y   D. 10y + x
   E. *None of these answers*

3. A certain radio costs a merchant $72, which includes overhead and selling expenses. At what price must he sell it if he is to make a *profit* of 20% on the selling price?   3.____

   A. $86.40   B. $90   C. $92   D. $144
   E. *None of these answers*

4. A formula for infant feeding requires 13 oz. of evaporated milk and 18 oz. of water. If only 10 oz. of milk are available, how much water, to the nearest ounce, should be used?   4.____

   A. 7 oz.   B. 14 oz.   C. 15 oz.   D. 21 oz.
   E. *None of these answers*

5. A 5-quart solution of sulfuric acid and water is 60% acid. If a gallon of water is added, what percent of the resulting solution is *acid*?   5.____

   A. 33 1/3%   B. 40%   C. 48%   D. 50%
   E. *None of these answers*

6. A wooden cone such as that shown in the figure at the right has its entire surface painted. Now suppose that it is cut into two parts with a saw, exposing a plane (flat) unpainted surface. All of the following figures could represent the cut (unpainted) surface EXCEPT   6.____

   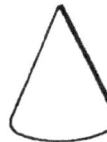

   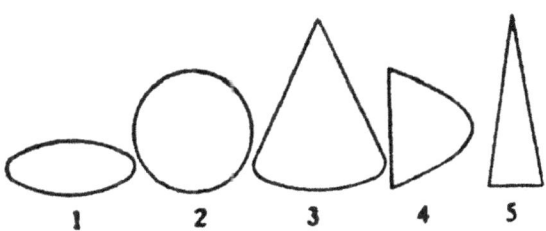

7. In a certain triangle ABC the three angles are represented by 2x, 3x - 10 and 3x + 30. What kind of triangle is ABC?   7.____

   A. Acute   B. Isosceles   C. Obtuse   D. Right
   E. *None of these answers*

8. Two triangles are each equilateral. Which of the following characteristics *always* belongs to these two triangles?

    A. Congruence   B. Equal areas   C. Equal perimeters
    D. Similarity   E. *None of these answers*

9. The base of an isosceles triangle is 16 and each of the equal sides is 10. Find the area of the triangle.

    A. 160   B. 80   C. 36   D. 24
    E. *None of these answers*

10. Given a circle A whose diameter is 2 ft and a rectangular piece of tin B, 10 ft by 4 ft. Find, correct to the near-est square foot, the tin that will be left after the great-est possible number of circles of the size of A have been cut from B.

    A. 0 sq. ft.   B. 2 sq. ft.   C. 9 sq. ft.   D. 20 sq. ft.
    E. *None of these answers*

SOLUTIONS TO PROBLEMS

1. Answer (D) $\frac{rs}{r+s}$ Formula: $\frac{\text{Time worked}}{\text{Time required}} =$ Part of job done

   Let x = number of days needed when A and B work together.
   Then x/r (part of job completed by A when working with B) + x/s (part of job completed by B when working with A) = 1 (the complete job).

   Then sx + rx = rs; x(s+r) = rs; x = $\frac{rs}{r+s}$

2. Answer (D) 10y + x
   Let us assume that the number is 53. Then 5 is the tens digit (y) and 3 is the units digit (x). 53 = 10 (5) + (3) - 53. Statement (D) is CORRECT.

3. Answer (B) $90 Formula: Selling price = Cost + Profit Let x = selling price; therefore, .20x = profit.
   By substitution, x = $72 + .20x or x - .20x = $72 or 80x = $7200 or x = $90.

4. Answer (B) 14 oz. Let x = amount of water to be added. Then 13:18 = 10:x or 13x = 180 or x = 13.8 oz. or 14 oz. (to the nearest ounce).

5. Answer (A) 33 1/3 %. Explanatory note: The quantity of solution x the percentage of solution yields the quantity in solution. Therefore, 5 qts. x 60% = 3 qts of acid. Since 1 gallon of water or 4 qts. is added, the total quantity of solution is now 9 qts., with 3 qts of acid included. Using the formula,

   $\frac{\text{quantity of acid}}{\text{quantity of solution}} \times 100$ percent of acid, $\frac{3}{9} \times 100 = 33$ 1/3%. quantity of solution

6. Answer (C)   By inspection

7. Answer (D) Right
   2x + (3x - 10°) + (3x + 30°) = 180° or 8x + 20° = 180° or x = 20°. Angle 2x = 40°; angle 3x - 10° = 50; and angle 3x + 30° = 90°. Since the triangle contains a right angle, it must be a right triangle.

8. Answer (D) Similarity
   The triangles are similar since each angle of each triangle is equal to 60° (a.a.a. = a.a.a.).

9. Answer (E) None of these answers
   In isosceles triangle ABC, draw altitude BD; now AD = DC = 8 (since the altitude of an isosceles triangle is also the median).
   Let x = BD; then $(AB)^2 = (AD)^2 + (BD)^2$ (right triangle).
   By substitution, $10^2 = 8^2 + x^2$ or $x^2 = 36$, x = 6.
   Since the area of a triangle = 1/2 base x altitude, we have 1/2 x 16 x 6 = 48, which is the area of the triangle.

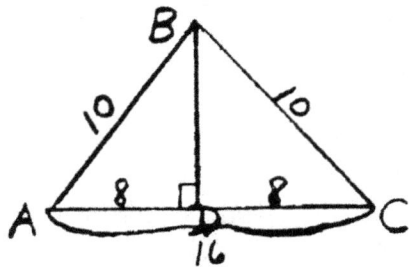

10. Answer (C) 9 sq. ft. The largest number of circles that can be cut along the length of the rectangular piece of tin is 5, and the largest number of circles that can be cut along the width is 2, since the diameter of the given circle is 2 ft. Therefore, the maximum number of circles that can be cut is 10 (5 x 2). To find the area of the tin that will be left, we must find the area of the rectangle and the area of the 10 circles. Then sub-tract the area of the ten circles from the area of the rectangle. Or, briefly stated, area of tin = area of rect-angle - area of 10 circles. Formula: Area of circle = πr^2.

By substitution, area of each circle = $\frac{22}{7} \times 1 \times 1 = 3.14$ sq.ft

The area of all 10 circles = 31.4 sq. ft.

Formula: Area of rectangle - base x altitude. By substitution, 10 x 4 = 40 sq. ft. (area of rectangle).

∴ 40 sq. ft. - 31.4 sq. ft. = 8.6 sq. ft. or 9 sq. ft. (area of tin left to the nearest sq. ft.).

TEST 5

DIRECTIONS: Each question or incomplete statement is followed by several suggested answers or completions. Select the one that BEST answers the question or completes the statement. *PRINT THE LETTER OF THE CORRECT ANSWER IN THE SPACE AT THE RIGHT.*

1. The number of diagonals, d in a polygon of n sides is given by the formula $d = \frac{n^2 - 3n}{2}$. if a polygon has 90 2 diagonals, how many sides has it?

    A. 8   B. 10   C. 12   D. 15   E. 20

    1._____

2. A train left Albany for Buffalo, a distance of 290 miles, at 10:10 a.m. The train was scheduled to reach Buffalo at 3:45 p.m. If the average rate of the train on this trip was 50 miles per hour, it arrived in Buffalo

    A. about 5 minutes ahead of schedule
    B. on time
    C. about 5 minutes late
    D. about 13 minutes late
    E. more than a quarter of an hour late

    2._____

3. The expression a^x means that a is to be used as a factor x times. Therefore, if ax is squared, the result is

    A. $a^{(x2)}$ B. b. a^{2x} C. $2a^{2x}$ D. $2a^x$
    E. *None of these answers*

    3._____

4. The number of telephones in Adelaide, Australia, is 48,000. If this represents 12.8 telephones per 100 of population, the population of Adelaide, to the nearest thousand, is

    A. 128,000   B. 375,000   C. 378,000   D. 556,000
    E. *None of these answers*

    4._____

5. One end of a ladder 32 feet long is placed 10 feet from the outer wall of a building that stands on level ground. How far up the building, to the nearest foot, will the ladder reach?

    A. 28 feet   B. 29 feet   C. 30 feet   D. 31 feet
    E. *None of these answers*

    5._____

6. The length of a rectangle is 3 inches greater than its width and its area is 88 square inches. An equation that may be used to find the width w of the rectangle is:

    A. $3w^2 = 88$
    B. $w^2/3 = 88$
    C. $w^2 + 3w - 88 = 0$
    D. $w^2 - 3w = 88$
    E. *None of these answers*

    6._____

7. On a certain map the scale is given as 1" = 1 mile. A boy copies the map, making each dimension three times as large as the given dimensions. On his map how many miles will 6 inches represent?

    A. 2 miles   B. 3 miles   C. 6 miles   D. 18 miles
    E. *None of these answers*

8. A boy travels on his bicycle at the rate of 6 miles per hour and his sister on hers at the rate of 5 miles per hour. They start at the same time and place and travel -over the same road in the same direction. After traveling for 3 hours the boy turns back.
How far from the starting point has his sister traveled when they meet?

    A. 16 miles   B. About 16.4 miles   C. About 16.9 miles
    D. 17 miles   E. *None of these answers*

9. The equation $2x - y - 4 = 0$ is represented graphically be-low. Which, if any, of the following statements is *false*?

    I. As x increases, y increases.
    II. When $x = 0$, $y = -4$; when $y = 0$, $x = 2$.
    III. The angle marked is greater than 45.
    IV. The graph, if continued, would pass through the point $x = 15$, $y = 26$.

    A. I   B. II   C. III   D. IV
    E. *None of these*

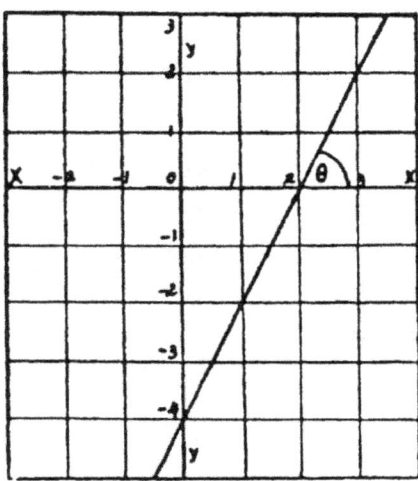

10. If an event can succeed in p ways (all equally probable) and fail in q ways, the probability that the event will succeed is $\frac{p}{p+q}$. Which, if any, of the following state ments is TRUE?

    I. The probability of drawing a glass marble in a single draw from a bag containing 8 glass marbles and 12 clay marbles is 2/3.
    II. The letters x, y and z can be arranged in 6 different orders: xyz, zyx, yxz, etc. If one of these arrange-ments is chosen at random, the probability that z will be the middle letter is 1/6.
    III. If one of the integers from 8 to 15 inclusive is chosen at random, the probability that the integer is even is equal to the probability that it is odd.
    IV. The probability that a man, aged 40, will live to reach the age of 70 is 4/7.

    A. I   B. II   C. III   D. IV
    E. *None of these*

SOLUTIONS TO PROBLEMS

1. Answer (D) 15 Given d = 90 and the formula $d = \dfrac{n^2 - 3n}{2}$

   $\therefore 90 = \dfrac{n^2 - 3n}{2}$

   $180 = n^2 - 3n$ or $-3n - 180 = 0$ or $(n + 12)(n - 15) = 0$ $n = -12$ (invalid), $n = 15$

2. Answer (D) About 13 minutes late.
   Given distance = 290 miles and average rate = 50 miles per
   hour $\text{Time} = \dfrac{\text{Distance}}{\text{Rate}} = \dfrac{290}{50} = 5\dfrac{4}{5}$ hours or 5 hours, 48 minutes

   10:10 a.m. + 5 hours, 48 min. = 3:58 p.m. Scheduled time of arrival given as 3:45 p.m.
   $\therefore$ 13 minutes late.

3. Answer (B) $a^{2x}(a^x)^2 = a^{2x}$ (by inspection)

4. Answer (B) 375,000 $\text{Ratio} = \dfrac{\text{Number}}{\text{Population}}$

   Given: Number = 48,000 and Ratio $\dfrac{12.8}{100}$

   $\therefore \dfrac{12.8}{100} = \dfrac{48,000}{x}$ or $12.8x = 48,000 \times 100$ $X = 375,000$

5. Answer (C) 30 feet
   The area of a right triangle is formed. $x^2 + 10^2 = 32^2$ or $x^2 + 100 = 1024$ or $x^2 = 924$ $x = 30.3$ or 30 ft. (to the nearest foot)

   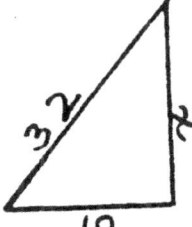

6. Answer (C) $w^2 + 3w - 88 = 0$
   w = width of rectangle w + 3 = length of rectangle
   Area = length x width or (w + 3)(w)
   $\therefore w^2 + 3w = 88$ or $w^2 + 3w - 88 = 0$

7. Answer (A) 2 miles 3:1 = 6:x or 3x = 6 or x = 2 miles

4 (#5)

8. Answer (B) About 16.4 miles   Distance coverd after 3 hours
   Boy - 6 x 3 = 18 miles
   Girl - 5 x 3 = 15 miles
   Distance between them - 3 miles

   x = distance traveled by the girl after first 3 hours
   3 -x = distance traveled by the boy during this time

   $\therefore \dfrac{x}{5} = \dfrac{3-x}{6}$ (the element of Time is eliminated here since it is the same for both the girl and the boy)

   6x = 15 - 5x or 11x =15 x = 1.4 miles .

   $\therefore$ the girl (sister) traveled 15 + 1.4 or 16.4 miles

9. Answer (E) None of these The following coordinates of x and y may be obtained from the graph

X	0	1	2	3
y	-4	-2	0	2

   a. As x increases, y increases. TRUE (by inspection)
   b. When x = 0, y = -4; when y = 0, x = 2. TRUE (by inspection)
   c. The angle marked 6 is greater than 45°.   TRUE
      A right angle is formed by the straight line 2x - y - 4 = 0, the X axis, and the line x = 3. The leg opposite angle 6 consists of 2 units and the adjacent leg of 1 unit. 8 would be 45 if the legs were equal (the acute angles of an isosceles right tri-angle are each 45). The angle must be more than 45 since the leg opposite the angle 6 is the greater.
   d. The graph, if continued, would pass through the point
      x = 15, y = 26.   TRUE
      The coordinates of a point which lies on a graph will satisfy the equation of the graph
      2x - y - 4 = 0 or 2(15) - (26) -4=0 or 30 - 30 = 0 0=0

10. Answer (C) III
    P_{even} = 4 = 8, 10, 12, 14; q_{even} = 4 = 9, 11, 13, 15

    $\dfrac{p}{p+q} = \dfrac{4}{4+4} = \dfrac{1}{2}$

    P_{odd} = 4 = 9, 11, 13, 15; q_{odd} = 4 = 8, 10, 12, 14

    $\dfrac{p}{p+q} = \dfrac{4}{4+4} = \dfrac{1}{2}$

    $\therefore$ c is true inasmuch as $\dfrac{1}{2} = \dfrac{1}{2}$

SCIENCE READING COMPREHENSION
EXAMINATION SECTION
TEST 1

DIRECTIONS: This section consists of several reading passages, each followed by questions based on the text. Each question consists of a statement followed by several suggested answers, only one of which is correct. After reading each passage, choose the letter of the BEST answer among the suggested answers, basing our answer upon what is stated or implied in the passage, and on your own understanding of science. *PRINT THE LETTER OF THE CORRECT ANSWER IN THE SPACE AT THE RIGHT.*

Questions 1-3.

In order to determine the exact day of the week that a certain date fell, apply the following formula. To the day of the month add the figure corresponding to the month (see Month Table below), the year of the century, the number of leap years since the beginning of the century (divide the last two figures of the year by four), and the number corresponding to the century (see Century Table below). Divide this sum by 7, and the remainder will give the value for the day of the week, which can be obtained from the Day Table below.

MONTH TABLE				CENTURY TABLE		DAY TABLE	
Month	Value	Month	Value	Century	Value	Day of Week	Value
Jan.	0 (6)	July	6	1752-1799	5	Sunday	1
Feb.	3 (2)*	Aug.	2	1800-1899	3	Monday	2
Mar.	3	Sept.	5	1900-1999	1	Tuesday	3
April	6	Oct.	0	2000-2099	0	Wednes.	4
May	1	Nov.	3			Thurs.	5
June	4	Dec.	5			Friday	6
						Saturday	0

*Use figure in parentheses for Leap Years only.

1. On what day of the week was July 4, 1942? 1.____
   A. Friday   B. Saturday   C. Thursday   D. Wednesday

2. On what day of the week did January 1, 2000 fall? 2.____
   A. Friday   B. Monday   C. Saturday   D. Sunday

3. On what day of the week was Christmas 1799? 3.____
   A. Monday   B. Sunday   C. Tuesday   D. Wednesday

Questions 4-5.

In a gear system, gear A is the driver, meshing with gear B. Gear B, in turn, meshes with gear C. All gears mesh externally.

4. When gears A, B, and C have, respectively, 32, 128, and 64 teeth, and gear A rotates at 150 rpm, how fast does gear C rotate? 4.____
   A. 37 ½ rpm   B. 75 rpm   C. 300 rpm   D. 600 rpm

5. If the driver has t teeth and the gear to which it meshes has two-thirds as many teeth, and the third gear in the system has one-half as many teeth as the gear with which it meshes, how fast and in what direction does gear A turn when gear B rotates clockwise at 1,200 rpm? 5.____
   A. Clockwise, 800 rpm   B. Clockwise, 1,800 rpm
   C. Counter-clockwise, 800 rpm   D. Counter-clockwise, 1,800 rpm

Questions 6-9.

The figure shown in the diagram at the right is made of pieces of plastic, each piece half a centimeter thick and one centimeter wide.

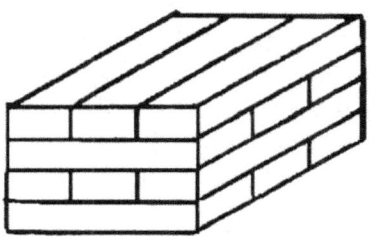

6. What is the volume of the figure? 6.____
   A. 12 cu cm   B. 18 cu cm   C. 27 cu cm   D. 36 cu cm

7. How many pieces are touched by at least 8 other pieces? 7.____
   A. 1   B. 2   C. 3   D. 4

8. If all the pieces had been cut from one strip of plastic, how long a piece of ½ cm x 1 cm material would have been required? 8.____
   A. 15 cm   B. 18 cm   C. 27 cm   D. 36 cm

9. What is the TOTAL surface in square centimeters of all the pieces? 9.____
   A. 10   B. 18   C. 72   D. 120

Questions 10-13.

In the present experiment, White Rock chicks were used. The alkanolamine of 2,4-D was administered orally through a pipette. In the first experiment, data for which are given in Table 1, one part of the alkanolamine was diluted with 19 parts of water. The dosages recorded are in terms of the acid equivalent. Five chicks (each weighing approximately 50 gm at the beginning) were used in each group. The chicks were weighed, and then were given the appropriate dose (Table 1) three times a week on alternate days for a period of four weeks, making a total of 12 doses. As the chicks gained in weight, the amount administered was adjusted in order to maintain the original dosage. At the end of four weeks, they were again weighed. The table shows the percentage increase in weight for the four-week period.

TABLE 1
EFFECT OF ALKANOLAMINE 2,4-D ON WHITE ROCK CHICKS

Dosage (mg of acid/kg of body weight)	Increase in Weight at End of Four Weeks (%)
0.00 (control)	456
.28	444
2.80	469
28.00	427
280.00	373

The differences between the control group and those given dosages of 0.28, 2.80, and 28.00 mg/kg were not significant at the 5% level. The difference between the control group and the group given a dosage of 280 mg/kg was barely significant at the 5% level.

Next, experiments were started to determine the lethal dose of the alkanolamine of 2,4-D, when diluted 1:9 with water. Each chick of a group of 5 (each averaging 166 gm) was given one dose of 380 mg/kg of body weight. These chicks survived.

Each chick of another group of 5 chicks (average weight, 111 gm) was given a dose of 765 mg/kg of body weight. All of these chicks died.

10. The lethal dose of diluted 2,4-D for small chicks is between
    A. 2.8 mg/kg and 28 mg/kg
    B. 28 mg/kg and 280 mg/kg
    C. 280 mg/kg and 380 mg/kg
    D. 380 mg/kg and 765 mg/kg
    10.____

11. In the first experiment, the LARGEST total dose administered to any one chick was approximately _____ mg.
    A. 300 B. 550 C. 1,120 D. 3,360
    11.____

12. The alkanolamine of 2,4-D is
    A. a cumulative poison
    B. an antidote
    C. not a cumulative poison
    D. not an organic compound
    12.____

13. Chicks might be killed by feeding on plants which had been sprayed with 2,4-D. Which of the following is the LEAST tenable? This statement
    A. cannot be judged as probably true or probably false on the basis of the information given
    B. is probably false
    C. is probably true
    D. might be true under certain conditions, false under other conditions
    13.____

Questions 14-17.

The diagram below shows the daily insolation in cal cm^{-2} day^{-1} received at the earth's surface in the absence of an atmosphere.

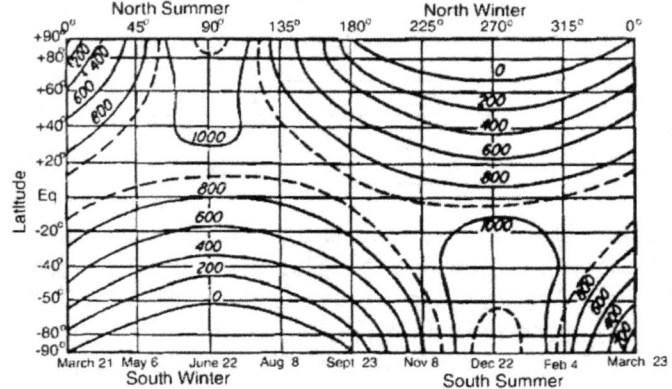

14. During the northern summer, the North Pole receives the maximum daily insolation. This might be accounted for by the
    A. declination of the sun's axis toward the earth
    B. ice and snow of that region reflecting more of the sun's rays
    C. length of the Arctic summer day
    D. soil of that area absorbing heat more rapidly

14.____

15. The total radiation received by the southern hemisphere during the southern summer is greater than the amount received by the northern hemisphere during its summer. This is probably BEST accounted for by the fact that
    A. during the southern summer the earth is nearer the sun than during the northern summer
    B. fewer observations of insolation are taken in the southern hemisphere than in the northern hemisphere
    C. the northern summer is shorter than the southern summer
    D. the southern hemisphere contains less land and more water than the northern

15.____

16. Assuming a 40% loss in insolation due to atmospheric conditions at the equator on June 22, how many calories of insolation would reach an area of one square foot in that one day? (1 cm = .3937 inches)

    A. $\dfrac{144(800)(.60)}{(.3937)^2}$
    B. $\dfrac{(12)^2(.3937)^2(800)}{.40}$

    C. $\dfrac{(.3937)^2(.60)}{(144)(800)}$
    D. $(800)(.40)(.3937)(12)$

16.____

17. Assuming atmospheric absorption to be constant, which of the following locations (time and latitude) is likely to be the WARMEST?
    A. January 1, +40°
    B. July 1, -40°
    C/ March 1, +60°
    D. May 1, -40°

17.____

Questions 18-20.

A glance at the five leading causes of death in 1900, 1910, and 1945, years representing in some measure the early and late practice of physicians now inactive, shows a significant trend. In 1900 these causes were (1) tuberculosis, (2) pneumonia, (3) enteritis, typhoid fever, and other acute intestinal diseases, (4) heart diseases, and (5) cerebral hemorrhage and thrombosis. Ten years later, the only change was that heart disease had moved from fourth to first place, tuberculosis now being second, and pneumonia third. In 1945, however, the list had changed profoundly. Heart diseases were far out in front; cancer, which had come up from eighth place, was second; and cerebral hemorrhage and thrombosis, third. Fatal accidents, which had been well down the list, were now fourth, and nephritis was fifth. All of these are, of course, composites rather than single diseases, and it is significant that, except for accidents, they are characteristic of the advanced rather than the early or middle years of life.

18. On the basis of the paragraph, which of the following statements is MOST tenable?
    A. A cure for cancer will be found within this decade.
    B. Many of the medical problems of today are problems of the gerontologist (specialist in medical problems of old age).
    C. Older persons are more accident-prone than are younger persons.
    D. Tuberculosis has been all but eliminated.

18.____

19. Which of the following trends is LEAST indicated in the paragraph?
    A. As one grows older, he is more subject to disease.
    B. Pneumonia has become less common.
    C. Relative to mortality rates for acute intestinal diseases, the mortality rate for cancer has increased.
    D. The incidence of heart diseases has increased.

19.____

20. Which of the following statements is MOST NEARLY correct?
    A. Such mortality trends are caused by decreased infant mortality.
    B. The data reported are a function of improved diagnosis and reporting.
    C. The mortality data are based on the records of physicians who practiced continuously from 1900 to 1945.
    D. There appears to be a greater change in the mortality patterns from 1910 to 1945 than in the decade ending in 1910.

20.____

Questions 21-24.

When suspensions of finely chopped liver tissue of normal dogs are kept under aseptic conditions (with 1% sodium fluoride or thymol), it is observed that after 18-22 hours there is a progressive decrease in the amount of its lipid content. This decrease, which may amount to 20% of the total lipid originally present, usually is maximal after 30 hours or less. Subsequently, it was shown that, if the suspensions are kept in the incubator under the same conditions for longer periods of time (i.e., 48-120 hours), their fat content is progressively restored until the initial values of total lipid are reached again.

The present note deals with the effect of some pancreatic extracts upon the phenomenon of lipodieresis. it has been shown that, when suspensions of liver tissue taken from depancreatized dogs are used, the phenomenon of lipodieresis never occurs; that is, the lipid content of livers from depancreatized dogs always remains about constant during the whole period of autolysis (Table 1).

TABLE 1
LIPODIERESIS IN LIVER TISSUE OF DEPANCREATIZED DOGS

Dog No.	Hours-	Liver Lipids in Weight %				
		0	18	48	76	120
2	5-gm. sample	12.7	12.3	12.7	12.8	12.2
4	5-gm. sample	26.5	26.0	26.2	26.1	26.4
5	5-gm. sample	19.2	19.1	19.1	19.1	19.2
6	5-gm. sample	23.2	23.0	23.1	23.1	23.1

However, the addition of a small amount of pancreatic extract to the same suspensions of liver tissue from depancreatized dogs restores the phenomenon of lipodieresis and the subsequent reappearance of fat. See Table 2.

Dog No.		Liver Lipids in Weight %				
	Hours-	5	18	48	76	120
1	5-gm. liver + 5 mg. lipocaic	12.72	12.11	12.14	12.10	12.63
2	5-gm. liver + pancr. extract	26.50	18.21	23.43	23.90	26.72
2	5-gm. liver + 50 mg. lipocaic	26.52	21.82	23.77	25.68	26.16
4	5-gm. liver + pancr. extract	19.21	14.02	16.59	18.77	19.04
4	5 gm. liver + 50 mg. lipocaic	19.21	14.50	17.05	18.92	19.11
5	5 gm. liver + pancr. extract	23.10	17.01	21.60	22.07	23.12
5	5 gm. liver + 50 mg. lipocaic	23.12	17.20	21.05	21.60	22.90

We have also examined the effect of that pancreatic extract having apparently lipotropic activity (so-called "lipocacic").

21. So far as their lipid content is concerned, liver suspensions of normal and of depancreatized dogs, when incubated for varying periods of time,
    A. behave in a similar manner
    B. behave in the same manner
    C. do not behave in a manner capable of being compared
    D. do not behave in the same manner

21.____

22. With the addition of pancreatic extracts to the liver suspensions of depancreatized dogs, the lipid content
    A. decreases
    B. decreases, then increases
    C. increases
    D. increases, then decreases

22.____

23. As compared with the pancreatic extract first used, lipocaic appears to act in 23.____
    A. a different manner and less effectively
    B. a different manner and more effectively
    C. the same manner but less effectively
    D. the same manner but more effectively

24. The word *lipid* refers to 24.____
    A. a starch compound
    B. certain fats
    C. lymph nodes
    D. pigmentation of the liver

KEY (CORRECT ANSWERS)

1.	B	11.	B
2.	D	12.	C
3.	D	13.	C
4.	B	14.	C
5.	C	15.	A
6.	B	16.	A
7.	B	17.	D
8.	D	18.	B
9.	D	19.	A
10.	D	20.	D

21. D
22. B
23. C
24. B

TEST 2

DIRECTIONS: This section consists of several reading passages, each followed by questions based on the text. Each question consists of a statement followed by several suggested answers, only one of which is correct. After reading each passage, choose the letter of the BEST answer among the suggested answers, basing our answer upon what is stated or implied in the passage, and on your own understanding of science. *PRINT THE LETTER OF THE CORRECT ANSWER IN THE SPACE AT THE RIGHT.*

Questions 1-3.

The effect of germination of water extracts of several different plant materials including sweetclover was tested. Sweetclover hay that had been cut when the plants were about 18"-24" high was used in the tests herein reported. Portions of the hay were cut into short lengths and placed in flasks with varying proportions of water. The corn seeds were then placed in the flasks and soaked in the sweetclover-water mixture for 24 hours. At the end of the soaking period, 5 seeds from each concentration of sweetclover extract were placed on an agar medium in Petri dishes in quadruplicate. The plates were incubated at room temperature. After 3 days the root and top growth of the corn seedlings were measured and compared with those of seeds soaked in distilled water. The results with sweetclover are shown in Table 1.

TABLE 1
INFLUENCE ON GERMINATION AND GROWTH OF SOAKING
CORN SEEDS FOR 24 HOURS WITH SWEETCLOVER EXTRACT

	Parts of Plant Material to Distilled Water	Germination (%)	Seedling Growth After 3 Days (Length in cm)*	
			Tops	Roots
Sweetclover	1:5	33	0.3	0.8
Sweetclover	1:10	52	0.5	0.9
Sweetclover	1:20	75	0.7	1.7
Sweetclover	1:80	92	1.8	3.8
Sweetclover	1:100	87	1.6	4.0
Control		95	2.8	6.4

*Based on the number of germinated seeds

The results with corn seeds soaked in different concentrations of coumarin in distilled water are shown in Table 2.

TABLE 2
THE INFLUENCE OF GERMINATION AND GROWTH OF SOAKING CORN
SEEDS IN COUMARIN SOLUTION FOR 24 HOURS

Grams of Coumarin in 100 ml of Water	Germination (%)	Seedling Growth After 3 Days (Length in cm)	
		Tops	Roots
0.125	0	0	0
0.062	0	0	0
0.031	12	0.3	0.4
0.015	42	0.4	0.5
0.007	90	1.2	4.2
None	95	2.9	7.6

1. The effect of sweetclover infusion was to _____ growth.
   A. accelerate   B. inhibit   C. promote   D. stop

2. As compared with a dilution of 1 part of sweetclover to 10 parts of water, a dilution of 1 part of sweetclover to 100 parts of water had what effect on the growth of corn seedlings?
   A. Decreased effect   B. Increased effect
   C. No effect   D. Same effect

3. In the second part of the experiment, was coumarin an important factor in affecting growth?
   A. Insufficient information given   B. No
   C. Yes   D. Yes, for roots only

Questions 4-5.

Let us use the symbol Δ instead of the customary sign indicating the operation of addition, ∇ to indicate subtraction, $\perp$ to indicate division, and $\top$ to indicate multiplication.

4. If a given chemical compound can be purchased for $1.59 per pound with a 15% discount for purchasing in lots of 100 pounds or more, which is the solution to the purchase price for 111 pounds?
   A. $(111 \top 1.59) \top (1.00 \nabla .15)$ B. $(1.59 \top 111) \perp (0.15)$
   C. $(1.59 \top .15) \top 111$ D. $111 \top 1.59 \top 15 \top 100$

5. What is the value of $[a^2 \nabla b^2 \Delta c^2 \nabla (a \nabla b)^2] \perp c^2$?
   A. $(a \Delta b) \top (a \nabla b) \perp c^2$ B. $(a \nabla b) \top 2 \top b$
   C. $c^2 \Delta 2 \top a \top b \perp c^2$ D. $1 \Delta (2 \top b) \top (a \nabla b) \perp c^2$

Questions 6-8.

In the course of experiments on the biosynthesis of labeled drugs, we encountered some difficulty in growing young *Digitalis lanata* plants in a sealed atmosphere. Excess moisture in the atmosphere of the terrarium was considered as one of the major factors detrimental to their growth. Consequently, a device for controlling the excessive humidity was devised. The necessity of preventing loss of any $C^{14}O_2$ from the terrarium required the construction of an air-tight unit such as that illustrated in Figure 1.

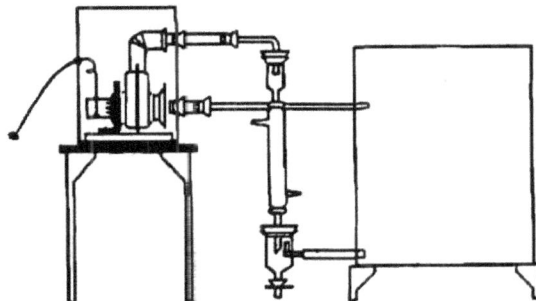

Figure 1

It consists of a motor-driven blower houses in an air-tight 9" x 12" battery jar covered with a circular piece of glass plate and sealed with a 50/50 mixture of beeswax and rosin.

6. The air drawn from the terrarium
   A. is dry
   B. contains moisture
   C. is pure
   D. contains carbon monoxide

7. The excess moisture is
   A. drained off
   B. evaporated
   C. saved
   D. wiped off

8. The air is drawn through the
   A. condenser into the motor blower
   B. motor blower into the condenser
   C. motor blower into the terrarium
   D. terrarium into the condenser

Questions 9-12.

Worthcar Farm mice weighing 20-25 gm and bearing 15-day-old transplants of sarcoma 180 (with some variation in size) were injected intravenously with 0.25 cc of a 1:14 dilution of saturated fluorescein in normal saline and killed at various times after injection by crushing the cervical cord. The animals were opened, the tumors hemisected, and both animals and tumors examined under ultraviolet light. Sixty-eight mice (136 tumors) were studied in groups at intervals from less than 1 minute after injection up to ½ hour, and at ½ hour intervals to 7 hours. The findings in the various groups are summarized in Table 1.

TABLE 1
DISTRIBUTION OF FLUORESCEIN IN SARCOMA 180 AT INTERVALS
AFTER INTRAVENOUS ADMINISTRATION

	Fluorescence	
	Animal Tissues*	Tumors**
Under 12 min.	Marked	Non-uniform fluorescence, tending to be higher on periphery
12 min. – 3 hrs.	Marked early to none at 3 hrs., with some variability	Uniform marked fluorescence
3-7 hrs	None	Marked fluorescence in necrotic areas; tended to decrease by 7 hrs.

* Fluorescence was present at all times in the colon, gallbladder, and urinary bladder – the normal routes of excretion of fluorescein
** In a few animals with spontaneous mammary carcinoma, this tumor showed essentially the same sequence of changes in distribution of fluorescein as the transplanted sarcoma 180.

Microscopic sections of all tumors showed the presence of irregular areas of necrosis.

9. The distribution of fluorescein in sarcoma 180 after a constant intravenous dose is determined by the length of time between injection and observation and by the amount of
   A. dilution   B. dosage   C. fluorescence   D. necrosis

10. A major factor determining the distribution of fluorescein in the tumors at any given time after injection is the _____ into and out of poorly vascularized areas.
    A. slowness of condensation
    B. slowness of diffusion
    C. swiftness of condensation
    D. swiftness of diffusion

11. Relative staining of viable and non-viable portions of tumors with fluorescein must be considered a phenomenon of
    A. dose duration
    B. fluorescence
    C. necrosis
    D. staining

12. The tumors were
    A. removed and prepared for microscopic examination
    B. removed and split, staining one half and not the other
    C. split along the mesial plane
    D. split and stained differentially

Questions 13-16.

Pure samples of dandelion and willow pollen were removed from a brood comb of a colony in the spring. A sample of mixed pollen, largely composed of dandelion, willow, maple, plum, alder, and a few other plants which were unidentified was obtained also. From 0.1 to 0.2 gm of each sample was moistened with water and ground in a small mortar with powdered glass until many of the pollen grains had been crushed. The material was diluted approximately 1:10 with 95% ethyl alcohol to precipitate the proteins, centrifuged, and the supernatant (extract) poured off. The extraction was repeated several times until the supernatant gave a negative nin-hydrin test. The extracts were concentrated by evaporation almost to dryness and diluted to approximately 500 microliters with water. The free amino acids in these extracts were determined qualitatively by partition chromatography on filter paper. Separation was accomplished on two-dimensional chromatograms, using 50 and 250 microliters of each extract.

The residue from the alcoholic extraction was analyzed qualitatively for the amino acids in the proteins. Half of the residue from each sample was hydrolyzed in 5N NaOH and the remaining half in 5N H_2SO_4. Hydrolysis was carried on for 10 hours in small ampules in an autoclave at 120°C. The hydrolysates were then neutralized; extracted with 95% ethyl alcohol, and processed in the same manner as above. Aliquots of 50 microliters of each hydrolysate were used for the separation of the amino acids on two-dimensional chromatograms. Table 1 contains a list of the amino acids identified in the samples.

TABLE 1

Amino Acids and Amides	Dandelion		Willow		Pollen Mixture	
	Free Amino Acids	Protein Hydrolysate	Free Amino Acids	Protein Hydrolysate	Free Amino Acids	Protein Hydrolysate
Alanine	++	+	++	+	++	+
β-Alanine			+		+	
α-Almino-η-butyric acid			+	+	+	+
Arginine	+	+	+	+	+	+
Asparagine	+		++		+++	
Aspartic acid	+	+	+	+	+	+
Cystine		+		+	+	+
Glutamic acid		+	+	+	+	+
Glutamine	+		+		++	
Glycine	+	+	+	+	+	+
Hydroxyproline	+	+	+	+	+	+
Isoleucine and/or leucine	+	+	+	+	+	+
Lysine		+		+	+	+
Methionine	+	+	+	+	++	+
Proline	+++	+	++	+	+++	+
Serine	+	+	+	+	++	+
Threonine		+		+	+	+
Tryptophane			+		+	+
Tyrosine		+	+	+	+	+
Valine	+	+	+	+	+	+

(++) and (+++) indicate relative quantities of the compounds appearing on the same chromatogram.

13. The study is a
    A. qualitative analysis
    B. qualitative summary
    C. quantitative analysis
    D. quantitative summary

14. If either of two amides is present in the proteins, it is converted to its amino acids during the hydrolysis and is, therefore, lacking in the hydrolysates. One of these amides is
    A. β-Alanine
    B. asparagine
    C. threonine
    D. tryptophane

15. The other amide referred to in the previous question is
    A. cysteine
    B. glutamic acid
    C. glutamine
    D. glycine

16. How many of the amino acids and amides appeared in both dandelion and willow pollen both as free amino acids and as protein hydrolysates?
    A. 10
    B. 12
    C. 14
    D. 17

6 (#2)

Questions 17-19.

As a result of the valiantly critical spirit which engendered the heresies, we have overcome the notion that mathematical truths have an existence independent and apart from our own minds. It is even strange to use that such a notion could ever have existed. Yet this is what Pythagoras would have thought – and Descartes, along with hundreds of other great mathematicians before the 19th century. Today mathematics is unbound; it has cast off its chains. Whatever its essence, we recognize it to be as free as the mind, as prehensile as the imagination. Non-Euclidean geometry is proof that mathematics, unlike the music of the spheres, is man's own handiwork, subject only to the limitations imposed by the laws of thought.

17. According to the paragraph, mathematical truth is   17._____
    A. a structure of human imagination   B. an eternal verity
    C. proven by non-Euclidean theorems   D. the product of heresy

18. Non-Euclidean mathematics is   18._____
    A. a departure from the mathematics of Descartes
    B. Pythagorean in character
    C. prehensile and consummate
    D. the basis for modern musical harmony

19. Mathematical truth is   19._____
    A. an ideal toward which mathematicians strive
    B. limited by logic
    C. unlimited in scope
    D. unreal and does not exist

Questions 20-22.

Let us set up a number system with the numbers _, X, Δ, _X, XX, ΔX, _Δ, X, ΔΔ, and –XX, corresponding, respectively, to the numbers 0 to 9 inclusive.

20. What is the sum of XΔ, _Δ, and XX?   20._____
    A. ΔΔ   B. XXΔ   C. --X   D. ΔΔX

21. Which of the following values is equal to the fraction XΔ/X--X?   21._____
    A. Δ/ΔXΔ   B. X/XX   C. XX/XXX   D. XΔ/ΔXΔ

22. Solve ΔΔ times XX divided by Δ.   22._____
    A. XXΔ   B. ΔXX   C. XΔX   D. ΔΔΔ

Questions 23-26.

Two groups of subjects were used. Group A learned List 1; Group B did not. The data for List 2 are the percentages that the number of repetitions required to learn the second list when it was preceded by the first list, were of the number required to learn it when it was not preceded by any other list.

TABLE 1

Condition	Example of Pairs in List 1		Example of Corresponding Pairs in List 2		Repetitions to Learn List 2 When List 1 Was Repeated		
					2 times	5 times	10 times
1	dev	zic	dev	fev	115	114	110
2	lex	sep	lex	sef	103	101	81
3	xal	yif	fes	yif	110	84	60
4	bes	lup	bef	lup	85	65	45
5	rax	pes	wum	foz	100	105	85

23. The data in this table show that
    A. in condition 5, when List 1 is repeated twice to one group, both groups learn List 2 in the same number of trials
    B. none of the other three conclusions given here can be drawn from the data in Table 2
    C. the second most difficult condition in general for Group A is condition 5
    D. when xal-yif, as an example of pairs in List 1, is repeated 5 times to Group B, Group A learns the second list quicker

24. For Group A, the MOST favorable condition for learning is when
    A. all words in Lists 1 and 2 are different
    B. all words in Lists 1 and 2 are short
    C. first words of pairs are similar and the second words are the same
    D. first words of pairs are the same and the second words are similar

25. On the basis of the above data, which of the following conditions makes learning List 2 MOST difficult when List 1 is repeated 10 times to Group A?

	List 1		List 2	
A.	nif	zut	nif	zek
B.	nif	zut	nif	zuf
C.	zut	nif	zek	nif
D.	zut	nif	zuf	nif

26. Which of the following conditions makes learning List 2 LEAST difficult when List 1 is repeated 5 times to Group A?

	List 1		List 2	
A.	niz	pes	kal	gof
B.	pes	ril	kal	ril
C.	pes	ril	pog	ril
D.	ril	pes	ril	pef

KEY (CORRECT ANSWERS)

1.	B	11.	A
2.	A	12.	C
3.	C	13.	A
4.	A	14.	B
5.	D	15.	C
6.	B	16.	A
7.	A	17.	A
8.	B	18.	A
9.	D	19.	B
10.	D	20.	D

21. B
22. C
23. A
24. C
25. A
26. C

SCIENCE READING COMPREHENSION
EXAMINATION SECTION
TEST 1

DIRECTIONS: This section consists of several reading passages, each followed by questions based on the text. Each question consists of a statement followed by several suggested answers, only one of which is correct. After reading each passage, choose the letter of the BEST answer among the suggested answers, basing our answer upon what is stated or implied in the passage, and on your own understanding of science. *PRINT THE LETTER OF THE CORRECT ANSWER IN THE SPACE AT THE RIGHT.*

Questions 1-3.

A hydrogen ion scale is used as a means of expressing the alkalinity or acidity of a solution. The units on this scale are called pH values. Values of pH greater than 7.0 denote alkalinity, and of pH less than 7.0 denote acidity. To get an idea of the magnitude of the units, it may be stated that a solution which has a pH of 5.0 is ten times as acid as one with a pH of 6.0. A similar relationship holds on the alkaline side of the scale.

1. How much more alkaline is a solution which has a pH of 10.0 than one which has a pH of 8.0?   1.____
   A. 0.5   B. 2.0   C. 10.0   D. 100.0

2. A solution having a pH of 7.0 is   2.____
   A. acid
   B. acid or alkaline, depending on which has been added to give it a pH of 7.0
   C. alkaline
   D. neither acid nor alkaline

3. From the statement, one may conclude that the   3.____
   A. higher the pH, the greater the acidity of the solution
   B. lower the pH, the greater the acidity of the solution
   C. lower the pH, the greater the alkalinity of the solution
   D. point pH = 7.0 is an average value

Questions 4-7.

The modern method of determining mean sea level is to establish a tide gauge and operate it for a considerable period of time. Figure 1 shows a schematic diagram of the installation, and you will note that the recording instrument is mounted on the table or bench inside the tide-gauge house, and that the bench and instrument are placed over the float well so that a vertical wire leading from the float to the recording instrument will hang in the center of the well and keep the float from dragging on the sides of the well. Two counter-weights show in the diagram. One is in a bight in the wire leading from the float over a spool on the gauge and through suitable pulleys to the counter-weight and then to an anchorage in the roof. The other furnishes the power for the take-up spool to keep the paper wound up properly and to relieve some strain on the clock that controls the feeding of the paper over the main roller along an element of which the recording pencil moves back and forth.

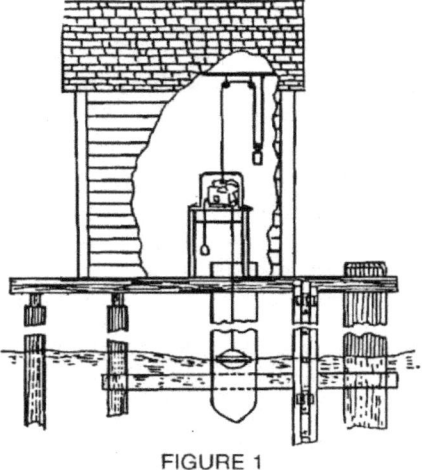

FIGURE 1

In a close-up of the recording gauge, we would notice two clocks, one causing the paper to feed over the main roller at the rate of one inch per hour and the other producing the time marks at hourly intervals on the curve traced by the recording pencil. A fixed pencil traces a datum line the length of the curve as the paper passes under it.

The curve is traced by means of a pencil which is made to move along an element of the main roller by means of a spirally-grooved shaft which in turn is directly connected to the spool over which the wire passes in leading from the float to the counter-weight. This counter-weight keeps the wire taut at all times and prevent slippage on the spool, which is grooved and carries several turns of wire at one time to insure sufficient friction between the wire and the spool.

The tide staff is simply a long board, graduated in feet and tenths from the bottom upward, and is mounted in a vertical position on some suitable structure so that its zero is well below the lowest expectable low stage of the tide at that station. This staff is read daily at the time the gauge is inspected and serviced, and the staff reading is noted directed on the curve at the point indicated by a manually-made jog, similar to an hourly time mark, put in the curve at the time the staff reading was taken. These staff readings serve to define the height of the datum line on the curve with respect to the zero of the staff gauge.

At suitable intervals of time, the staff is connected, by means of spirit leveling, with the bench marks on shore. These are set at suitable locations on shore and near the tide station. They serve to furnish the permanent points to which the observations are referred.

4. "Mean sea level" refers to the sea surface's 4._____
    A. amount of fluctuation   B. average height
    C. greatest height   D. lowest point

5. A tide gauge produces a graphic record of the 5.____
   A. fall of the surface of the water
   B. height of the bench marks
   C. rise and fall of the surface of the water
   D. rise of the surface of the water

6. Which of the following is LEAST essential in recording mean sea level? 6.____
   A. Intervals on the graph paper
   B. Location of the bench marks
   C. Size of the float
   D. Time of recording

7. To measure mean sea level, it is essential to have 7.____
   A. a mechanical timepiece
   B. a method for recording time
   C. at least one clock
   D. two clocks

Questions 8-10.

Sixty newly-hatched loggerhead turtles placed in an open pit on the beach milled around but showed no oriented movements in the direction of the water. When vision of the surf was permitted by placing them on the open beach, they entered the water immediately. Four animals, released on the beach on a quiet, moonless night when the surf was absent, failed to find the water; but when released later, at the same point on the beach, after the moon had risen, they crawled quickly into the ocean.

A group of five animals placed on the beach at night were observed to follow a beam from a flashlight as it was moved around on the beach surface. Confusion of orientation was produced in a group of fifty turtles by releasing them on the beach on a moonlit night and by stimulating them simultaneously by a spot of light directed near them on the sand. About half of the animals followed the spot of light as it was moved about, and the other half crawled to the sea. Some individuals could be induced to reverse their direction of crawl, even after getting into the water, by moving the light from the edge of the ocean up onto the slope of the beach.

Gravity as a stimulus was compared with light directly by releasing the animals on an inclined plane with a lighted window at the top. The results are shown in Table 1.

TABLE 1
NUMBER OF TURTLES RESPONDING POSITIVELY TO
SIMULTANEOUSLY PRESENTED LIGHT AND GRAVITATIONAL STIMULATION

Angle of Incline	Number of Animals Tested	Number Showing Positive Geotropic Response	Number Showing Positive Phototropic Response	Number Showing Ambiguous Response*
6°	16	1	8	7
10°	6	1	3	2
13°	11	2	8	1
Total	33	4	19	10

*This group includes inactive animals as well as four animals which moved in no particular direction around the release point on the inclined plane.

8. The purpose of the experiments was to determine the critical stimulus or stimuli for
    A. direction of the migration
    B. learning to swim
    C. leaving the nest
    D. various types of illumination

    8._____

9. The experiments show that the critical stimulus for newly-hatched loggerheads in their movement from the nest to the sea is normally
    A. gravity
    B. light reflected from the surf
    C. moonlight
    D. moving light

    9._____

10. Under the conditions of the experiments, the following was found to be relatively ineffectual:
    A. Geotropism
    B. Photokinesis
    C. Phototropism
    D. Photokinesis and phototropism

    10._____

Questions 11-12.

The following diagram shows a pump.

11. In the operation of the pump, when the handle is raised, valve B is _____ and valve C is _____.
    A. closed; closed
    B. open; closed
    C. closed; open
    D. open; open

    11._____

12. Water is discharged from the pump through 1
    A. D
    B. F
    C. G
    D. an opening not shown in the diagram

    12._____

Questions 13-15.

In order to prevent loss of potency by injection in aqueous solution as well as contamination by traces of alcohol, a simple drying technique was devised by which anterior lobes of glands (*Rana pipiens*) were oven-dried at 94°C, for 48 hours, and stored in desiccators until injected. A preliminary experiment conducted on 6 nonbreeding frogs collected in Wisconsin in November demonstrated that as few as 4 dried anterior pituitaries (from female donors) will induce ovulation, although as many as 7 or more may be needed on some frogs. Subsequent tests in January (25 frogs injected) and March (17 frogs injected) showed dried anterior pituitaries to be as effective as fresh glands in inducing ovulation.

Glands removed from freshly caught frogs (*R. pipiens*) and dried in mid-January were compared in ovulation-inducing capacity with glands removed and dried in mid-March. The recipients, females in the pre-breeding condition, were injected during the last week of March. All recipients, furthermore, were tested for ovulation by stripping and shown to be negative prior to injection. Control frogs did not ovulate throughout the duration of the experiment, terminated the last of April. Whereas an average of 4 January glands were necessary to cause at least 50 percent ovulation (within one week after injection), 1-3 March glands induced ovulation in frogs in the same stage of breeding activity (see Table 1).

TABLE 1
OVULATION-INDUCING CAPACITY OF DRIED FEMALE ANTERIOR
PITUITARIES FROM JANUARY AND MARCH FROGS TESTED
BY RESPONSE OF MARCH FROGS

Gland Source By Date	Number Glands Per Frog	Number Frogs Injected	Number Showing At Least 50% Ovulation	% Showing At Least 50% Ovulation
January	2	9	0	0
	3	10	3	30
	4	6	4	66
March	1	6	4	66
	2	6	4	66
	3	5	5	100

13. Desiccation of the anterior pituitary probably _____ its potency.
    A. alters
    B. decreases
    C. does not alter
    D. increases

14. The number of donor glands required to induce ovulation between January and March
    A. decreases
    B. decreases, then increases
    C. increases
    D. increases, then decreases

15. Between January and March, the gonadotropic potency of the anterior pituitary
    A. decreases
    B. decreases, then increases
    C. increases
    D. increases, then decreases

Questions 16-18.

Gannets (*Morus bassanus*) were selected as the best available species for this experiment on bird navigation since they are large white birds, easily observed from an airplane, and since they are strictly marine and virtually never fly more than a very short distance inland. Thus, we could be sure that the 17 gannets which we released more than 100 miles from the nearest salt water were in completely unknown territory. Nine of them were followed from an airplane, the remainder being controls against the possibility that the presence of the airplane 1,500'-2,000' above the bird would influence its homing performance. Since both groups showed roughly the same speed (average 99 miles/day) and the same percentage of returns (63% of those released in good physical condition), it seemed clear that the airplane had no detrimental effect on their homing.

The performance of gannets as to speed and percentage of returns is compared, in Table 1, with other species which have been transported in sufficient numbers to equivalent distances to permit a valid comparison.

TABLE 1

	Returns (%)	Avg. Speed (Miles/Day)
Herring gull (inland releases)	97	90
Swallow	67	141
Gannet	63	99
Leach's petrel	61	38
Starling	54	17
Noddy and sooty tern	52	114
Common tern (inland releases)	29	109

Figure 1 shows the actual routes flown by 9 gannets followed for portions of their return flight ranging from 1 to 9 ½ hours and from 25 to 230 miles. Five of these birds were back at their nests after the following periods of time: No. 10, 70 hours; No. 22, 45 hours; No. 23, 45 hours; No. 25, 24 hours; and No. 78, 75 hours. The rest (Nos. 3, 8, 21, and 24) did not return

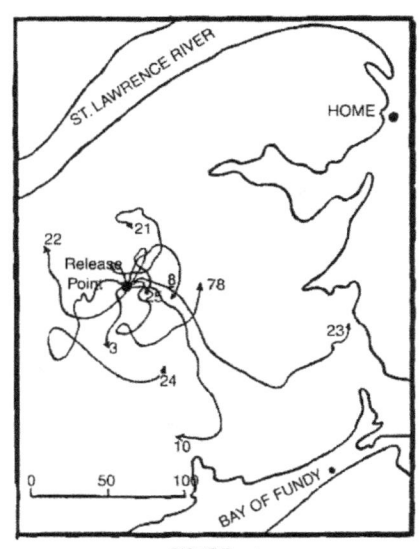

FIGURE 1

Flight paths of homing gannets as observed from an airplane. The birds were captured at their nests on a small island marked "home," transported rapidly to the release point, which was in completely unknown territory, and followed as far as possible after release. The arrowhead indicates each bird's direction of flight when last seen.

16. According to the table, one of the best species for experiments on bird navigation is probably the
    A. common tern
    B. gannet
    C. herring gull
    D. starling

17. The flight paths of the gannets indicate
    A. exploration of feeding places
    B. good orientation
    C. observation of landmarks
    D. possible spiraling

18. The evidence from this experiment suggests that, in reaching their nests, birds may rely on
    A. the direction of the wind
    B. the position of the sun
    C. their sensitivity to the earth's magnetic field
    D. unidentified environmental cues

Questions 19-20.

The lead type of storage cell consists of lead plates immersed in dilute sulfuric acid. When the lead cell is charged, the active deposit on the positive plate is lead peroxide. This plate has a reddish-brown color. The active substance of the negative plate is spongy lead. (The positive plate is the one of higher potential – the one from which the current flows in the discharge.) When the cell is discharging, lead sulfate is formed on both plates.

When the cell is being charged, the density of the acid increases; when it is discharging, the density decreases. Therefore, a test of the density of the acid affords a simple way of telling when the cell needs charging. The curves in Figure 1 show the changes that take place in the voltage of the terminals on charge and discharge, and the changes in the density of the acid on discharge.

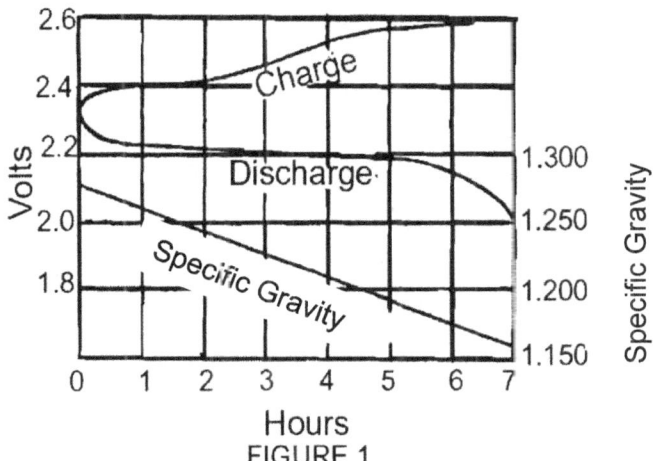
FIGURE 1

19. When the cell begins discharging,
    A. lead peroxide is no longer formed on the positive plate
    B. the current begins flowing to the positive plate
    C. the positive plate is no longer of higher potential
    D. the positive plate loses its reddish-brown color

20. Figure 1 shows that the
    A. cell can general current for a little over 13 hours
    B. cell cannot be recharged
    C. density of the acid is changing
    D. specific gravity of the acid is not dependent on voltage charges

Questions 21-25.

In the course of a comprehensive investigation dealing with the influence of heredity on the carotene content of corn, crude carotene values were determined on the grain from all possible single cross combinations of 10 inbred lines of yellow dent corn, all of the same general maturity class and grown during the last season. A 7 x 7 triple lattice design was used in the field experiment, thus providing for analysis three replicate samples of grain for each single cross. In the field experiment, the soil type and fertilizer treatment were the same on the three plots.

The corn was harvested at maturity, and the shelled corn was air-dried at room temperature for 10 days and stored in airtight containers at 0°C until it was analyzed. Carotene estimations were made by the official A.O.A.C. method, modified by the use of Hyflo Supercel and magnesium oxide, 3:1, as the chromatographic adsorbent.

Seed was not available for the Iowa I205 x Ohio 28 cross; hence, the carotene value for this combination was missing from the data. The range of yields of the other single cross combinations tested was from 71 to 123 bushels/acre.

The average difference between the highest and lowest of the three carotene values for the individual single crosses was of the order of 1 percent, the values given in Table 1 being the means for three duplicate estimations.

TABLE 1											
CAROTENE CONTENT OF CORN											
(mg./lb – 15.5 percent moisture basis)											
		Nebraska 6	Wisconsin 8	Illinois M14	Illinois A	Indiana WF9	Ohio 28	Wisconsin 32	Ohio 51A	Wisconsin 22	Iowa I205
Nebraska	6		1.91	1.64	1.50	1.41	1.30	1.48	1.09	1.08	.67
Wisconsin	8	1.91		1.68	1.27	1.27	1.17	1.31	1.01	.88	1.07
Illinois	M14	1.64	1.68		1.26	1.23	1.03	.93	1.17	.84	.70
Illinois	A	1.50	1.27	1.26		.97	.95	.95	.93	.79	.66
Indiana	WF9	1.41	1.27	1.23	.97		.93	.98	.79	.74	.62
Ohio	28	1.30	1.17	1.03	.95	.93		.88	.66	.72	-
Wisconsin	32	1.48	1.31	.93	.95	.98	.88		.79	.73	.58
Ohio	51A	1.09	1.01	1.17	.93	.79	.66	.79		.60	.53
Wisconsin	22	1.08	.88	.84	.79	.74	.72	.73	.60		.69
Iowa	I205	.67	1.07	.70	.66	.62	-	.58	.53	.69	
Least significant difference between single crosses = .19 mg.											

21. Which of the single cross combinations tested showed the HIGHEST per acre yield?
    A. Insufficient data are given to answer the question
    B. Ohio 28 and Iowa I205
    C. Wisconsin 8 and Illinois M14
    D. Wisconsin 8 and Nebraska 6

21.____

22. On the average, the crosses involving which line produced corn of the HIGHEST carotene content?
    A. Illinois A   B. Iowa I205   C. Nebraska 6   D. Ohio 51A

22.____

23. The use of an experimental design which provided for repetition of the experiment would
    A. be desirable only with reference to the inbred lines of corn
    B. help to control soil type and fertilizer treatment
    C. probably give identical results
    D. provide more adequate experimental evidence

23.____

24. The experiment reported here shows that
    A. carotene is probably the most important nutritive factor in the development of new corn hybrids
    B. different strains of yellow corn do not vary widely in carotene content
    C. the carotene content of corn must be estimated on a percent moisture basis
    D. the genetic constitution of corn may be largely responsible for its carotene content

24.____

25. The experiment reported indicates that the carotene content of the stored corn is
    A. affected by temperature
    B. associated with genetic factors
    C. influenced by humidity
    D. related to its weight

25.____

KEY (CORRECT ANSWERS)

1.	D	11.	B
2.	D	12.	A
3.	B	13.	C
4.	B	14.	A
5.	C	15.	C
6.	C	16.	C
7.	B	17.	D
8.	A	18.	D
9.	B	19.	A
10.	A	20.	C

21. A
22. C
23. D
24. D
25. B

TEST 2

DIRECTIONS: This section consists of several reading passages, each followed by questions based on the text. Each question consists of a statement followed by several suggested answers, only one of which is correct. After reading each passage, choose the letter of the BEST answer among the suggested answers, basing our answer upon what is stated or implied in the passage, and on your own understanding of science. *PRINT THE LETTER OF THE CORRECT ANSWER IN THE SPACE AT THE RIGHT.*

Questions 1-2.

Suppose an ancient culture had a number system of only two digits. One of these was x, the equivalent of our zero; and the other was 1, equivalent to our one. Thus, their counting was 1, 1x, 11, 1xx, 1x1, 11x, 111, 1xxx, etc., corresponding to our numbers 1, 2, 3, 4, 5, 6, 7, 8, etc.

1. Which of the following is equivalent to our number 13?　　　　　　　　　　1.____
   A. 1111　　　　B. 11x1　　　　C. 111x　　　　D. 1x1x

2. What is the value of 1xxxxx?　　　　　　　　　　　　　　　　　　　　　　2.____
   A. 32　　　　　B. 50　　　　　C. 81　　　　　D. 100,000

Questions 3-7.

Fourth day parasite counts were accumulated on 499 White Rock chicks inoculated at 6-8 days of age with 16×10^6 parasitized red cells. Analysis by sex showed that for 222 females the counts averaged 62.3% (S.E. = 1.2), whereas for 227 males the counts averaged 53.8% (S.E. = 1.2).

To determine whether the sex difference in parasite counts could be experimentally increased, male and female sex hormones of proven activity in chicks were administered. Ninety infected chicks were divided into 3 equal groups. Each chick in group A was injected intramuscularly with 0.1 mg. of testosterone propionate in 0.1 cc. of corn oil daily for 6 days, beginning on the day before the inoculation. Chicks in group B were similarly injected with 0.1 mg. of aestradiol benzoate, and each of the controls in group C received 0.1 cc. of corn oil alone daily for the same period. The difference in parasite counts in the two sexes was not significantly increased by the administration of male or female sex hormones under the conditions of these experiments.

The incidence of exoerythrocytic schizonts in the capillary endothelium of the brain of chicks examined at various intervals after inoculation of sporozoites is presented in Table 1.

TABLE 1
INCIDENCE OF EXOERYTHROCYTIC SCHIZONTS IN THE CAPILLARY ENOTHELIUM
OF THE BRAIN OF CHICKS EXAMINED 6-12 DAYS AFTER THE
INTRAMUSCULAR INJECTION OF SPOROZOITES OF P.GALLINACEUM

	6th-10th Day		11th Day		12th Day	
	No. Examined	% Positive	No. Examined	% Positive	No. Examined	% Positive
Females	61	65.6	41	90.2	40	92.5
Males	67	43.3	55	69.1	57	91.2
diff.* S.E. diff		2.59				Not significant

$\dfrac{\text{* diff.}}{\text{S.E. diff}}$ represents the ratio of the observed difference to its Standard Error. Values greater than 2.00 are considered significant.

Parasite-count differences between the males and females were observed also in 418 blood-inoculated chicks treated with a suppressive level of quinine hydrochloride (Table 2).

TABLE 2
FOURTH-DAY PARASITE COUNTS OF INFECTED
CHICKS TREATED WITH QUININE

	Number Treated	Average Count	Chicks Showing Count of 30% and Above	
			Number	%
Females	212	7.28%	15	7.1
Males	206	4.60%	5	2.4
$\dfrac{\text{diff.}}{\text{S.E. diff}}$		2.55%		2.3

3. Differences in infections of the chicks are attributable to the
   A. age of the chicks
   B. method of statistical analysis
   C. sex of the host
   D. type of inoculation

4. As compared with the males, the female chicks showed higher parasite counts
   A. and earlier endothelial invasion
   B. and later endothelial invasion
   C. after the experimental period
   D. prior to the experimental period

5. As compared with the females, the male chicks were _____ protected by quinine.
   A. almost equally
   B. less effectively
   C. more effectively
   D. not

6. Statistical significance is represented by
   A. a comparison of percentages in terms of expected variation due to sampling
   B. comparison of female and male chicks
   C. percentage of parasite counts among infected chicks
   D. percentage of positive reactions after intramuscular injections

7. The null hypothesis, the use of which is implied by the fourth-day parasite counts of infected chicks treated with quinine, was
   A. inadequate
   B. not helpful
   C. proved untenable
   D. shown to be acceptable

Questions 8-10.

Early twentieth century world's records for running were as follow:
- 100 yards — 9.4 seconds
- 220 yards — 20.3 seconds
- 440 yards — 46.4 seconds
- 880 yards — 1 minute 49.2 seconds
- mile — 4 minutes 1.4 seconds
- 2 miles — 8 minutes 42.8 seconds
- 3 miles — 13 minutes 32.4 seconds

8. Which graph BEST illustrates the relation between speed and distance? (Distance is measured from left to right, and speed on the ordinate.)

   A.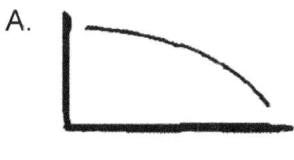
   B.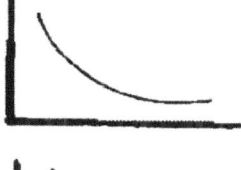
   C.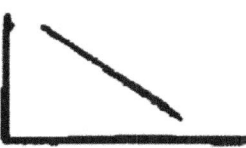
   D.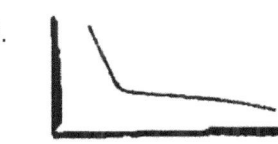

   8.____

9. How many times faster (speed) is the record for the 100-yard dash than for the mile?
   A. 1 ½ B. 15 C. 25 D. 50

   9.____

10. About what would be the speed for the half-mile run?
    A. 10 miles per hour
    B. 15 miles per hour
    C. 20 miles per hour
    D. 25 miles per hour

    10.____

Questions 11-13.

Suppose that you have a number of solid aluminum blocks of the shape shown in the diagram. Each is a right angle with sides 1 ½ inches long, cut from material ½ inch thick.

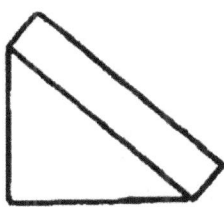

11. How many cubic inches of water will one such block displace?
    A. 0.2500 B. 0.5625 C. 1.1250 D. 2.2500

    11.____

12. What is the total surface area in square inches of one of these blocks? 12.____
   A. 2.25 + √4.5   B. 3.75
   C. 3.75 + √1.125 D. 4.50

13. What would be the MAXIMUM number of such blocks which could be put 13.____
    in a space 9 inches high, 9 inches long, and 9 inches wide?
    A. 81   B. 729   C. 1,296   D. 2,592

Questions 14-15.

In the gear system shown at the right, A and C are on the same shaft, but can rotate independently. Gear B is the driver.

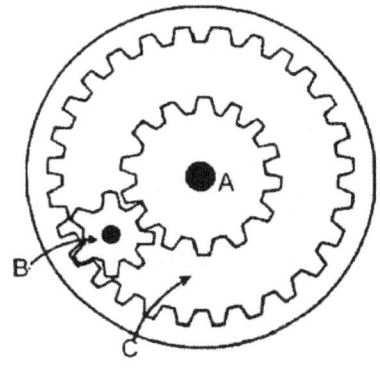

14. Suppose gear A had 20 teeth, gear B had 16 teeth, and gear C had 64 teeth. 14.____
    The ratio of revolutions per minute of gear A to gear C would be
    A. 1:1   B. 4:1   C. 5:4   D. 16:5

15. When gear A is turning clockwise, gears B and C, respectively, are turning 15.____
    in what directions?
    A. Clockwise, clockwise   B. Clockwise, counterclockwise
    C. Counterclockwise, clockwise D. Counterclockwise, counterclockwise

Questions 16-19.

Pteroyltriglutamic acid (*teropterin*) was administered in daily dosses varying from 10 to 150 mg. intramuscularly and in other patients from 20 to 500 mg. intravenously. Pteroyldiglutamic acid (*diopterin*) was given in amounts from 50 to 250 mg. intramuscularly and from 20 to 300 mg./day orally.

There have been no reactions following intravenous administration of either substance. No important local reactions following intramuscular injection of pteroyltriglutamic acid have been observed.

Systemic reactions have not been observed. No important changes in pulse, respiration, or temperature were noted, nor have there been any significant long-term variations in blood pressure. There have been no allergic reactions of either major or minor degree.

Twenty-seven of the patients with advanced neoplastic disease have died, and, of these, 13 were examined post mortem. Exclusive of 11 patients with acute leukemia from whom biopsies of bone marrow were obtained, there were 11 patients from whom biopsies of the tumor were obtained both before treatment was instituted and after treatment had been carried out for a period of at least a few weeks. Study of the gross and histological material available from these patients revealed no change in organs and tissues which could be regarded as a deleterious effect of the substances employed. In no instance was there any evidence of pancytopenia, agranulocytosis, degeneration of the kidneys, liver, or myocardium, or any suggestion of a polyarteritis.

16. Apparently, the action of the acids was 16.____
    A. helpful   B. nontoxic   C. not helpful   D. toxic

17. Which statement is possible NOT true? No significant local reactions 17.____
resulted from
    A. intramuscular injection of diopterin
    B. intramuscular injection of teropterin
    C. intravenous injection of diopterin
    D. intravenous injection of teropterin

18. Conclusions from the experiment should be based on the 18.____
    A. clinical evidence
    B. clinical, laboratory, and post-mortem studies
    C. laboratory results
    D. post-mortem studies

19. Neoplastic disease is associated with 19.____
    A. a marked decrease in white blood cells
    B. a new kind of blood plasma
    C. some blood transfusions
    D. tumorous growth

Questions 20-22.

    A regular hexagon is inscribed in a circle. The area of a circle is πr^2, where r is the radius of the circle. Each of the six triangles is an equilateral triangle.

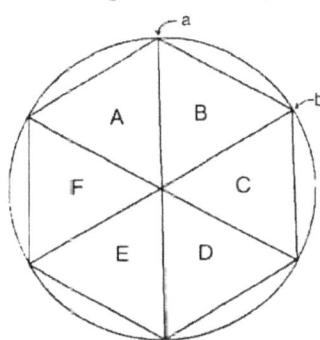

20. If r = 10 centimeters, what is the distance from a to b? 20.____
    A. $\pi\sqrt{10}$ centimeters   B. 10 centimeters
    C. 10π centimeters   D. 100π centimeters

21. What is the area of triangle E, when the diameter of the circle is one meter? 21.____
   A. $\frac{1}{8}\sqrt{3}$ square meter
   B. $\frac{1}{16}\sqrt{3}$ square meters
   C. ¼ square meter
   D. ½ square meter

22. About what percent of the area of the circle is covered by the hexagon? 22.____
   A. 78%   B. 83%   C. 88%   D. 93%

Questions 23-25.

   A new record for population increase in the United States was set in 1947. The excess of births over deaths exceeded 2,400,000. About 3,900,000 babies were born in the United States in 1947 (population, 140,000,000). This was the highest birth rate in at least 25 years, and was 50 percent above the figure for 1933, when the birth rate dropped to its lowest level. It was the fourth year – each time within the instant decade – that more than 3,000,000 babies were born during any one year.
   In recent years, there has been a remarkable reduction in infant mortality. The rate has been reduced by one-third since 1939, and by one-half since 1930. About as many infants died in 1947 as in 1933.

23. Infant mortality rates for 1947 as compared with 1933 23.____
   A. cannot be estimated from the information given
   B. were about the same
   C. were higher
   D. were lower

24. The birth rate per thousand population in 1933 was about 24.____
   A. 13   B. 18   C. 25   D. 35

25. Which of the following statements is BEST supported by the paragraphs? 25.____
   A. The low infant mortality rate in 1947 contributed considerably to the record population increase.
   B. 1947 showed the highest birth rate recorded for the United States.
   C. 1947 showed the lowest infant mortality rate recorded for the United States.
   D. The 1947 infant mortality rate was five-sixths lower than in 1930.

KEY (CORRECT ANSWERS)

1.	B	11.	B
2.	A	12.	C
3.	C	13.	C
4.	A	14.	D
5.	C	15.	D
6.	A	16.	B
7.	C	17.	A
8.	B	18.	B
9.	A	19.	D
10.	B	20.	B

21. B
22. B
23. D
24. B
25. A

SCIENCE READING COMPREHENSION EXAMINATION SECTION

DIRECTIONS: This part consists of several reading passages, each followed by a series of statements. Read the passage and then classify each of the statements under one of the following categories:
A. The statement is warranted by information given in the passage.
B. The statement is true but not warranted by the passage.
C. The statement is contradicted by the passage.
D. The statement is contradicted by established evidence but not by the passage.

PRINT THE LETTER OF THE CORRECT ANSWER IN THE SPACE AT THE RIGHT.

SAMPLE PASSAGE

In vertebrates circulation is effected by two systems, the vascular system and the lymphatic system. The vascular system consists of vessels that distribute the blood. Blood is composed of a liquid plasma in which float various elements, chiefly red and white cells. The lymphatic system in mammals is essentially a network of vessels which carry lymph, a liquid plasma containing floating white blood cells. Both systems are closely associated but the lymphatic plays a relatively passive role; so it is the vascular system that one ordinarily has in mind when speaking of the circulatory system.

The essential elements of the vascular system are the heart, for the propulsion of blood, the arteries which carry blood away from the heart to the tissues of the body, and the veins which carry blood from the tissues back to the heart. The arteries divide and subdivide to form smaller and smaller arteries which finally merge into exceedingly delicate tubes, the capillaries. These capillaries permeate the tissues of the body and then deliver the blood to the smallest veins which pass it on to larger and larger veins and finally to the heart. Consequently, the blood flows through a closed system of blood vessels from the heart and back to the heart.

Statements 1-4.

1. Blood platelets are structures found in the blood.   1.____

2. Both the vascular system and the lymphatic system transport fluid through vessels.   2.____

3. Valves in the arteries control the flow of blood.   3.____

4. Blood cells are found only in the blood.   4.____

ANSWER KEY TO SAMPLE PASSAGE
1. B   2. A   3. D   4. C

TEST 1

PASSAGE

Compared with other animals, mammals are recent forms of life. Fossils indicate that the earliest mammals appeared about 60 million years ago. Prior to the end of the Mesozoic Era and the dawn of the Cenozoic Era, the warm humid climate had favored the giant reptiles. Topographic changes altered the climate of continents, resulting in seasonal temperature variations and differences in the precipitation in various continental areas. The earliest mammals were small and included forerunners of the squirrel, rat, and mouse, including the little ancient horse, Eohippus. It had five toes. Mammals increased in size and became more abundant. Hoofed mammals including ancient species of rhinoceros and camel roamed the forests and grasslands in great herds. Later, flesh-eating mammals such as the sabre-toothed cats flourished and destroyed large number of hoofed mammals. Near the end of the Cenozoic Era, further cooling of the climate resulted in the Glacial Age. Then prehistoric elephants, called mastodons and mammoths, migrated to Africa through Europe, Asia, and North America. Many species of ancient mammals perished long ago, but a large number served as the ancestral stock of the mammals of today. Modern mammals vary greatly in size. They are for the most part land animals although some are adapted to life in the sea. Some few are capable of flight.

Statements 1-6.

1. Giant reptiles lived during the Mesozoic Era. 1.____
2. The small early mammals destroyed the giant reptiles. 2.____
3. One of the few early mammals which has survived to the present day is the opposum. 3.____
4. The whale is a fish. 4.____
5. Modern horses have 5 toes. 5.____
6. Flesh-eating mammals have hoofs. 6.____

KEY (CORRECT ANSWERS)

1. A
2. C
3. B
4. D
5. D
6. C

TEST 2

PASSAGE

If the volume which a certain number of gas molecules occupies remains constant, the pressure exerted by the gas increases if its temperature is raised. If the pressure exerted by this number of gas molecules remains the same as the temperature is increased, the volume the gas occupies increases. If the temperature of these gas molecules remains constant, the pressure exerted by the gas increases if the volume occupied by the gas becomes smaller. Equal volumes of all gases at S.T.P. contain the same number of molecules.

Statements 1-6.

1. When a gas is collected over water, the amount of pressure due to water vapor varies according to the temperature. 1.____

2. Increase in temperature decreases the density of a gas, if the pressure is kept constant. 2.____

3. At constant volume, an increase in temperature of a given mass of gas decreases the pressure exerted. 3.____

4. Different gases expand or contract at different rates. 4.____

5. At constant temperature, the pressure exerted by a given number of gas molecules varies inversely with the volume. 5.____

6. The volume of a certain amount of dry gas varies directly with the Kelvin temperature, provided the pressure remains constant. 6.____

KEY (CORRECT ANSWERS)

1. B
2. A
3. C
4. D
5. A
6. B

TEST 3

PASSAGE

Boron atoms are small, their atomic radii being only 0.80 Angstroms. Their valence electrons are quite tightly bound, giving boron a relatively high ionization energy for a Group III element. It is a metalloid which forms only covalent bonds with other atoms. At low temperatures, boron is a poor conductor of electricity; but as the temperature is raised and its electrons have more kinetic energy, the conductivity of boron increases. This behaviour is typical of a semiconductor.

Silicon atoms with four valence electrons, crystallize with a tetrahedral bond arrangement similar to that of carbon atoms in diamond. Its ionization energy and electronegativity are fairly high. It is a metalloid and forms covalent bonds with all other elements, except possibly the halogens. It is a semiconductor. Unlike carbon silicon forms only single bonds.

Statements 1-6.

1. Silicon forms silicon-silicon bonds or silicon-hydrogen bonds in preference to siliconoxygen bonds.   1.____
2. Boron has the highest electronegativity of the Group III elements.   2.____
3. Boron forms only covalent bonds.   3.____
4. The conductivity of silicon decreases with increasing temperature.   4.____
5. The electrical conductivity of metals decreases with an increase in temperature.   5.____
6. The valence electrons of silicon are held loosely.   6.____

KEY (CORRECT ANSWERS)

1. D
2. B
3. A
4. C
5. B
6. D

TEST 4

PASSAGE

There are several practical methods of softening water. Hard water containing HCO_3^- ions may be softened by boiling. The metal ions precipitate as carbonates. Sodium carbonate when added to hard water precipitates the metal ions responsible for hardness. Certain natural minerals known as zeolites have porous three-dimensional networks of silicate-aluminate groups that act as large fixed ions carrying negative charges. Metallic ions such as Na+ are attached to these complexes to form giant molecules. If hard water is permitted to stand in contact with sodium zeolite, the ions responsible for hardness replace the Na^+ ions. The exhausted zeolite may be regenerated. Synthetic ion-exchange resins of organic nature are of two types, acid-exchange resin or cation exchanger and base-exchange resin or anion exchanger. Combinations of these two types make possible the removal of both positive or negative ions in solution in water. Water so treated is called demineralized water and is now being used for many processes that formerly required distilled water.

Statements 1-6.

1. Temporary hard water may be softened by boiling.   1.____

2. Soluble solids may be entirely removed from water by the use of ion-exchange resins.   2.____

3. Temporary hard water cannot be softened by the use of sodium carbonate.   3.____

4. An application of the Law of Mass Action enables the exhausted zeolite to be regenerated.   4.____

5. A cation exchanger has large negatively charged organic units whose neutralizing ions in water solution are H_3O^- ions.   5.____

6. Other precipitating agents such as borax and trisodium phosphate are sometimes used to soften hard water.   6.____

KEY (CORRECT ANSWERS)

1. A
2. D
3. C
4. B
5. B
6. B

TEST 5

PASSAGE

An acid, defined in its narrower sense, is a substance with contains hydrogen, and yields hydrogen ions as the only positive ions in water solution. In the more general modern sense, an acid is a proton donor. Acids are covalent molecular substances which ionize in water solution. Nonmetallic oxides that combine with water to form acids are called acid anhydrides. Bases are substances which combine with the hydrogen ions from acids. The hydroxide ion is the most common base. The hydroxides of the active metals are ionic substances, those which are very soluble form solutions which are strongly basic. Ammonia dissolves in water to form a solution with a low concentration of ammonium ions. Metallic oxides of active metals are basic anhydrides.

Statements 1-6.

1. Sodium hydroxide forms a water solution which is strongly basic.   1.____

2. Water is amphiprotic, it may either gain or lose protons.   2.____

3. An acid is a proton acceptor.   3.____

4. All bases are hydroxides of active metals.   4.____

5. The number of acids represented in the equation: $HC_2H_3O_2 + H_2O = H_3O + C_2H_3O_2^-$ is two.   5.____

6. Acids are NOT ionic compounds.   6.____

KEY (CORRECT ANSWERS)

1. A
2. B
3. C
4. D
5. A
6. A

TEST 6

PASSAGE

The formation of body cells is called mitosis. After a cell has been formed it enters a period of growth and other activities called the interphase which is often referred to as the resting cell. At the end of this stage, the cell begins nuclear division or mitosis, the four stages of which are known as prophase, metaphase, anaphase, and telophase. In prophase the chromatin net condenses into double ribbons. These are the chromosomes. These become shorter and thicker until they appear as distinct rodlike bodies. The nuclear membrane gradually disappears and numerous fine threads composing the spindle form from poles above and below the nucleus. During the last part of prophase, the nuclear membrane and other parts of the nucleus are no longer visible. The next stage, the shortest of the four stages, is the metaphase. The chromosomes having arranged themselves along the imaginary center of the cell referred to as the equator are pulled apart lengthwise into two identical halves. During the next stage, the anaphase, the two sets of chromosomes move along the spindle thread in opposite directions toward the respective poles. Late in the anaphase in a plant cell, a cell plate forms across the middle of the spindle, which splits the cell into two halves. During the next stage, each of the new cells will form a wall along this cell plate. In an animal cell, indentations appear in the outer membrane and gradually deepen cutting the cell in half. Anaphase ends when the chromosomes have reached their poles. The final or telophase stage includes the formation of two daughter nuclei. The spindle fibers disappear gradually. The rod-shaped chromosomes reverse the process of shortening and become long, loosely tangled threads that again have the appearance of a chromatin network. The other nuclear contents reappear and become surrounded by a nuclear membrane. As each daughter cell is reorganizing, division of the cell in the region of the equator is completed.

Statements 1-6.

1. During anaphase, a wall forms along the cell plate in plant cells. 1.____

2. Metaphase is an easy stage to identify but the hardest to find in tissue prepared for microscopic study because it is the shortest of the four stages. 2.____

3. Chromosomes are pulled apart lengthwise into two identical halves during metaphase. 3.____

4. During interphase a cell carries on its normal activities including growth until maturity is reached and the process of mitosis starts. 4.____

5. In the reproductive cells of the human being there are 46 chromosomes. 5.____

6. Chromosomes first emerge as distinct rodlike bodies during metaphase. 6.____

KEY (CORRECT ANSWERS)

1. C
2. B
3. A
4. A
5. D
6. C

TEST 7

PASSAGE

Muscles produce movement. Voluntary muscles are under the control of our will. Involuntary muscles are never controlled by our will. They help in the operation of our digestive, respiratory, circulatory, and excretory systems.

The involuntary muscles are composed of spindle-shaped cells with one nucleus known as unstriated or smooth muscle. They form the walls of many internal organs such as the stomach and the layers of such muscle contract in waves to churn the food or pass it along. Artery walls also contain layers of smooth muscle.

Striated or skeletal muscle cells are long cylindrical cells with many nuclei (voluntary muscles). Such cells do not run the entire length of most muscles but are bound together in small bundles by sheaths of connective tissue. The small bundles are held together by a heavier sheath which encloses the entire muscle. They are bound to muscles and bone by tendons.

Cardiac muscle (heart) is similar to striated muscle when viewed under the microscope. The cells, however, are branched and contain special bands of material at intervals.

Statements 1-6.

1. Some muscles such as those in the eyelids and diaphragm are both voluntary and involuntary. 1.____

2. Smooth muscles are not controlled by the nervous system. 2.____

3. Heart muscle resembles voluntary muscle in appearance under the microscope. 3.____

4. Smooth muscle is bound together into small bundles by connective tissue sheaths and these bundles are enclosed by a heavier sheath enclosing the entire muscle. 4.____

5. Tendons connect muscles to bones. 5.____

6. Voluntary muscle cells have a single nucleus. 6.____

KEY (CORRECT ANSWERS)

1. B
2. D
3. A
4. C
5. A
6. C

TEST 8

PASSAGE

Elements of Group V, a family of non-transion elements, increase in metallic properties as their atomic number, atomic weight, and atomic size increase. Nitrogen and phosphorus are typical nonmetals showing such nonmetallic properties, such as covalent bonding with other atoms and are found in the negative ions of acids. Bismuth is a typical metal in its properties. Arsenic and antimony are metalloids. Each of these elements has five electrons in its outer shell. Two of these fill the first orbital of the outer shell. If the other three electrons are shared, the element has an oxidation number of +3. Nitrogen and the other members of this family also attain an oxidation number of +5 by forming a double bond and two single bonds with three atoms. Nitrogen is the most stable member of the family. Phosphorus is so active that one form of it will catch fire spontaneously in the air.

Statements 1-6.

1. Bismuth is the most metallic element in Group V.   1._____

2. Phosphorus forms hydrated positive ions in solution.   2._____

3. If an element of this family shares the two electrons which fill the first orbital of the outer shell, it has an oxidation number of +2.   3._____

4. Nitrogen's stability is due to the strength of the triple bond between the atoms in its molecule.   4._____

5. All elements of the family will burn when heated in air   5._____

6. Nitrogen has the smallest atomic radius.   6._____

KEY (CORRECT ANSWERS)

1. A
2. C
3. D
4. B
5. B
6. A

TEST 9

PASSAGE

Natural radiation may be used to determine the age of extinct or preserved animals or plants. One type of carbon, carbon 14, has an unstable nucleus and, therefore, is radioactive. It exists in the atmosphere as a result of cosmic rays striking nitrogen atoms which are converted to carbon 14. A low but constant level of radioactivity is maintained in living plants and animals through the carbon atoms involved in the carbon-dioxide-oxygen cycle. When living things die, the carbon atoms in their cells are no longer replaced and the radio-activity of the carbon atoms slowly diminishes. Half of the carbon 14 in a dead organism will be converted to the more common, non-radio-active carbon 12 in 5,570 years. The age of ancient specimens made of wood may be determined by comparing the radioactivity of the specimen with that of wood in living trees.

Artificial radioactive particles produced by atomic reactors and explosions may be carried all over the world. Strontium 90 is produced in some nuclear explosions. It has a half-life of 27 years. It may be taken up by plants and ingested by animals. Since it is chemically similar to calcium it accumulates in bones and can destroy tissue, cause cancer and death. Radioactive wastes from atomic re-actors must be dumped and constitute another international problem of contamination and danger from artificially produced radiation.

Statements 1-6.

1. The age of the earth may be determined by the study of radioactive substances found in the earth. 1.____

2. Carbon 14 cannot be produced in atomic reactors. 2.____

3. Carbon 14 is only found in living organisms. 3.____

4. The half-life period of carbon 14 is 5,570 years. 4.____

5. Carbon 14 is much more dangerous than strontium 90 because carbon 14 has a much longer half-life. 5.____

6. An article which has 1/2 the radioactivity of a specimen from a living tree is approximately 2,300 years old. 6.____

KEY (CORRECT ANSWERS)

1. B
2. D
3. C
4. A
5. D
6. C

TEST 10

PASSAGE

A study of traits in fruit flies has led scientists to believe that certain differences in inheritance are related to the sex chromosomes. Certain characteristics appear more frequently in one sex than in the other. These are called sex-linked traits. A cross was made between a red-eyed male fruit fly and a white-eyed female fruit fly. The result was 50% red-eyed females and 50% white-eyed males. Another cross using red-eyed females and white-eyed males produced 100% red-eyed offspring. Hence red-eyes are dominant over white-eyes. Furthermore, the Y-chromosome did not carry a factor for eye color so that whatever trait for eye color was on the X chromosome, when it united with the Y chromosome, appeared in the offspring. In the case of the first cross, the recessive factor appeared in males and in the second the factor for red-eyes appeared. The females could only be white eyed when both X chromosomes contained the gene for white eyes. If the X chromosome in a male had the gene for white eyes, the trait appeared, because the Y chromosome contained no gene for eye color. In man, hemophilia and color blindness are sex-linked.

Statements 1-6.

1. In fruit flies, red eyes are dominant over white eyes.

2. Because of sex linkage, no male fruit flies can be white eyed.

3. In human beings, only males are color blind.

4. Crossing a normal male with a female who is a carrier for hemophilia may result in the production of a normal (non-bleeder) male.

5. The mating of a red-eyed male with a white-eyed female produces 50% white-eyed females and 50% red-eyed males.

6. The descendants of a red-eyed male and a red-eyed female are all red-eyed females.

KEY (CORRECT ANSWERS)

1. A
2. C
3. D
4. B
5. C
6. C

TEST 11

PASSAGE

The two essential parts of the flower concerned with sexual reproduction are the stamens and the pistil. The stamen consists of a slender filament supporting the sac, known as the anther. Pollen grains, the male reproductive cells, develop in four pollen sacs in each anther. When the pollen is ripe, the anther splits. The transfer of the pollen is known as pollination. The pistil consists of a sticky top called the stigma, a stalk known as the style, and a swollen base or ovary which contains the ovules. The ovule is attached to the ovary wall by a slender stalk through which nourishment reaches the ovule during its development. The walls of the ovule are composed of two layers, or integuments. A tiny hole, the micropyle, leads through the integuments to the interior. An oval embryo sac occupies most of the interior of the ovule. It contains 8 nuclei at the time of fertilization. Three of these, the antipodals, lie in a group at the end of the embryo sac farthest from the micropyle. Near the center are the two polar nuclei. The largest nucleus at the end of the sac, nearest the micropyle, is the egg or female nucleus. On either side of the egg is a synergid.

When the pollen grain is ripe and leaves the anther it contains one generative nucleus and one tube nucleus. After the pollen grain reaches the stigma it develops a pollen tube, the generative nucleus dividing and forming two sperm nuclei. When the tube reaches the embryo sac in the ovule the sperm nuclei are discharged. One of the sperm nuclei unites with the egg in a union known as fertilization. The fertilized egg then becomes a zygote.

Statements 1-6.

1. Imperfect flowers on different plants are a guarantee of cross-pollination   1._____

2. The ovule contains two synergids.   2._____

3. The endosperm is formed by the union of one of the sperm nuclei with the polar nuclei.   3._____

4. Nourishment reaches the ovule through the tiny opening known as the micropyle.   4._____

5. Plant cells have only one nucleus.   5._____

6. The ovary develops into a fruit, after fertilization has occurred.   6._____

KEY (CORRECT ANSWERS)

1. B
2. A
3. D
4. C
5. C
6. B

TEST 12

PASSAGE

Maturation is a series of changes which the primary sex cells undergo to form gametes. Gametes are the two mature sex cells which unite to form a fertilized egg. The union of two dissimilar gametes is called fertilization. The nucleus of every cell contains chromosomes which are made up of genes, the trait determining structures. Each particular type of plant and animal has a definite number of chromosomes arranged in pairs. Every body cell of the fruit fly has 8 chromosomes (4 pairs). During fertilization when the sperm and egg nucleus fuse this diploid of chromosomes must be kept constant for the species.

The primary male sex cell becomes larger during maturation. Similar chromosomes of a pair come together and line up. The chromosome pairs separate and the cell divides. The daughter cells which are of the same size each have one member of a pair of chromosomes. This process is called reduction division and the number of chromosomes present in the cells (daughter) is known as the haploid number. The two new cells divide again by mitosis, the chromosomes splitting lengthwise. These cells then change shape, develop a tail and thus become sperm. The formation of eggs is similar to sperm formation. However, when the primary female sex cell undergoes reduction division, the cytoplasm divides unequally forming a large and a small daughter cell, the smallest cell being known as the polar body. In the next division, mitosis, the large cell again divides unequally but each of the two cells has the same number of chromosomes. The polar body also divides by mitosis so that there are now three polar bodies. These are useless and degenerate, resulting in only one true egg cell.

Statements 1-6.

1. Polar bodies are produced during the formation of sperm. 1._____

2. Primary sex cells have the diploid number of chromosomes. 2._____

3. A zygote has the haploid number of chromosomes. 3._____

4. Mitosis does not occur during the process of maturation. 4._____

5. The fertilized egg cell divides repeatedly without growth immediately following fertilization in a process known as cleavage. 5._____

6. More sperm cells are produced from a mature male primary sex cell than are eggs produced from a mature female primary sex cell. 6._____

KEY (CORRECT ANSWERS)

1. C
2. A
3. D
4. C
5. B
6. A

TEST 13

PASSAGE

Biologists believe that bacteria were among the first forms of life on earth. Long before there were any plants capable of carrying on photosynthesis, certain lowly bacteria probably synthesized sugar by obtaining energy from inorganic iron and sulfur compounds, instead of the sun.

Later when green plants began building up stores of organic compounds, other kinds of bacteria began using them as a food supply. Still other bacteria invaded the tissues of plants themselves as well as the bodies of animals.

Bacteria have survived through the ages and have increased their numbers until they are today the most abundant form of life. They live, invisibly, almost everywhere. They thrive in the air, in water, in food, in the soil, and in the bodies of host plants and animals. In fact, any environment which can support life in any form will have its population of bacteria.

Statements 1-6.

1. Today, bacteria are the most abundant form of life.   1.____

2. Originally bacteria were able to synthesize sugar by utilizing the sun's energy.   2.____

3. Most bacteria are harmful; therefore, our main problem is to kill bacteria.   3.____

4. The extensive deposits of iron ore we are using today are the result of bacterial action   4.____
   during ancient geological times.

5. Bacteria were among the first forms of life.   5.____

6. Nitrogen-fixing bacteria synthesize ammonia.   6.____

KEY (CORRECT ANSWERS)

1. A
2. C
3. D
4. B
5. A
6. D

TEST 14

PASSAGE

The small intestine is the most vital of all digestive centers. The upper ten inches constitute the duodenum, the second portion, the jejunum, is about seven and a half feet in length. The lower portion, the ileum is about 15 feet long and joins the large intestine.

The intestinal glands secret a fluid which contains erepsin which changes peptids to amino acids. Maltase, lactase, and sucrase are other enzymes. They split the respective polysaccharides into glu-cose. Pancreatic fluid is discharged into the small intestine through the pancreatic duct which leads to a common opening with the bile duct. This fluid contains trypsin which changes proteins, peptones, and proteoses to peptids; amylase which changes starch to maltese; and lipase which changes fats to fatty acids and glycerine. The liver secretes bile which emulsifies fats and activates lipase. Absorption takes place in the small intestine. The great number of villi (finger-like projections containing blood vessels and lacteals) bring the blood and lymph close to the digested food and increase the absorption surface of the intestine enormously.

Statements 1-6.

1. The small intestine is about 23 feet long.   1._____

2. Bile and pancreatic fluid are introduced into the small intestine through an opening in the duodenum.   2._____

3. Trypsin changes proteins into their simplest form, the amino acids.   3._____

4. Absorption occurs only in the small intestine.   4._____

5. Fatty acids and glycerine are absorbed by the lymphatics in the villi.   5._____

6. The bile helps make the contents of the small intestine more acidic.   6._____

KEY (CORRECT ANSWERS)

1. A
2. B
3. C
4. D
5. B
6. D

TEST 15

PASSAGE

A nerve impulse is known to be an electrochemical impulse which brings about a change in the nerve processes. When a nerve impulse passes along a nerve, carbon dioxide is liberated. A nerve impulse causes a muscle to contract by indirect stimulation. The impulse, traveling along the axon of a motor nerve, ends at the motor end plates at the tips of brushlike structures. Here the impulse causes the release of a minute amount of a chemical called acetylcholine. This substance transmits the impulse to muscle fibers, which begin a series of chemical reactions resulting in contraction. Following the brief period of contraction, the nerve releases cholinesterase which neutralizes acetylcholine causing the muscle fibers to relax.

Statements 1-6.

1. A nerve impulse is a flow of electricity. 1._____

2. Cholinesterase neutralizes acetylcholine. 2._____

3. Carbon dioxide liberated in the nerve causes the muscle to contract. 3._____

4. The nerve impulse to a muscle fiber travels along an axon. 4._____

5. Muscle fibers contract under the influence of acetylcholine and then relax after neutralization, all in 0.1 second or less. 5._____

6. A nerve impulse causes a muscle to contract by direct stimulation. 6._____

KEY (CORRECT ANSWERS)

1. D
2. A
3. C
4. A
5. B
6. C

TEST 16

PASSAGE

Valence means the combining capacity of an element. Chemical bonds are produced when valence electrons are either transferred from the outer shell of one atom to the outer shell of another atom, or are shared with electrons in the outer shell of another atom. The formation of chemical bonds usually enables an atom to acquire a chemically stable outer shell consisting of an octet of electrons.

There are two types of bonding. 1. Ionic bonding in which electrons are actually transferred from the outer shell of one atom to the outer shell of a second atom. The resultant particles are ions-atoms or groups of atoms with an unbalanced electrostatic charge. 2. Covalent bonding, in which two atoms share a pair of electrons, and form molecules.

Statements 1-6.

1. A chemically stable outer shell consists of an octet of electrons. 1.____

2. A polar covalent bond is formed when two unlike atoms share a pair of electrons. 2.____

3. Covalent bonds result in atoms with an unbalanced electrostatic charge. 3.____

4. Lead achieves an oxidation state of +2 by transferring its outermost S electrons. 4.____

5. Lithium acquires an outer shell consisting of an octet of electrons when it combines with chlorine. 5.____

6. The H-H bond in the H_2 molecule is nonpolar covalent. 6.____

KEY (CORRECT ANSWERS)

1. A
2. B
3. C
4. D
5. D
6. B

TEST 17

PASSAGE

Amphibia means, literally, "having two lives." It refers to the fact that the frog and its relatives (salamanders and newts) are, for the most part, aquatic, fishlike animals when young, but land-dwellers when they become adults. This series of changes is a metamorphosis. In this transition many strange combinations of gills and lungs, fins and legs occur.

In general, the Amphibia are distinct from other vertebrate animals in the following ways:

(1) body covered by a thin, flexible skin without scales, fur, or feathers; (2) feet, if present, often webbed;
(3) immature or larval forms, vegetarian; adults usually carnivorous;
(4) heart two-chambered in larvae, but three-chambered in adults;
(5) metamorphosis occurring, i.e., from tadpole to adult frog.

Statements 1-6.

1. Frogs are different from other amphibians in that they lack tails in the adult stage.　　1.____

2. The tadpole is the larval stage of the frog.　　2.____

3. Adult amphibia always have feet.　　3.____

4. Eggs of amphibia are fertilized internally.　　4.____

5. Gills may be found on animals with legs and fins may occur accompanied by lungs.　　5.____

6. The heart of the adult frog has two auricles.　　6.____

KEY (CORRECT ANSWERS)

1. B
2. A
3. C
4. D
5. A
6. B

280

TEST 18

PASSAGE

Water molecules are covalent molecules. The electrons are unevenly distributed, causing the oxygen end of the molecule to be more negative, and the hydrogen end more positive. Electrovalent compounds are composed of ions. Water dipoles exert an attracting force on these ions, weakening their bonds. The ions enter solutions as hydrated particles, that is, loosely bonded to water dipoles. Polar covalent molecules may ionize in water solution as hydrated ions. Strong electrolytes ionize completely (practically), weak electrolytes only slightly. Water ionizes very slightly, forming hydrogen ions and hydroxide ions. Hydrogen ions are never free in water solutions but are hydrates in the form of hydronium ions.

Statements 1-6.

1. A 1 molal solution of an electrolyte raises the boiling point and lowers the freezing point to the same degree as does a 1 molal solution of a non-electrolyte. 1.____

2. The water molecule is non-linear and, therefore, polar. 2.____

3. Electrovalent compounds dissociate into ions when they undergo melting. 3.____

4. Hydronium ions are hydrated hydrogen ions. 4.____

5. Since water is composed of covalent molecules, it does not ionize. 5.____

6. Increasing the dilution of a concentrated solution of a weak electrolyte increases the degree of ionization of the electrolyte. 6.____

KEY (CORRECT ANSWERS)

1. D
2. B
3. B
4. A
5. C
6. B

TEST 19

PASSAGE

Spermatophyta, a phylum of the plant kingdom includes all plants which produce seeds. A seed is an embryo plant covered by one or more protective seed coats. Food stored in a seed nourishes the young plant until it is established in its new location. A seed is a packaged plant ready for delivery. A seed may travel through the air, on water, be carried by animals, or lie dormant for many months. When conditions are favorable, the coat gets soft, and the young plant emerges. The plumule becomes the leaves. The hypocotyl becomes the stem and roots. Gymnospermae are the more primitive and older seed plants and their seeds are not enclosed in a fruit. They flourished in the early stages as far back as the carboniferous period. The angiospermae are flowering plants and are divided into the monocots and the dicots. The monocots produce a single seed leaf while the dicots have two.

Statements 1-6.

1. All plants produce seeds.   1.____
2. A seed contains stored food.   2.____
3. The seed plants have gained domination of the earth.   3.____
4. Gymnosperms are of no value to our civilization.   4.____
5. Flowering plants produce fruit which enclose the seed.   5.____
6. The plumule synthesizes all the food needed for the seed to germinate. 6.____

KEY (CORRECT ANSWERS)

1. C
2. A
3. B
4. D
5. B
6. C

TEST 20

PASSAGE

A colloidal suspension is a two-phase system consisting of a dispersed phase and a dispersing medium. The dispersed substance is known as the internal phase, and the dispersing medium is known as the external phase. The colloidal state is one of subdivision rather than chemical nature. There is no fine line of demarcation between solutions and colloidal suspensions, and between colloidal suspensions and temporary suspensions. Colloids fall into an inter-mediate position between molecular size and visible size, and range in diameters from 10 to 1,000 Angstroms. The subdivision of materials results in a great increase in specific surface and results in the phenomenon of adsorption. Adsorption is both specific and selective.

Statements 1-6.

1. A colloidal suspension may be made by grinding corn starch in a mortar and then mixing thoroughly with water. The water is the internal phase. 1.____

2. Activated coconut charcoal used in gask mask canisters will selectively adsorb most toxic gases in preference to oxygen and nitrogen. 2.____

3. Coarse suspensions (temporary suspensions) may be made into colloids by reduction in the size of suspended particle. 3.____

4. A colloidal dispersion of gas in gas is possible. 4.____

5. A particle whose diameter is approximately 1×10^{-6} centimeters is in the colloidal dimension range. 5.____

6. Adsorption is due to the chemical nature of the colloidal particle rather than to its relatively large amount of surface. 6.____

KEY (CORRECT ANSWERS)

1. C
2. B
3. A
4. D
5. A
6. B

TEST 21

PASSAGE

The lungs of a bird lie in the back against the ribs in the anterior region of the body cavity. The capacity of the lungs is greatly increased by a system of air sacs which extend from the lungs into the chest area and the abdomen and connect with cavities in the larger bones. Air is drawn through the nostrils in the beak and down the traches and its lower divisions (bronchi) to the lungs and air sacs by relaxation of the thoracic and abdominal muscles. Contraction of these muscles forces the air out. Though the lungs are small, the rapid respiration rate fills them often.

The bird's respiratory system is also its principal temperature-regulating system. It has no sweat glands. Most excess heat is discharged from the body through the lungs.
Statements 1-6.

1. The bird's lungs are in the front of its chest. 1.____

2. Birds often pant on a hot day indicating that the air sacs assist in heat elimination. 2.____

3. Birds have no sweat glands. 3.____

4. The bird's song is produced in the throat where the song box is located. 4.____

5. Air sacs are found connected to cavities in the bones. 5.____

6. The diaphragm separates the bird's body cavity into a chest and abdominal section. 6.____

KEY (CORRECT ANSWERS)

1. C
2. B
3. A
4. D
5. A
6. B

TEST 22

PASSAGE

Carbohydrates, fats, and proteins are organic nutrients containing carbon and having originally been formed by living cells. Carbohydrates are primarily fuel foods and make up more than half of your total diet. They are oxidized rapidly to supply energy for body activity, such energy value being measured in Calories.

A saccharide is any one of a group of carbohydrates which includes the sugars and starches. A saccharide unit is called a hexose and is composed of six atoms of carbon and six molecules of water.

Monosaccharides, the simple sugars, are composed of one hexose molecule. Disaccharides consist of two hexose molecules and require conversion to simple sugars before absorption into the blood. Starches are polysaccharides which consist of many hexose molecules joined together. One class of carbohydrates, the celluloses, come from plant cell walls and are indigestible in man. Carbohydrates are stored in the liver of man as glycogen or animal starch. If it were not for the liver, we would have to eat a small quantity of food continuously. Excess sugar, carried by the blood, is converted to glycogen in the liver. When the level of blood sugar decreases, the glycogen is converted back to sugar.

Statements 1-6.

1. Celluloses are polysaccharides.   1.____
2. Glycogen supplies the blood with disaccharides when they are needed.   2.____
3. Carbohydrates yield more energy than other organic nutrients of equal weight. 3.____
4. A Calorie is an energy unit.   4.____
5. Carbohydrates usually constitute more than 50% of one's diet.   5.____
6. Protein foods may be used to yield energy.   6.____

KEY (CORRECT ANSWERS)

1. B
2. C
3. D
4. A
5. A
6. B

TEST 23

PASSAGE

Rhizopus is the genus name for this member of the Phycomycetes. This mold (bread mold) starts as a microscopic spore which grows on the surface of bread forming a network of silvery, tubular hyphae. Within a few days, the mold grows over the surface of the bread, forming a cottonlike mass of hyphae, the mycelium. This is composed of several distinct kinds of hyphae. Those hyphae spreading over the surface of the food supply are called stolons. At intervals along the stolons, clusters of tiny rootlike hyphae, or rhizoids, penetrate the food supply and absorb nourishment. Rhizoids secrete digestive enzymes which act on the sugar, starch, and other carbohydrates in the bread. These digested foods are then absorbed into the hyphae of the mold. After a few days of growth on the bread surface, black knobs appear among the hyphae of the bread mold. Each black knob is a spore case or sporangium which is produced at the tip of a special ascending hypha or sporangiophore. Each sporangium is a thin-walled case containing thousands of black spores. When it dries out, its wall splits releasing the spores.

Statements 1-6.

1. A hypha is an elongated structure composed of many cells.   1.____
2. A spore is a sexual reproductive cell.   2.____
3. Rhizoids absorb nourishment.   3.____
4. Spore cases are produced at the tips of rhizoids.   4.____
5. A mycelium is a mass of hyphae.   5.____
6. Although certain fungi are colored blue or green, they do not contain chlorophyll.   6.____

KEY (CORRECT ANSWERS)

1. B
2. D
3. A
4. C
5. A
6. B

TEST 24

PASSAGE

The energy required to remove an electron from an atom is ionization energy, and is usually expressed in electron-volts. Low ionization energy is characteristic of a metal, while high ionization energy is characteristic of a nonmetal. An intermediate ionization energy is characteristic of a metalloid. Within groups of elements, the ionization energy generally decreases with increasing atomic number. Ionization energy is a periodic property, increasing from Group I to Group VIII.

Statements 1-6.

1. The ionization energy of magnesium is greater than that of sodium. 1.____

2. The ionization energy of sodium is greater than that of potassium. 2.____

3. There is a decrease in ionization energy between Groups II and III in Periods 2 and 3. 3.____

4. Ionization energy varies uniformly from atom to atom within a series. 4.____

5. Apparent irregularities occur in ionization energy between the last transition element and Group III because of extra stability of completed sublevels. 5.____

6. The ionization energy of neon is greater than that of fluorine. 6.____

KEY (CORRECT ANSWERS)

1. A
2. C
3. B
4. D
5. B
6. A

TEST 25

PASSAGE

A substance which loses electrons is said to be oxidized. A substance which gains electrons is said to be reduced. Both processes occur simultaneously. In such oxidation-reduction reactions, electrons are transferred completely between ionic substances and partially between covalent substances. Oxidation numbers may be assigned to each element according to certain rules. Elements un-combined in compounds, have an oxidation number of zero. In ionic compounds, the oxidation number corresponds to the ionic valence. Oxygen in a compound, generally, has an oxidation number of -2. Hydrogen usually has an oxidation number of +1.

1. In the reaction, $CuO + H_2 = Cu + H_2O$, the substance which is oxidized is the hydrogen. 1.____

2. The total number of electrons lost by the reducing agent is equal to the total number of electrons gained by the oxidizing agent during an oxidation-reduction reaction. 2.____

3. In a compound, an element cannot have an oxidation number of zero. 3.____

4. In Al_2O_3 the oxidation number of the Al is +2. 4.____

5. The oxidation number of hydrogen in H_2 is +1. 5.____

6. A substance which is oxidized is a reducing agent, while a substance which is reduced is an oxidizing agent. 6.____

KEY (CORRECT ANSWERS)

1. A
2. B
3. D
4. C
5. C
6. A

---

300 BASIC PRINCIPLES OF THE BIOLOGICAL SCIENCES

CONTENTS

		Page
I.	GEOGRAPHIC DISTRIBUTION	1
II.	ECOLOGICAL RELATIONSHIPS	1
III.	TAXONOMY	3
IV.	MODIFICATION OF SPECIES	3
V.	GENETICS AND HEREDITY	6
VI.	EMBRYONIC DEVELOPMENT	8
VII.	MORPHOLOGY AND PHYSIOLOGY	8
VIII.	ORGANIZATION	11
IX.	PROTOPLASM AND CELLS	11
X.	ENERGY, MATTER AND LIFE	14
XI.	PALEONTOLOGY	15
XII.	APPLIED BIOLOGY	16

300 Basic Principles of the Biological Sciences

I. GEOGRAPHIC DISTRIBUTION
1. Living things are not distributed uniformly or at random over the surfaces of the earth, but are found in definite zones and local regions where conditions are favorable to their survival.
2. Stretches of water act as barriers to purely terrestrial animals, and stretches of land bar the migrations of the inhabitants of water.
3. Life exists from the depths of the ocean to the mountain heights.
4. Each species of animal or plant tends to extend its range until some impossible barrier is encountered.
5. The distribution of any group of land animals will depend upon three factors – first, upon the region where the group happened to originate; second, upon the connections which this region then and later happened to have with other land masses; and third, upon the fate of the group in the different regions to which it obtained access.
6. Discontinuous widespread distribution is characteristic of old groups of animals and means that they formerly occupied also much of the intervening space.
7. Most regions that are surrounded by barriers are devoid of a very great variety of species of animals or plants. However, the larger the area isolated, the greater the variety of forms.
8. For most species of organism, periods of great scarcity of individuals' alternate with waves of great abundance, and the peaks of the waves succeed each other in a regular cycle.
9. When new species are introduced into a country, few individuals or species will find themselves in the same balance as in their old home. For the majority, conditions will be unfavorable; they will fail to gain a footing and some will disappear. If the introduced species chances to be better suited, especially if it is removed from its old enemies and parasites, its numbers will increase often far beyond anything possible to it in its native country; not infrequently its abundance will force it into changed habits.
10. In general, the natural flora and fauna of a region is the most luxuriant that it can support.
11. New species of plants and animals appear at some definite point on the earth and then spread out from that location as a center.

II. ECOLOGICAL RELATIONSHIPS
   A. Environment and Living Things
      1. The environment acts upon living things, and living things act upon their environment.
      2. The environment of living things changes continually.
      3. All living things are continually engaged in an exacting struggle with their environments.
   B. Life Necessities
      1. Food, oxygen, certain optimal conditions of temperature, moisture, and light are essential to the life of most living things.
      2. Life, as we know it, is dependent upon complex chemical compounds of carbon, nitrogen, hydrogen, oxygen, and other elements.
      3. Water is essential to all living things because protoplasmic activity is dependent upon an adequate water supply.

4. Life may exist under conditions of light from bright sunlight to the complete darkness of caves or of depths of soil or water.
5. The range of temperature for life activities is very narrow as compared with the range of possible temperatures. There is a minimum temperature below which, and a maximum temperature above which, no life processes are carried on. The temperature range for life processes is from many degrees below 0°C. to nearly the boiling point of water.

C. Limiting Factors
1. Life is wholly confined to the surface of the planet earth and to a few miles above and below its surface (as far as our certain knowledge goes) and no one single form of life is able to span even these limits.
2. Living organisms cannot live in the upper levels of the atmosphere because of deficiency of oxygen for respiration, deficiency of pressure upon the exterior of the body, and intense cold.
3. The numbers of any species depend, on the one hand, upon its rate of reproduction and growth, and on the other, upon its death rate from accident, enemies, and disease.

D. Interdependence
1. All plants and animals are engaged in a constant struggle for energy.
2. Every living species is continually producing a multitude of individuals, many more than can survive, varying more or less among themselves, and all competing against each other for the available energy.
3. Change in the numbers of organisms in communities may be rapid even though the environmental conditions apparently alter slowly and gradually.
4. The existence of organisms depends upon their interrelations with the environment which includes both the inorganic world and other organisms.
5. A balance in nature is maintained through interrelations of plants and animals with each other and with their physical environment.
6. When the balance of nature is disturbed, disastrous results often follow.
7. The first forms of life were altogether independent, but evolution has resulted in the general interdependence of organisms,
8. Certain associations of plants and animals are the result of a struggle for survival; for example, community or social life, parasitism and symbiosis.
9. All gradations of association occur in intimate associations between organisms, from those which are mutually beneficial to the individuals concerned (symbiosis) to those in which one member secures all the advantage at the expense of the other (parasitism).
10. Commensalism usually evolves, not in the direction of mutualism, but toward parasitism.
11. The parasite-host relationship is usually specific and requires not only marked adaptation on the part of the parasite but often also an adjustment on the part of the host.
12. It is indispensable to successful parasitic existence that the relationship be so adjusted that means are provided for the escape of the parasites or their offspring in order that new generations in new hosts may obtain.
13. True parasites secure their nourishment from the host plant or animal without exerting an injurious effect; pathogens damage the host by invading the tissues, multiplying there and producing infection.
14. A characteristic of many parasites is that they have alternate hosts.

15. Saprophytic organisms are responsible for decay by which process the necessary raw materials for growth of new organisms are released from dead matter.
16. The continuance of higher forms of life in anything like the present kinds and numbers would be impossible without bacteria and molds. They break down the complex carbohydrate and protein substances of dead plants and animals into simpler substances which may then be used again by living plants.
17. All the higher forms of terrestrial life are dependent either directly or indirectly on the soil bacteria for their nitrogen supply.
18. Life depends for its primal food supply upon chlorophyll-bearing plants and, for its sustained supply, upon bacteria. The whole of life, considered chemically, is one cyclic process from chlorophyll-bearing plant to bacteria and so again to chlorophyll-bearing plant.
19. The oxygen of the atmosphere is removed by animals and returned by chlorophyll-bearing plants.
20. The nutritional processes of different classes of organisms supplement each other in such a manner that they result in a nutritional balance among living things.

E. Soil and Soil Minerals
1. Plants and animals are directly or indirectly dependent on the soil.
2. All plant and animal life, along with the climate and varying weather, play an active part in helping to form and to change the soil.
3. Parent material for the development of soils is formed through the physical disintegration and chemical decomposition of rock particles and organic matter.
4. Only the topsoil, with its rich organic matter, its porous structure, and its living organisms, can hold the water and provide the minerals necessary to the life of most plants.

III. TAXONOMY
1. The present variety in living forms has resulted from the modifications through long periods of time of simpler and less varied ancestral types, and by degeneration in many groups of organisms from more complex organisms.
2. Similar organisms are grouped together because they are believed to be related through common descent.
3. Evolutionary relationships in organisms are formulated on the basis of structural similarity.
4. In all organisms, increasing complexity of structure is accomplished by an increasing division of labor.
5. In general, living things give evidence of a definite progression from simple to complex forms.
6. The greater the similarity in structure between organisms the closer is their kinship; the less the similarity in structure, the more remote is their common ancestry.

IV. MODIFICATION OF SPECIES
A. General
1. All life comes from preceding life.
2. One of the most "constant" features of natural phenomena is variability, but variability is always within definite limits.
3. Living things, even of the same kind, are never exactly alike, not even with regard to single traits (characteristics) such as color or shape.
4. Organisms which have no means of reproduction other than asexual show very little variation.
5. The evolution of the earth and the living things inhabiting it has resulted from the operation of natural forces.

6. Living things alter their types; present species have not always existed, but have originated by descent from others which in turn were derived from still earlier ones, and so down to the first living forms.
7. The forms of living things have changed slowly but steadily in the past except for those resulting from mutations,
8. Evolution has needed enormous lapses of time for its operations.
9. The existing forms of life on the earth are not all the forms of life which have existed; there has been a great variety of animals and plants which have passed away.
10. The crises of evolution when they occur are not crises of variation but of selection and elimination; not strange births but selective massacres. The germ plasm has gone on throwing up mutations at about the same rate age after age.
11. Most of the species of modern animals are of relatively recent origin; having evolved from others in the past and probably continuing to evolve into other species of animals.
12. As nature progressed in the production of new forms, new potentialities also were added.
13. Variation and heredity together are responsible for the appearance and the continuation of the processes of evolution.
14. In organisms, the more similar the body structures and their mode of origin, and the greater the number of such structures, the closer the relationship of the organisms.
15. If two or more groups of organisms have similar homologous structures they have descended from similar ancestors or from the same common ancestor.
16. Analogous structures in plants and animals serve to carry on similar functions but they are not similar in basic plan or mode of origin.
17. Adult organisms that differ greatly from one another but which show fundamental similarities in embryological development have originated from similar ancestors.
18. Similarity between organisms suggests common ancestry; the nature of the differences between them indicates which is the more primitive type.
19. The embryos of different animals, in addition to being more like each other as development is traced backward, show also a widening contrast with their parents and their adult destiny.
20. The greater the period that has elapsed since two stocks diverged, the greater the difference in the terminal products.
21. In organisms inhabiting similar environments evolution has often produced convergence - the molding of unrelated stocks into similar forms by the needs of their way of life.
22. Animals of diverse origin living among similar surroundings tend to become, at least superficially, alike and they often develop parts that have the same function.
23. Isolation of a piece of land or a body of water from the rest of the world always permits its animal and plant inhabitants to evolve along their own peculiar lines and each race involved tends to become more uniform.
24. New types of living things arise through variations in previously existing kinds.
25. Plants and animals in the course of their generations are changed and molded to meet the requirements of their existence, and the individuals and types best adapted to their life situations are the ones that survive.
26. During the main evolution of any stock, for each type of organism that lives on to be ancestral to the next evolutionary phase, there are considerable numbers thrown off to live a few tens of thousands of years and die without descendants.

27. Every species of organism is subject to certain checks or controls in the form of enemies and only those members that are most capable of avoiding their enemies survive to reproduce new offspring and thereby transmit many of their characters to their offspring.

B. Mutations
1. The genes of all organisms are subject to change, such changes producing heritable modifications in organisms called mutations.
2. The history of organisms shows that evolution and race divergence has been the result of mutations.
3. All heritable variations which are not the result of recombinations of genes are mutations, which are changes in genes, in some cases induced by environmental agents.
4. New kinds of living things have arisen through mutation.
5. Any hereditary change that follows the laws of Mendelian heredity is due to a gene mutation.
6. Mutations occur independently of the activities of individuals as more or less haphazard hereditary variations.

C. Adaptations
1. All living things are slowly changing, both structurally and functionally, in response to changes in their physical environments.
2. The surface of the earth and the atmosphere surrounding the earth are undergoing constant changes; therefore in order to survive, organisms must migrate, hibernate, aestivate, build artificial shelters, or otherwise become adapted to these changes.
3. Species not fitted to the conditions about them do not thrive and finally become extinct.
4. The organisms most likely to survive and reproduce are those that are structurally and physiologically best fitted to their environments.
5. Some of the differences between related groups of organisms separated by a geographical barrier are due to adaptive responses to slightly different environmental factors.
6. In higher plants and in the higher air-breathing vertebrates, a progressive emancipation from life in water and an adaptation to life on dry land is traceable.
7. The chief difference in the structure of organisms from the lowest to the highest are resultant of the means adopted to perform certain functions under different exigencies imposed by the environment and mode of life.
8. Protective adaptations aid survival.
9. The biological functions of color are to conceal, to disguise, or to advertise.
10. Chlorophyll-bearing plants are adapted for food making.
11. In a living organism, adaptation of action and adaptation of structure are necessary for survival.
12. Every living organism possesses some body parts which are adapted for the life it leads.
13. Each species of living organism is adapted, or is in the process of becoming adapted, to live where it is found.
14. The power of living things to change is definitely restricted; specialization reaches the limit of efficiency prescribed by mechanical or chemical laws.
15. The more highly specialized an organism is, the more likely it is to become extinct if its environment changes.

16. An adaptive character may give its possessors a definite advantage over other members of the species, and so in the course of generations, due to the elimination of the non-possessors of this character, and of the conferring of this character upon others by heredity, becoming a character of all the members of the species.
17. Animals and plants lacking some means of mechanical support are debarred from terrestrial life.
18. In the water, free swimming organisms are very light becuase their specific gravity is only slightly greater than that of the medium in which they live.
19. Water-living organisms do not merely dilute their weight but counteract it by accumulating lighter substances inside themselves.
20. Those organisms which cannot adjust themselves to their environment lose out in the struggle for existence.

V. GENETICS AND HEREDITY
  A. General
    1. Living things come only from living things.
    2. The germ plasm of animals and plants passes on from generation to generation and there has been a continuous stream from the first organism to the present living organisms.
    3. The fundamental function of the germ plasm is the perpetuation of the species; the body or somoplasm serves as the vehicle for the germ plasm.
    4. Every cell originated from a cell and every chromosome from a chromosome.
    5. The genes in the chromosomes of eggs and sperms are the physical basis of heredity.
  B. Chromosomes
    1. All cells within one multi-cellular individual, except the gametes in animals and the spores in plants, are characterized by the same chromosomal content, as they all originated by cell division from a common cell.
    2. All individuals of a unicellular species, except asexual species, contain the same set or "similar sets" of chromosomes.
    3. Each kind of living thing has its characteristic chromosome complement, and the constancy of that complement is preserved at each cell division. Different species show the utmost diversity in number, size, and form of chromosomes.
    4. The number of chromosomes in the somatic cells of all the individuals of a species is a constant, except in chimeras, gynandromorphs, etc.
    5. In the maturation of the sex cells at the pairing of the chromosomes, except for the single sex chromosomes in some organisms, the two members of each pair come originally, one from the paternal line and one from the maternal line.
    6. In fertilization in most bi-sexual organisms, the egg contributes half (+ 1 or -1) the specific number of chromosomes to the zygote as does also the sperm.
    7. The separation of homologous chromosomes at reduction division in the germ cell is a matter of chance, the separation in any one pair occurs absolutely without reference to what had occurred in any other pair in the cell.
  C. Genes
    1. The hereditary characteristics possessed by any organism depend wholly upon the genes that were transmitted to it in the reproductive cells received from its parents.
    2. The hereditary characters in all organisms are determined by the genes which are carried in the chromosomes.
    3. Living things reproduce offspring which possess the genes of their ancestors though these offspring do not necessarily resemble any one of these ancestors.

4. In most cases, a character is not determined by a single gene, but by the interplay of two or more genes; in this interaction the genes may interfere with, modify, counteract, or reinforce each other.
5. Genes that lie in the same chromosome tend to remain together in reduction division so that the characters which they determine are linked in inheritance.
6. The greater the distance two genes lie apart in the chromosome the more often will they separate and cross over when a chromosome fragments and part of it adheres to another chromosome.
7. The sex chromosome may carry the genes for a number of characters other than sex. Such characters are sex linked.

D. Meiosis
1. Meiosis or "chromosome reduction" from the diploid to the haploid number occurs at some stage in all organisms in which sexual processes take place; and when followed by the return to the diploid number of chromosomes at fertilization, it keeps the number of chromosomes constant for the species.
2. In plants and animals subject to parthenogenetic development (development from unfertilized germinal cells), reduction of the number of chromosomes does not occur.
3. During the process of maturation in an egg or a sperm, corresponding maternal and paternal chromosomes, with their genes, go to different cells in the reduction division so that each secondary oocyte or spermatocyte receives one, but not both, of these chromosomes with its genes.
4. No relation exists between the common origin of chromosomes from the same gamete and their later distribution during chromosome reduction. Chance alone seems to determine how the chromosomes are distributed.
5. The heredity of an individual organism produced by sexual means is determined by what occurs to the chromosomes in the reduction division in maturation and in fertilization.
6. In plants the gamete-bearing phase of the life cycle is haploid; the spore-bearing phase is diploid. The reduction division occurs during spore formation.

E. Mendel's Laws
1. Since the genes of the two parents combine at random in the germ cells and since the germ cells meet at random in fertilization, the individuals of any generation occur in certain predictable ratios.
2. In the second and later generations of a hybrid, every possible combination of the parent character occurs, and each combination appears in a definite proportion of the individuals.
3. Every individual organism is composed of distinct hereditary characters which are transmitted by distinct hereditary factors (genes). In a hybrid the different parental genes are combined. When the sex cells of the hybrid are formed the two parental genes separate again, remaining quite unchanged and pure, each sex cell containing only one of the two genes of one pair.
4. All individuals of the first generation of hybrids, the F_1 generation, are uniform in appearance in alternative inheritance. Only one of the two parental characters, the stronger or the dominant one, is shown; in intermediate inheritance a mixture of the parental characteristics is shown.
5. In a cross of the F_2 generation of hybrids the genes which determine the characters are segregated in the gametes so that a certain percent of the offspring possess the dominant character alone, a certain percent the recessive character alone, while a certain percent are again hybrid in nature.

6. In polyhybrid crossings (F individuals with two or more pairs of hereditary characters) all possible combinations of the parental characters are shown in characteristic ratios.
7. Sex is inherited; it follows a given distribution of the chromosomes according to definite Mendelian ratios.
8. Animals resemble each other more and more closely the farther back we pursue them in embryological development.
9. The life history of the individual tends in a very general way to recapitulate the history of the race.
10. Acquired characters are not inherited.
11. Fluctuating variations found within a pure line are not inherited and cannot change the character of the offspring permanently.
12. Heredity supplies the native capacities of an organism; environment determines to a large extent how fully these capacities will be developed.
13. Cells within an organism are dependent upon their immediate cellular environment as well as their genes, in the process of becoming what they finally become.
14. Many hereditary characters are subject to non-genetic or environmental variation in expression.
15. Inbreeding in animals or plants results in a uniform strain.
16. Reversion occurs only when different varieties of plants or animals are crossed, or in subsequent generations following a cross, never in genetically pure stocks.
17. Hybridization gives variation, isolation gives fixation, and fixation gives speciation.
18. New types of organisms, different enough to be regarded as new species, may result from a cross.

VI. EMBRYONIC DEVELOPMENT
1. All embryos start from a single fertilized egg cell and grow through division and redivision into the form of the organism which produces the egg cell.
2. Similarities in the embryological development of organisms show hereditary relationships between these organisms and the closer two species are related the longer they parallel one another in development.
3. The action of "organizers" (probably chemical in character) produced in the developing embryo causes the developing egg, which at first acts as a whole, to produce specialized parts which develop independently.

VII. MORPHOLOGY AND PHYSIOLOGY
A. Physical Support and Movement
1. In many multicellular organisms body form is secured and maintained either by the consistency of the tissues and the internal pressure of body fluids, or by the secretion of special substances which are formed into supporting structures.
2. A characteristic of living organisms is the power of independent motion, either of protoplasm within the cell or of the body as a whole.
3. The power of contraction which results in movement is possessed by all protoplasm to a greater or lesser degree.
4. The difference in motion and locomotion between animals and plants is one of degree.

B. Material for Growth and Replacement
1. Growth and repair are fundamental activities for all protoplasm.
2. Plants and animals utilize similar food substances but they are obtained in different ways.

3. The carbohydrate foods made by the chloroplasts of chlorophyll-bearing plants are the original source of all energy used by plants themselves (except by the autotrophic bacteria) as well as that used by animals.
4. Starches, fats and proteins are produced by plants and it is upon these that all animals depend primarily for food.
5. The food requirements of every living thing are: fuels capable of yielding, when oxidized, the supply of energy without which life cannot continue; materials for growth and for replacement for the slight wearing away of the living tissue involved in any activity; minerals, the necessary constituents of cell structures, of cell products, and of the bathing fluid of cells; the vitamins or "accessory" food factors.
6. An animal cannot live without proteins. They are necessary in cell growth and maintenance; so are necessities in the diets of animals. Plants are able to use carbohydrates and nitrates to build up the proteins necessary for growth and maintenance of their cells.
7. Digestion in plants and animals is carried on by enzymes, or organic catalysts, which are made by the organisms themselves and which take part in and speed up the chemical reactions but do not undergo any permanent chemical change themselves.
8. Digestion accomplishes two things: it makes food soluble in water, thus enabling the nutrients to pass through membranes and thereby reach and enter the cells; it reduces complex nutrients (fats, proteins, and carbohydrates) to simple building materials which in turn can be rebuilt into whatever living material or structural feature is necessary at the place of use.
9. All cells contain autolytic enzymes that at death are capable of producing digestive changes which result in the final disintegration of the body,

C. Respiration and Release of Energy
1. Cellular respiration (aerobic decomposition) occurs in all living cells and all organisms possess structures by means of which it can be carried on. Its first step is intake of oxygen either directly from the air or dissolved in water, its final product is carbon dioxide, and free energy is released. In the cells it is accomplished at ordinary temperatures by the intervention of special enzymes.
2. Anaerobic decomposition (fermentation) is accomplished at ordinary temperatures by the intervention of special enzymes, dissimilation occurs in the absence of oxygen, its final products are carbon dioxide and alcohol, and free energy is released.
3. The respiratory process of both plants and animals involves exactly the same gaseous exchange and accomplishes the same function the release of energy.
4. Oxygen free in the atmosphere or dissolved in water supplies the respiratory needs of practically all living organisms, except for a few parasitic and anaerobic animals, and a number of bacteria and fungi which can extract the oxygen needed for their energy production from the organic substances on which they feed.
5. Carbon dioxide set free during the respiration of both plants and animals is absorbed by plants and used as a raw material of photosynthesis.

D. Internal Transportation
1. Circulation is carried on in all living organisms. With increase in size and complexity of the body of an organism there goes a corresponding elaboration of the transportation (circulatory) system.

E. Disposal of Wastes
   1. In organisms the end products of metabolism, water, carbon dioxide, and nitrogenous compounds are either stored in the cells as insoluble crystals; are eliminated in solution by diffusion, or osmosis (excretion); are incorporated into useful cell products (secretion); or are recombined into food substances within the organism.

F. Integration of Activities
   1. All living things respond to stimuli in their environment.
   2. The nature of the response made by a cell to a stimulus is determined by the nature of the responding protoplasm, as well as by the kind of stimulus.
   3. In general, the extent of a response is rather definitely fixed for any given nerve cell. If a cell responds at all, it does so to its full capacity.
   4. From the simple to the complex organisms there is an increasingly elaborate coordination of receptivity of stimuli and response to stimuli.
   5. The multitude of interrelated neurons of the nervous system of higher animals forms a complex system through which every organ of the body is in connection with every other organ.
   6. Every animal comes into the world with a certain inherited endowment of congenital behavior.
   7. All animals can modify to some extent their inherent modes of reaction.
   8. Inherent reactions in animals are unlearned, independent of intelligence, and more or less inflexible in their operation; under natural conditions they are usually beneficial to the individual or the race.
   9. The intelligence shown by the members of a phylum of higher animals usually bears a direct relation to the stage of development of the special sense organs and to the proportionate size of the brain.
   10. Much of the behavior of living animals depends on their nervous organization, and they exhibit a great variety of behavior because the nervous organization varies in complexity.
   11. The secretions of the endocrine glands are absorbed directly into the blood stream from the gland tissue that produces them and are absorbed from the blood by the tissues of the organs whose activities are regulated by these substances.
   12. In animals certain waste products as well as vitamin and endocrine substances exert regulatory effects on the activities of various organs in the body.

G. Reproduction
   1. Reproduction is a fundamental biological process that provides for the continuance of life on the earth by providing new individuals.
   2. The ability and necessity of members of a species to produce other individuals like themselves is essential for the welfare and maintenance of the species, since no living thing can maintain itself for an unlimited period of time.
   3. Reproduction in all organisms is a process of growth in which a single cell or a group of cells is separated from the parent body and develops into a new individual.
   4. All the modes of reproduction of organic life are alike in their nature, varying only in complexity of development; they fall into two general categories, asexual and sexual reproduction.
   5. The most primitive method of reproduction employed by organisms is the splitting of the whole body into two halves, each of which grows into a complete new individual.

6. Asexual reproduction in organisms may be brought about by fission (simple division, by external or internal budding, or by sporulation.
7. Offspring produced asexually are almost always like the parent; they will have exactly the same or similar chromosomes and the same gene complex.
8. Alternation of generations or a somewhat parallel process is characteristic of all higher plants, but is comparatively uncommon with animals.
9. Sexual reproduction is an almost universal method of reproduction and occurs in representatives of every phylum of plants and animals.
10. All sexually reproduced individuals begin their careers as single fertilized cells.
11. The reproductive elements and their union in fertilization are fundamentally the same in plants and animals.
12. In sexual reproduction a male cell from one parent unites with a female cell from the other parent to produce the young (except in the few cases of self-fertilization).
13. Throughout the plant and animal kingdoms there is a general preference for cross-fertilization; an avoidance of the union of eggs with male elements from the same individual. In those animals and in the great majority of plants which are hermaphrodite, there are usually precautions to restrain self-fertilization.
14. In organisms which reproduce by sexual means fertilization serves two functions: stimulating the egg to develop, and introducing the hereditary properties of the male parent.
15. Sexual union in plants and animals affords a method of variation due to the combining of the egg and sperm, with their chromosomes and genes, at the time of fertilization.
16. The genes in the chromosomes of the egg and the sperm are the carriers of the structural characters of the parents to the next generation.
17. In the vast majority of organisms it is the male which has the unsymmetrical chromosome complement, and the sperms therefore are the determiners of sex.
18. Regeneration is almost universal among living things; from the simple to the more complex animals the abilities to regenerate lost parts and to reproduce asexually fall off, gradually and independently, as the body becomes more specialized.
19. In many organisms the number of young which are produced bears a definite relation to the chance of survival; the smaller the chance the more numerous the offspring.
20. The less the amount of parental care given to the offspring the greater is the need for the animal to be prolific.

VIII. ORGANIZATION
1. The smallest unit of living material capable of existing independently and of maintaining itself is the unit called the cell.
2. The cell is the unit of structure and function in all organisms.
3. Cells are organized into tissues, tissues into organs and organs into systems, the better to carry on the functions of complex organisms.
4. From the lower to the higher forms of life, there is an increasing complexity of structure, and this is accompanied by a progressive increase in division of labor.
5. In all organisms, the higher the organization the greater the degree of differentiation and division of labor and of the dependency of one part upon another.
6. In plants and animals, organs of the same structural plan are often applied to the most diverse functions.

IX. PROTOPLASM AND CELLS
A. General
1. Protoplasm is the physical basis of all life.

2. The distinctive properties of organisms depend upon the complexity of the molecular organization of protoplasm, the one essential constituent of every living thing.
3. The physical and chemical properties of plant and animal protoplasm are similar.
4. Many of the rhythmic changes of protoplasm, such as ciliary action, heartbeat, and rhythmic processes in cell division, are based upon reversible changes in the colloidal state.
5. Protoplasm is built only by protoplasm and every cell comes from a cell.
6. None of the materials present in living protoplasm leaves it when death ensues, for a given bit of protoplasm weighs exactly the same after death as when alive.
7. Life and protoplasm in a cell will remain indissolubly associated for an indefinite period of time unless the cell suffers an accident, or becomes diseased, or is unable to throw off the toxic waste substances that accumulate with age as a result of normal metabolism.
8. Carbon and nitrogen are the basic elements in the protoplasmic compounds.
9. Every cell consists essentially of a mass of protoplasm which is usually differentiated into a central portion, the nucleus, and an outer portion, the cytoplasm.
10. In cells the fundamental processes of food intake, digestion, regeneration of lost structures, and survival are controlled by the nucleus.
11. The nucleus of a cell always contains a complex of protein materials, chromatin, the specialized vehicle which transmits hereditary characters in organisms.
12. The size of cells bears no constant relation to the size of the animals or plants in which they are found.

B. Mitosis
1. The fundamental process of reproduction in all organisms whose cells possess nuclei is cell division which results in the precise distribution of the chromatin of the nucleus.
2. Cell division is the essential mechanism of reproduction, of heredity, and to a large extent, of organic evolution.
3. All cells arise through the division of previous cells (or protoplasm), back to the primitive ancestral cell (or protoplasm).
4. Growth and development in organisms is essentially a cellular phenomenon, a direct result of mitotic cell division, and it is always controlled and guided by the axiate organization of the cell.

C. Life Processes
1. The orderliness of the life processes of an organism is not an isolated orderliness, but one aspect of the orderliness of the universe.
2. Many of the processes of change in the universe are rhythmic, or periodic, and life processes constitute no exception to the rule.
3. The fundamental life processes are the same in all organisms.
4. All chemical processes that belong to life itself are processes that occur in solution.
5. The colloidal nature of the cell material as a whole furnishes the basis of some of the fundamental life processes.
6. Throughout the life of every organism there is a building up and a tearing down of protoplasm with constant transformations of energy.
7. An organism must have certain materials for its life processes and each organism must secure the required materials that it cannot build for itself.

8. All cells produce certain chemical compounds, secretions, which may be used in the processes going on within the cell, in cavities adjoining the cells, or at considerable distances from the cells where they are produced.
9. Enzymes, vitamins, and hormones are chemical regulators (stimulators and suppressors) of the reactions that occur in living organisms.

D. Photosynthesis
1. The work of the chlorophyll of all chlorophyll-bearing plants is essential to all living things.
2. All living things, except chemosynthetic bacteria, depend directly or indirectly on photosynthesis for food.
3. The forms of all chlorophyll-bearing plants are adapted for carrying on photosynthesis.
4. In the presence of sunlight the chloroplasts of chlorophyll-bearing plants convert carbon dioxide and water into intermediate substances, and these into sugar, and sugar into starch, and liberate oxygen; thus directly or indirectly producing practically all the food in the world.
5. In photosynthesis, the energy of sunlight is used to lift the carbon to an energy level from which, as it descends, it furnishes the energy for the building of many compounds and for the carrying on of life processes.
6. All the energy used by chlorophyll-bearing plants in their secondary building processes comes from compounds formed in photosynthesis.

E. Metabolism
1. The protoplasm of a cell carries on continuously all the general processes of any living body: the processes concerned in the growth and repair or upbuilding of protoplasm (anabolism) and the processes concerned with the breaking down of protoplasm and elimination of wastes from the cell (catabolism). The sum of all these chemical and physical processes is metabolism.
2. In cells a quantitative gradient in metabolic rate runs from the apical to the basal pole of the cell, and the various formed components of the cell are arranged in definite relation to the gradient.
3. When anabolism exceeds catabolism, as it does in all young animals, growth is inevitable.
4. Living organisms, during the growth period, increase the mass of the cell from within through the ingestion and utilization of food substances. When the cell reaches a maximum size, mitosis usually results.
5. All living things grow by intussusception or assimilation, making over the materials which are taken into the body into the kind of material of which the body is composed.
6. All living cells require oxygen to provide energy or to build new protoplasm.
7. All living things, except a few anaerobes and autotrophic bacteria, secure their energy by oxidizing food.
8. Oxidation (combustion) furnishes the essential source of heat in the animal body; and other factors remaining constant, the more heat so produced the warmer the animal body.
9. The amount of oxygen taken into the body of an organism and absorbed by the cells is directly proportional to the amount of energy released in the body.
10. Decomposition of the carbon compounds of organisms provides a replenishment of carbon in the atmosphere in the form of carbon dioxide. Thus carbon is continually subjected to a series of cyclic changes from living to non-living substances.

11. All plants, and a few simple animals, are able to recombine nitrogenous byproducts of respiration into proteins by re-synthesizing them anew with carbohydrate molecules.
12. Diffusion, the spread of fluids and their dissolved substances, throughout the protoplasm of a cell or the tissues of an organism is an important method of conveying oxygen from the surface of a cell to the interior, or digested foods from the place of digestion to the protoplasm that will use them, or substances that stimulate any activity to the organ that responds to them, or the waste materials from the place where they are formed to the place where they are stored or excreted.
13. Osmosis, the diffusion of molecules of a solvent (usually water) through a semi-permeable membrane (a layer of cells or the membrane of a single cell) from the point of higher concentration of the solvent to a point of lower concentration, with a stoppage of the flow of molecules of the solute, is a basic process in plant and animal physiology.
14. Turgor in cells is maintained by osmotic pressure; cell membranes are semi-permeable with respect to water and the substances dissolved in it and where the concentration of the solute is higher within the cell than outside, the entrance of water into the cell is accomplished mainly by osmosis.
15. Throughout the organic world there is a cyclic relation between death and the continuance of organic life.
16. Species can and do become extinct, but they usually live on for ages in spite of the death of individuals.

F. Characteristics of Living Things
1. Most living things differ from non-living things by being able to perform the control functions of irritability and spontaneous movement.
2. All living organisms (except viruses and bacteriophage) carry on the common life processes: reproduction, growth, nutrition, excretion, respiration, and irritability.
3. There is a definite size limit for each species of plant and animal.
4. The smaller an organism, the greater is the proportion of its surface to its weight, since surface increases as the square of its length, weight as its cube.
5. In most organisms, large size is accompanied by tissue differentiation and special organs for different kinds of work.
6. The bodies of most animals exhibit some degree of symmetry, either spherical, radial, or bilateral.
7. The bodies of most animals exhibit bilateral symmetry which is an adaptation for forward motion.
8. At every stage of development the individual is an integrated organism; all of its cells, tissues, and organs are correlated and act together as a unit
9. Individuality in an organism is maintained throughout Life in spite of the fact that the actual chemical constitution of the living substances composing it is constantly changing.
10. Except for those organisms which exhibit metagenesis, all living things are able in one way or another to produce new living things like, or nearly like, themselves.
11. All living things die, but life continues from age to age.

X. ENERGY, MATTER AND LIFE
1. The earth's position in relation to the sun is a determining factor of life on the earth.
2. The energy of solar radiation is continually working changes in the surface of the earth and the atmosphere surrounding the earth; all life on the earth is affected directly or indirectly by these changes.

3. Energy can be transformed into mass and mass into energy, but the sum total, mass plus energy, remains constant.
4. Energy and matter are not created or destroyed in the reactions associated with the life processes, but are passed on from organism to organism in endless succession.
5. The energy which makes possible the activity of most living things comes at first from the sun and is secured by the organism through the oxidation of food within its body.
6. Energy changes accompany all chemical changes in living organisms and every chemical change has physical concomitants.
7. Physically all animals are fundamentally mechanisms, driven by the energy liberated in the oxidation of food.
8. As long as life continues in any organism, energy is being released.
9. There are no elements in living matter which are not found in its lifeless environment; the energy by which life is operated is the same energy by which the simplest physical and chemical transformations are brought about.
10. There is a cycle, from inorganic substances in the air and soil to plant tissue, thence to animal tissue, from either of the last two stages via excretion or death and decay back to the air and soil. The energy for this everlasting rotation of life is furnished by the radiant energy of the sun.
11. The phenomena of life involve chemical change, so that wherever life processes are being carried on, chemical changes are taking place. However, chemical change may proceed without involving life.
12. All living organisms have other living things which compete with them for the available energy.
13. There are no living chemical compounds; life is a property of the coordinated association of the different organic and inorganic substances which make up protoplasm.

XI. PALEONTOLOGY
  A. Fossils
   1. Fossils, dated by the rocks in which they are found, reveal portions of the actual story of life's past changes by a progression of forms from simple to complex.
   2. Organisms whose fossils are found in any quantity lived and died in the period when the strata in which their remains are found were laid down.
   3. In fossilization, it is usually the hard parts of organisms that are preserved. Succession of Fossils
  B. Succession of Fossils
   1. The present is the key to the past; the succession of fossils in the rock shows a progressive series from simple to complex.
   2. When a large thickness of rocks shows every evidence of having been laid down steadily and continuously, year after year, it may well change its character. If it changes its character, the character of the animals and plants which live on and in it will change too.
   3. The fact of primary importance in the history of life displayed by the geological periods is the orderly succession of living forms.
   4. The older layers of rocks contain forms which are extremely unlike the now living animals and plants, while the more recent layers contain types more similar to our contemporary ones.

5. Each formation of sedimentary rock has its peculiar assemblage of fossils and there is a definite relation between the fossils found in rocks and the position of these rocks in the geologic timetable.
6. The most primitive and simplest forms of life exist in the oldest rocks, and organisms found in younger and younger rocks represent higher and higher forms.
7. Fossilization is the fate of very few animals and plants. The great majority of dead things simply decay and disappear and their material is returned to the general circulation of nature to be built up into the bodies of new organisms.

XII. APPLIED BIOLOGY
  A. Diseases
   1. All communicable diseases are caused by micro-organisms.
   2. For each disease caused by an organism a specific microbe exists.
   3. Viruses require living cells for their growth and they multiply only within living cells.
   4. Infection by micro-organisms is possible only under the following conditions:
      (a) The infecting organism must enter the host in sufficient numbers;
      (b) It must enter by an appropriate avenue;
      (c) It must be virulent;
      (d) The host must be receptive.
   5. For most species of organisms the great checks on increase in numbers are enemies, disease, and competition between individuals of the same species and of one species with another for food and other necessities of life.
   6. A parasitic organism harms its host in various ways and to various degrees, by actively attacking the tissues, by shedding poisons (toxins) which are distributed throughout the body of the host, by competing with the host for food, or even by making reproduction of the host impossible.
   7. Every influence exercised by micro-organisms upon man and his environment, whether beneficial or detrimental, is the result of a chemical change in the substances from which they secure their nutrition or of a chemical product synthesized from their nutrients.
   8. The antitoxins produced by the body of an organism are specific.
   9. Most cases of fermentation, souring, and putrefaction are brought about by living micro-organisms.
   10. Certain one-celled organisms escape adverse conditions by forming highly resistant spores which often survive until conditions are again favorable.

CHEMICAL NOTES AND RESOURCES

TABLE OF CONTENTS
                                                                    Page

GLOSSARY OF CHEMICAL TERMS
- Absolute temperature ... Alkali — 1
- Alkylation ... Aniline — 2
- Anion ... Base — 3
- Base-formers ... Carat — 4
- Carbogen ... Chemical Equilibrium — 5
- Chemical Symbol ... Concentrated — 6
- Condensation ... DDT — 7
- Decomposition Reactions ... Drier — 8
- Dross ... Emulsifier — 9
- Emulsion ... Exposure — 10
- Exothermic ... Formula Weight — 11
- Fourdrinier Machine ... Heat of Formation — 12
- Heat of Neutralization ... Inert Substance — 13
- Inhibitor ... Kindling Temperature — 14
- Kinetic Energy ... Mass Action (Law Of) — 15
- Matte ... Monoclinic — 16
- Monomer ... Nitrogen Cycle — 17
- Nitrogen Fixation ... Oxidation — 18
- Oxygen-Carbon Dioxide Cycle ... Pickling — 19
- Pigment ... Proteins — 20
- Proton ... Resin — 21
- Rhombic ... Solder — 22
- Solubility Product Constant ... Supersaturated — 23
- Surface-Active Agent ... Thermoplastic Type of Plastics — 24
- Thermosetting Type of Plastics ... Vapor Tension — 25
- Vat Dyes ... Wetting Agents — 26
- X-Rays ... Zirconium — 27

CHEMICAL LAWS
- Avogadro's Hypothesis ... Law of Conservation of Energy — 27
- Law of Conservation of Matter (Mass) ... Periodic Law (Moseley's) — 28

GLOSSARY OF COMMON SUBSTANCES
- Alum ... Carbonic Acid Gas — 29
- Caustic potash ... Hypo — 30
- Kaolin ... Quicksilver — 31
- Rochelle Salt ... Zinc White — 32

CHEMICAL ELEMENTS AND SYMBOLS
- Actinium ... Lanthanum — 33
- Lead ... Tungsten — 34
- Uranium ... Zirconium — 35

PERIODIC TABLE OF THE ELEMENTS — 36

CHEMICAL NOTES AND RESOURCES
GLOSSARY OF CHEMICAL TERMS
A

ABSOLUTE TEMPERATURE

Temperature on the Absolute scale whose zero is -273Centigrade.

ABSORPTION

A soaking up throughout the mass.

ACCELERATOR

Chemical additive which hastens or increases the speed of a chemical reaction. Used, for example, to improve the vulcanization of natural and synthetic rubber and latex compounds.

ACID

A water soluble chemical compound containing hydrogen replaceable by metals or basic radicals. An acid reacts with an alkali to form a salt and water. Example of acid: sulfuric acid, commonly used in storage batteries and many other applications.

ACID ANHYDRIDE

An oxide of a nonmetal capable of uniting with water to form an acid.

ACID-FORMERS

A property usually characteristic of those elements called nonmetals.

ACID SALT

A salt containing replaceable hydrogen.

ACID SULFITE

A salt formed by the union of a metal with the HSO ion.

ACRILAN

One of the synthetic fibers.

ADSORPTION

A condensation on the surface of a material.

ADSORPTION, ACTIVATED

That form of adsorption in which sufficient heat energy must be supplied before the film forms. This process is probably chemical in nature.

AERATED

Given an opportunity to dissolve or combine with air or some other gas.

AEROSOLS

Fog-like sprays.

AIR-SLAKED LIME

A mixture of calcium hydroxide and calcium carbonate formed by exploding calcium hydroxide to the air.

ALCOHOL

A compound containing an organic radical and one or more OH groups.

ALDEHYDE

An organic compound containing the CHO group.

ALIPHATIC

(Derived from Greek word for fat.) Pertaining to an open chain carbon compound. Usually applied to petroleum products derived from a paraffin base and having a straight or branched chain, saturated or unsaturated, molecular structure as distinguished from aromatic hydrocarbons which are built up from one or more benzene rings. Gasoline is a typical aliphatic hydrocarbon.

ALKALI

A compound that has the power to neutralize an acid and form a salt. Example: sodium hydroxide, referred to as caustic soda or lye. Used in soap manufacture and many other applications.

ALKYLATION
A process for rearranging straight chain hydrocarbons.

ALLOTROPISM
The ability of some elements to exist in more than one form.

ALLOY
A material composed of two or more metals.

ALPHA PARTICLES
Positively charged helium nuclei.

ALUM
The double sulfate of a monovalent and trivalent metal, containing a definite amount of water of hydration ($KAl(SO_4)_2 \cdot 12 H_2O$).

ALUMINOTHERMY
A thermite or similar reaction.

AMALGAM
An alloy of mercury with one or more other metals.

AMALGAMATION PROCESS
A process of extracting gold from ore by amalgamating the gold with mercury.

AMINO ACIDS
The "building blocks" from which the giant protein molecules are constructed.

AMMONIA (NH_3)
Nitrogen and hydrogen compound, a colorless gas liquefied by compression. Dissolves in water to form aqueous ammonia. Synthetic ammonia is main source of nitrogen for fertilizer and chemical production.

AMMONIUM ION, NH_4^+
This is a cation produced by the ionization of an ammonium salt.

AMMONIUM RADICAL, NH_4
An ammonium radical is a group of atoms which plays the role of a metal in certain salts (e.g., NH_4Cl).

AMORPHOUS
This is a substance without crystalline structure. The atoms or molecules are not arranged in a definite pattern.

AMPERE
An Ampere is one coulomb of electricity per second. That current which deposits .001118g. silver per second.

AMPHOTERIC
Referring to a compound which may ionize as a base in the presence of a strong acid, and as an acid in the presence of a strong base.

ANGSTROM UNIT (A)
$= 10^{-8}$ cm.

ANHYDRIDE
A compound, usually an oxide of a metal or a nonmetal, capable of uniting with water to form a base or an acid.

ANHYDROUS
Material from which the water has been removed.

ANILINE ($C_6H_5NH_2$)
One of the most important of organics derived from coal. Building block for many dyes and drugs.

ANION
An anion is a negatively charged ion. It is attracted to the anode (+electrode) during electrolysis.

ANODE
The positive terminal of an electric cell.

ANTIBIOTIC
A substance either synethesized chemically or produced by a microorganism, usually a mold or fungus, which kills other organisms, or retards, or completely represses their growth, normally without harm to higher orders of life. Antibiotics retain highly germicidial properties even in dilute concentrations.

ANTICHLOR
A chemical which acts against chlorine, such as a solution of sodium thiosulfate.

ANTIOXIDANT
A compound added to rubber and other substances to prevent deterioration by oxidation.

AQUA AMMONIA
A solution of ammonia gas in water.

AQUA REGIA
A mixture of concentrated nitric and hydrochloric acids capable of dissolving gold.

ARC-TYPE FURNACE
One that has an electric arc jumping the gap between carbon electrodes.

AROMATIC
Applied to group of hydrocarbons derived from or characterized by presence of the benzene nucleus (molecular ring structure). Sometimes called "cyclic solvents" or "cyclic hydrocarbons."

ASSOCIATION
A joining together of small molecules to form larger molecules.

ATOM
A chemical unit, the smallest part of an element which remains unchanged during any chemical reaction yet may undergo physical changes to other atoms as in atomic fission. Believed to be made up of a complex system whose electrically charged components are in rapid orbital motion.

ATOMIC NUMBER
A number identifying an element, equal to the number of protons in its atoms.

ATOMIC WEIGHT
The average relative weight of the atoms of an element compared with those of oxygen taken as a standard and given a value of 16.

B

BACITRACIN
One of the newer antibiotics.

BAKING SODA
The compound sodium hydrogen carbonate used in baking powders and for other purposes

BAROMETER
An apparatus for measuring atmospheric pressure.

BASE
A compound containing the hydroxyl group which, when dissolved in water, forms no negative ions but hydroxyl ions.

BASE-FORMERS
A property usually characteristic of metals.
BASIC ANHYDRIDE
An oxide of a metal capable of reacting with water to form a base. BASIC SALT
A salt containing replaceable oxygen or hydroxyl groups.
BENZENE (C_6H_6)
Major organic intermediate derived from coal or petroleum. Ring-shaped (cyclic) molecular structure makes it broadly useful as chemical building block.
BESSEMER CONVERTER
An egg-shaped converter which changes pig iron into steel by burning out impurities with an air blast.
BETA PARTICLES
Negatively charged particles, actually electrons, emitted by some radioactive materials.
BETATRON
One of the types of "atom-smashing" machines for bombarding atomic nuclei.
BINARY
Binary compounds are made up of only two elements.
BISQUE
A porous porcelain product that has been fired only once.
BLOCK TIN
Solid tin, as distinguished from tin-plate.
BOILING POINT
The temperature at which the vapor pressure of a liquid reaches atmospheric pressure.
BOTTLED GAS
Propane, butane, or a mixture of both, stored under pressure in steel cylinders and used as a fuel.
BREEDER REACTOR
A reactor which uses some fissionable material to produce energy and a greater quantity of fissionable material.
BRITISH THERMAL UNIT (B.T.U.)
The quantity of heat necessary to raise the temperature of one pound of water one degree Fahrenheit.
BROWNIAN MOVEMENT
The zigzag movement of colloidal particles through the medium in which they are suspended.
BUFFER
A suitable mixture of salt and acid (or salt and base) that regulates or stabilizes the pH of a solution.

<u>C</u>

CALCINE
A partially refined copper ore.
CALORIE
A unit for measuring heat, equal to the amount of heat necessary to raise one gram of water one degree Centigrade.
CALORIMETER
A vessel used in measuring the heat evolved in chemical or physical changes.
CARAT
A unit of weight used for gems, equal to 200 milligrams.

CARBOGEN

A mixture of oxygen with 5% to 10% of carbon dioxide.

CARBOHYDRATES

Compounds containing carbon, hydrogen, and oxygen, usually with the hydrogen and oxygen present in the ratio of two to one.

CARBONATED BEVERAGES

Beverages which contain dissolved carbon dioxide.

CARBOXYL

The COOH group in organic compounds as found in organic acids.

CARBURETOR

The second or middle chamber of a water gas apparatus in which the gas is often enriched by spraying in oil or by adding propane.

CATALYST

A substance which through acceleration or retardation changes the spread of a chemical reaction and effects a definite change in composition and/or properties of the end product. In paint manufacture, catalysts generally become part of the final product. In most uses, however, they do not.

CATHODE

The negative electrode or terminal.

CATION

(1) A positively charged ion. (2) The ion attracted to the cathode in electrolysis.

CAUSTIC

A substance that attacks skin, hair, or such materials by chemical action.

CELLULOSE ($C_5H_{10}O_{5n}$)

A carbohydrate which makes up the structural material of vegetable tissues and fibers. Purest forms: chemical cotton and chemical pulp. Basis of rayon, acetate and cellophane.

CEMENT

A mixture made from limestone and clay which, after mixing with water, sets to a hard mass.

CEMENTATION

A process formerly used for making steel by heating wrought iron in red-hot charcoal for a long period of time.

CENTIGRADE TEMPERATURE

Temperature on the Centigrade scale which has $0°$ for the freezing point of water and $100°$ for the boiling point at a pressure of 760 mm.

CHAIN REACTION

A reaction in which the material or energy which starts the reaction is also a product.

CHAMBER PROCESS

A process for making sulfuric acid in large lead chambers, using oxides of nitrogen to promote the necessary reaction.

CHECKERWORK

Loosely-stacked firebricks in a chamber providing a circuitous passage for fuel gas or air.

CHEMICAL CHANGE

A change which produces a new substance with new properties.

CHEMICAL EQUATION

A qualitative and quantitative expression of a chemical change.

CHEMICAL EQUILIBRIUM

A reaction in which the products unite to form the original reactants at the same speed at which the reactants are forming the product.

CHEMICAL SYMBOL
Either one or two letters used as an abbreviation for an element.

CHEMOTHERAPY
Use of chemicals of particular molecular structure in the treatment of specific disorders on the assumption that known structures exhibit an affinity for certain parts of cells of affected tissues and thereby eliminate the causative factors.

CHEMURGY
That branch of applied chemistry devoted to industrial utilization of organic raw materials, especially farm products, as in the use of pine tree cellulose for rayon and paper, and soy bean oil for paints and varnishes.

CHLORINATION
Adding chlorine to a material.

CHLOROMYCETIN
One of the antibiotics.

CHLOROPHYLL
Green coloring matter in leaves which acts as a catalyst for photosynthesis.

CHLORTETRACYCLINE
One of the antibiotics, formerly called aureomycin.

CHROMOPHORS
Certain groups whose presence results in compounds having a color.

COAL GAS
A fuel gas obtained by the destructive distillation of soft coal.

COKE OVEN CHEMICALS
Those organic compounds derived from bituminous coal in the production of metallurgical coke. This major chemical raw materials source provides a base for thousands of chemicals.

COLLOID
A particle in an extremely fine state of subdivision.

COMBINATION REACTIONS
Those in which one element reacts with another to form a compound.

COMBINING WEIGHT
The number of grams of an element that will combine with or replace 8 grams of oxygen or its equivalent.

COMBUSTION
Oxidation accompanied by noticeable light and heat.

COMMON-ION EFFECT
The addition of a substance containing an ion common to that already present, causing the reaction to be driven in a definite direction.

COMPONENT
One of a minimum number of substances necessary to give the composition of a system.

COMPOST
A product of the decay of plant material.

COMPOUND
A substance composed of two or more elements joined according to the laws of chemical combination. Each compound has its own characteristic properties different from those of its elements.

CONCENTRATED
Containing much of a material, the opposite of dilute.

CONDENSATION
(1) Changing a material such as vapor to a liquid;
(2) Increasing the size of very small particles up to colloidal size;
(3) A reaction between raw materials in the making of a plastic that results in the formation of water as one of the products.

CONTACT PROCESS
A process for making sulfuric acid in which the sulfur dioxide and oxygen come in contact with a catalyst.

COORDINATE VALENCE
A kind of chemical bonding somewhat similar to co-valence, but in which there is only one donor atom.

CORTISONE
A compound of animal origin, used particularly for athritis.

COSMIC RAYS
These are rays which come to the earth from somewhere in space, perhaps beyond the solar system.

COTTRELL PRECIPITATOR
A device for precipitating colloidal dust with electricity of high voltage.

COUNTERCURRENTS
Two currents proceeding in opposite directions through an apparatus.

COVALENCE
A kind of chemical bonding in which two atoms share an electron with each other. C.P.
Abbreviation for "chemically pure."

CRACKING
Breaking large or complex molecules into simpler, smaller molecules.

CRITICAL PRESSURE
The pressure of a system at its critical temperature.

CRITICAL SIZE
The smallest amount of fissionable material which can sustain a chain reaction.

CRITICAL TEMPERATURE
The highest temperature at which a liquid and its vapor can co-exist as separate phases.

CRYSTALLOID
A term applied to materials that crystallize easily and pass through a semi-permeable membrane without difficulty.

CRYSTALS
Solids separated from solutions having a definite shape or structure.

GULLET
Broken glass that is re-melted with raw materials in a new batch of glass.

CUPELLATION
A process of separating gold and silver from a base metal such as lead. An oxidizing flame converts the lead to the oxide(PbO), which is removed by a stream of air or is absorbed in the porous bottom of the reverberatory furnace. The silver-gold residue remains unchanged.

CYCLOTRON
One of the atom-smashing machines used to bombard the nuclei of atoms.

D

DACRON
One of the synthetic fibers.

DDT
Letters stand for dichloro-diphenyl-trichloroethane, an insecticide.

DECOMPOSITION REACTIONS

Those in which a compound is decomposed by heat, light, or electricity into simpler compounds.

DECREPITATION

The expulsion of water with a crackling sound when some crystals are heated.

DEHYDRATION

The removal of water from a substance.

DELIQUESCENCE

The process of picking up enough water to become wet.

DENSITY

Mass per unit volume, e.g., grams per cubic centimeter.

DESTRUCTIVE DISTILLATION

The process of heating wood, coal, bones, etc., in a closed vessel, resulting in a breaking down to simpler materials.

DETERGENT

An agent that removes dirt.

DEUTERIUM

An isotope of hydrogen of mass 2.

DEUTERON

The nucleus of the deuterium atom.

DEVELOPING

A process in photography in which the reduction of the silver compound, started by light, is promoted by the action of an alkaline, organic, reducing agent.

DIALYSIS

A process in which a semi-permeable membrane is used to separate colloidal particles from substances in true solution.

DIBASIC

A term applied to acids that have two replaceable hydrogen atoms.

DIESELENE

A petroleum fuel for Diesel engines.

DIFFUSION

The intermingling of liquids and gases.

DILUENT

A diluting agent, such as water in a solution, or turpentine in paint.

DIPOLES

Molecules with unbalanced charges so that one end may be positive and the other end negative.

DISINFECTANTS

Agents that kill, not merely arrest, the growth of bacteria.

DISSOCIATION

The separation of the ions of an electrovalent compound by the action of a solvent.

DISTILLATION

The process of evaporation followed by condensation of the vapors in a separate vessel.

DOUBLE REPLACEMENT REACTIONS

Those in which two compounds exchange ions to produce two new compounds.

DOUBLE SALT

A salt in which two metal atoms are combined with one acid radical or one metal is combined with two acid radicals, e.g., $KAl(SO_4)_2 \cdot 12 H_2O$.

DRIER

Catalysts, such as oxides of lead and manganese, added to paint to promote the drying of the paint.

DROSS
A powdery scum that floats on top of melted metal.

DUCTILITY
That property of a substance which permits its being drawn into wire.

DUTCH PROCESS
A process for making white lead using lead buckles, acetic acid, and decomposing tanbark or manure.

DYNAMITE
An explosive made by absorbing nitroglycerin in wood flour mixed with sodium nitrate.

DYNE
A unit of force. The force necessary to give a mass of one gram an acceleration of one centimeter per second per second.

DYNEL
One of the synthetic fibers.

EFFERVESCENCE
The process of giving off bubbles of gas from a liquid.

EFFLORESCENCE
The property of giving off water vapor to the air.

ELASTOMER
Actually, it is any flexible or elastic material but, in a more limited sense, a synthetic rubber or soft or rubbery plastic with some degree of elasticity at room temperature.

ELECTRIC POTENTIAL
Electrical pressure or voltage between terminals.

ELECTRODE
A terminal of an electric circuit where the current either enters or leaves.

ELECTROLYTE
A compound whose water solution conducts an electric current.

ELECTRON
A unit particle of negative electricity. Its mass is 1/1845 of the hydrogen atom.

ELECTRON VOLT
That quantity of energy which is equal to the kinetic energy of an electron accelerated by a potential difference of 1 volt.

ELECTRONEGATIVE ELEMENT
An element which has a tendency to take up electrons.

ELECTROPLATING
Deposition of metals on a surface by means of an electric current.

ELECTROTYPES
Copper plates from which the pages of a book are printed.

ELECTROVALENCE
Type of chemical bonding where one or more electrons are transferred from one atom to another.

ELEMENT
Solid, liquid or gaseous matter consisting of atoms of one type which cannot be further decomposed by chemical means. The atoms of an element may differ physically but do not differ chemically. Example: chlorine. Known elements: 101.

EMULSIFIER, EMULSIFYING AGENT
A chemical that mixes and disperses dissimilar materials to produce an emulsion and keep it stable. Casein, for example is a natural emulsi-fier in milk, keeping butter fat droplets emulsified.

EMULSION
Suspension of insoluble fine particles or globules of a liquid in another liquid.
ENDOTHERMIC
Pertaining to a reaction which absorbs heat.
ENERGY
The capacity for doing work.
ENZYME
An organic secretion that acts as a catalyst.
EQUATION
An expression which shows, by the use of symbols and formulas, the changes in arrangement of the atoms which occur during a chemical reaction.
EQUILIBRIUM
A reaction in which the products unite to form the original reactants at the same speed at which the reactants are forming the products.
EQUILIBRIUM (CHEMICAL)
A state in which a chemical reaction and the reverse reaction are taking place at the same rate. The concentrations (at equilibrium) of all substances remain constant.
EQUILIBRIUM CONSTANT
An equilibrium constant (K) is the ratio (number) obtained by dividing the product of the active concentrations of the substances produced in a reaction by the product of the active concentrations of the reactants, after equilibrium has been reached.
ERG
The work done by a force of one dyne per centimeter.
ESTER
A compound formed by the reaction between an acid and an alcohol.
ESTERIFICATION
The process of preparing esters by adding acid to an alcohol
ETHANE (C_2H_6)
A saturated hydrocarbon (maximum number of hydrogen atoms attached to each carbon) derived from petroleum or natural gas, important for organic synthesis. Ethylene derived from it.
ETHANOL (ETHYL ALCOHOL) (C_2H_5OH)
Organic compound derived through either a fermentation process or via synthesis from petroleum or natural gas. Wide use as solvent and for chemical synthesis.
ETHYLENE (C_2H_4)
Gaseous organic compound prepared in cracking of petroleum or by passing natural gas through heated tube. Removal of two hydrogen atoms from ethane component of petroleum or natural gas makes this unsaturated hydrocarbon of wide use as petrochemical base for numerous chemical reactions, notably plastic material manufacture.
ETHYLENE GLYCOL
Colorless liquid which is a useful humectant since it absorbs approximately twice its weight of water at room temperature and 100% humidity. A major use: anti-freeze. Among many other uses -chemical synthesis, as in producing alkyd resins.
EUTECTIC
A mixture of two or more substances with the lowest melting point.
EXPLOSIVE RANGE
A pair of percentages below or above which the gas will not form an explosive mixture with air.
EXPOSURE
In photography, the act of admitting light to the film or plate.

EXOTHERMIC
Pertaining to a reaction which liberates heat.
EXTRUDED
Forced through a die by pressure.

F

FAHRENHEIT TEMPERATURE

Temperature on the Fahrenheit scale with $32°$ as the freezing point of water and $212°$ as the boiling point at a pressure of 760 mm.

FAMILY OF ELEMENTS
A group of elements with more or less similar properties.
FATS
Glyceryl esters of certain organic acids.
FELDSPARS
Complex silicates, usually aluminum silicate with either sodium or potassium silicate.
FERMENTATION
A chemical reaction caused by living organisms or enzymes.
FERTILIZER
Plant food, or material, that contains compounds of the elements needed
by plants for growth.
FILTRATION

The process of removing suspended material from a liquid by allowing the liquid to pass through a material such as filter paper or a layer of sand.

FISSION
The disintegration of an atom into two nyclei with nearly equal mass.
FIXATION OF NITROGEN
A process in which atmospheric nitrogen is converted into useful compounds.
FIXING

In photography the operation of removing unchanged silver salts after the picture has been developed, thereby fixing the image on the film or plate.

FLOTATION (ORE)

A process in which crushed ore is agitated in water containing a fro-ther (pine oil) and a collector (potassium ethyl xanthate). The valuable mineral particles are attached to the froth and rise to the surface from which they are removed.

FLOTATION REAGENT

Chemical used in flotation separation of minerals. Added to pulverized mixture of solids, water and oil, causes preferential oil-wetting of certain solid particles, making possible the flotation and separation of un-wet particles.

FLUIDITY
The reciprocal of viscosity.
FLUORESCENT
Giving off light after exposure to sunlight.
FLOWERS OF SULFUR
Finely-divided sulfur formed by the condensation of sulfur vapors on a cool surface.
FLUX
A material added to unite with impurities to form an easily melted product.
FORMULA

A collection of chemical symbols indicating what elements and how many atoms of each are present in a compound.

FORMULA WEIGHT
The sum of the weights of the atoms in a formula.

FOURDRINIER MACHINE
A machine that converts a suspension of taper fibers into sheets.

FRACTIONAL CRYSTALLIZATION
Separation of two dissolved solids by evaporating until the less soluble solid separates while the more soluble solid remains in solution.

FRACTIONATION
The process of separating a mixture by careful evaporation, depending upon the materials having different boiling points.

FROTH-FLOTATION
A process for concentrating powdered ore by causing the good ore to cling to bubbles which float above liquid, while the worthless rocky material sinks to the bottom of the container.

FUNGICIDE
Any one of a group of chemicals used to prevent or inhibit the growth of fungi or bacteria. Among these are: plant fungicides, wood preservatives, mildew or mold preventives and disinfectants.

G

GALVANIZE
To coat iron or steel with zinc.

GAMMA RAYS
High energy X-rays emitted from a radioactive material.

GANGUE
Worthless material, rock or earth, present in an ore.

GEIGER COUNTER
A device used to detect the presence of radiation from radioactive material.

GEL
A jelly-like solid.

GENERATOR
In chemistry, the vessel in which a reaction occurs between chemicals.

GERMAN SILVER
An alloy containing copper, nickel, and zinc.

GRAM
Basic unit of weight in the metric system, equal to 1/1000 of the standard kilogram.

GRAM-EQUIVALENT WEIGHT
The weight of an element that will combine with or replace one gram of hydrogen.

GRAM-FORMULA WEIGHT
The number of grams of a substance that equal its formula weight.

GRAM-MOLECULAR VOLUME
The volume, 22.4 liters, occupied by one gram-molecular weight at any gast at S.T.P.

GRAM-MOLECULAR WEIGHT
That number of grams of any substance that equal its molecular weight, also called a MOLE of that substance

H

HALF-LIFE
The time required for one-half the atoms of a mass of radioactive material to decompose.

HALOGEN
The name given to the family of elements having seven valence electrons.

HEAT OF FORMATION
The heat which is given out or absorbed when a compound is formed from elements.

HEAT OF NEUTRALIZATION
The number of calories liberated in the formation of 18g. of water from hydrogen and hydroxyl ions.

HEAVY WATER
Water containing deuterium atoms in place of ordinary hydrogen atoms.

HEMOGLOBIN
The red coloring matter in blood.

HERBICIDE
A weed-killing agent. Most of these are specific in their action and therefore not intended for indiscriminate use. Label indicates particular purposes and gives directions for most effective application.

HOMOLOGOUS SERIES
A series of compounds each of which can be represented by a type of formula, such as C_nH_{2n+2}.

HUMIDITY, RELATIVE
The ratio of the actual amount of water vapor in atmosphere to the amount necessary for saturation at the same temperature.

HYDRATE
Crystals that contain water of hydration.

HYDRATED LIME
Calcium hydroxide, the product formed when water unites with calcium oxide.

HYDROCARBONS
Organic compounds composed solely of caron and hydrogen. Myriad variety of molecular combinations of C and H. Basic building block of all organic chemicals. Main chemical industry course of hydrocarbons: petroleum, natural gas and coal.

HYDROFORMING
The process of improving gasoline by heating it with hydrogen in the presence of a catalyst.

HYDROGENATION
The addition of hydrogen to a material.

HYDROLYSIS
The reaction of water with a salt to form the acid and the base of which the salt was a product; it opposes neutralization reactions.

HYDROPONICS
The science of gardening without the use of oil.

HYGROSCOPIC
Having a tendency to pick up water vapor.

I

INACTIVE SUBSTANCE
One which reacts, but not very readily, with other substances.

INDICATOR
A substance used to show, by means of a color change, whether an acid or a base is present.

INERT ELEMENT
An element of the zero group of the periodic table. Elements in this group have no chemical properties.

INERT SUBSTANCE
One which does not react at all with other substances under the usual conditions of chemical reactions.

INHIBITOR
(1) A material used to prevent or retard rust or corrosion.
(2) An agent which arrests or slows chemical action.

INORGANIC
Term used to designate chemicals that generally do not contain carbon. Source: matter, other than vegetable or animal. Example: chlorine is an inorganic chemical derived from salt.

INSECTICIDE
Any one of a group of chemicals used to kill or control insects.

INTERMEDIATE
An organic chemical formed as a "middle-step" between the initial material and the one or frequently several ultimate end products.

INVERSION
The combination of cane sugar with water to form two molecules of simple sugars.

ION
An atom or group of atoms which carries an electric charge.

ION-EXCHANGE RESINS
Granules of resins that absorb either positive or negative ions.

IONIC EQUILIBRIUM
The balance attained when the rate of dissociation equals the rate of association.

IOOTZATION
The formation of ions from polar compounds by action of a solvent.

IONIZATION CONSTANT
The product of the concentration of the ions divided by the concentration of the unionized molecules of solute (electrolyte).

IONIZATION POTENTIAL
The energy necessary to remove an electron from a gaseous atom to form an ion. This energy is expressed in electron volts.

IRRADIATION
Subjected to light, especially ultraviolet light.

ISOBARES
Atoms of the same atomic weight but having different atomic numbers are isobares.

ISOMERS
Compounds having the same composition but different structure.

ISOTOPE
One of two or more atomic species of an element differing in weight but having the same nuclear charge (atomic number). For example, in the element, chlorine, the atomic weight is the mean of the two isotopes making up the element.

K

KAOLIN
A fine, white clay composed of hydrated aluminum silicate.

KERNEL
All of the atom except the valence electrons.

KILN
A type of furnace used for producing quicklime, making glass, baking pottery, etc.

KILOCALORIES
Units equal to one thousand calories.

KILOGRAM
The standard of weight in the metric system equal to 1000 grams.

KINDLING TEMPERATURE
The lowest temperature at which a substance takes fire. This temperature varies with the physical state of the substance.

KINETIC ENERGY
Energy of motion.

KINETIC THEORY
The theory of matter which assumes that all molecules of matter are always in motion.

KNOCKING
A pounding sound produced in automobile engines by too rapid combustion of the mixture of gasoline vapor and air.

L

LAC OF SULPHUR
Precipitated sulfur.

LATENT HEAT
The heat absorbed or liberated in changing a mole of substance from one state to another at a fixed temperature, e.g., converting 18g. water to water vapor at 100° C.

LATEX
Original meaning: Milky extract from rubber tree. Now also applied to water emulsions of synthetic rubbers or resins. In emulsion paints, the film-forming resin is in the form of latex.

LAW, LeCHATELIER'S
A system in equilibrium, if disturbed by external factors such as temperature and pressure, will adjust itself in such a way that the effect of the disturbing factors will be reduced to a minimum.

LEHR
A cooling oven for annealing glass.

LIGNIN
Major non-carbohydrate constituent of wood and woody plants; functions as binder for the cellulose fibers. Removed from wood in pulp manufacture. Extracted from waste sulfite liquor. Research underway on chemical applications. Current use as adhesive base, for boiler water treatment and for road binders.

LIGNITE
A partially mineralized peat.

LIME
A term loosely used for all calcium compounds but properly belonging to calcium oxide, although often used for calcium hydroxide and calcium carbonate.

L.P.G., or LIQUEFIED PETROLEUM GAS
A compressed or liquefied gas comprised of pure propane, or a butane, or a combination of propane and butane; obtained as a by-product in petroleum refining or gasoline manufacture. Used in chemical synthesis.

LITER
The basic unit of volume in the metric system.

LITHOPANE
A paint base composed of barium sulfate and zinc sulfide.

LITMUS
A dye extracted from lichens which is used as an indicator.

LYE
A term used for either sodium hydroxide or potassium hydroxide.

M

MASS
The property of a substance (body) that determines the acceleration it will acquire when acted upon by a given force.

MASS ACTION, LAW OF
The speed of a chemical change is proportional to the concentration of the reacting substances.

MATTE
A mixture of sulfides produced in a partially refined ore.

MATTER
Anything which occupies space and has weight.

METALLURGY
The science of extracting and refining metals.

METALS
Elements with a luster that are good conductors of heat and electricity and are electropositive.

MERCERIZING
Treating stretched cotton with sodium hydroxide solution.

METAMORPHIC
Applied to rocks that have undergone a change in form due to heat or pressure.

METER
The basic unit of the metric system, equal to 39.37 inches.

METHANE (CH_4)
The simplest saturated hydrocarbon, chief component of most natural gas. Chemical raw material.

METHYL ALCOHOL (METHANOL, WOOD ALCOHOL) (CH_3OH)
Organic compound important for chemical synthesis; also used in denaturing alcohol; solvent and many other uses.

MILLILITER
One-thousandth of a liter.

MILK OF SULFUR
Precipitated sulfur.

MIXTURE
Two or more substances which, when combined, do not lose their identity and may be separated by mechanical means.

MODERATOR
A substance which slows down fast neutrons.

MOLAL SOLUTION
One mole of a substance dissolved in 1000g. of solvent.

MOLAR SOLUTION
One gram-molecular weight of a substance dissolved in enough solvent to make one liter of solution.

MOLE
That number of grams of a substance which is exactly equal to its molecular weight.

MOLECULAR VOLUME
The volume occupied by a mole of any gas at $0°$ C. and 760 mm pressure, e.g., 22.4 liters.

MOLECULAR WEIGHT
The sum of the weights of the atoms in a molecule.

MOLECULE
The chemical combination of two or more like or unlike atoms.

MONATOMIC
Molecules made up of one atom.

MONOBASIC ACID
An acid having one replaceable hydrogen atom per molecule.

MONOCLINIC
Referring to those crystals having one oblique axis.

MONOMER
A compound of relatively low molecular weight which, under certain conditions, either alone or with another monomer, forms various types and lengths of molecular chains called polymers or copolymers of high molecular weight. Example: styrene is a monomer which polymerizes readily to make the polymer, polystyrene.

MORTAR
A mixture of lime, sand, and water.

MOTHER LIQUOR
The liquid which is left after a crop of crystals has separated from a solution.

N

NAPHTHALENE ($C_{10}H_8$)
A white solid crystalline hydrocarbon found as a mineral and obtained from coal tar by distillation. Used as a moth repellent and a basic material in the manufacture of dyestuffs, synthetic resins, lubricants and other products.

NAPHTHENES
Hydrocarbons having a ring structure.

NASCENT
At the instant an element is liberated from a compound it is said to be in the nascent state. Nascent dryogen is probably atomic hydrogen.

NATIVE METAL
A metal found as an element, rather than as a compound, in the ground.

NATURAL GAS
A combustible gas composed largely of methane and other hydrocarbons with variable amounts of nitrogen and non-combustible gases; obtained from natural earth fissures or from driven wells. Among other things, used as a fuel, in the manufacture of carbon black and in chemical synthesis of many products.

NEON (Ne)
A rare gaseous element which forms no chemical compounds and is derived by fractional distillation of liquid air. Used mostly in luminescent electric tubes.

NEUTRALIZATION
The union of hydrogen ions of an acid with hydroxyl ions of a base to form water.

NEUTRON
A neutral particle found in the atom.

NIACIN ($C_6H_5O_2N$)
The anti-pellagra factor of the vitamin B complex; present in animal tissues, in fish, milk and green leafy vegetables.

NITER (KNO_3)
A white salt widely distributed in nature and formed in soils from nitrogenous organic bodies by the action of bacteria. Used in making gunpowder, medicinals and other products.

NITRIC ACID (HNO_3)
A colorless to yellowish fuming liquid with powerful corrosive properties. Manufactured by several methods, it is used in organic synthesis, in etching metals and ore flotation, in the manufacture of explosives, medicines, and other products.

NITROCELLULOSE
A powerful explosive made by treating cellulose with nitric and sul-furic acids.

NITROGATION
Adding of nitrogen compounds to the soil.

NITROGEN CYCLE
The cycle of changes through which nitrogen passes, starting with nitrates in the soil which become, in turn, plant proteins, animal proteins, dead matter, ammonia, nitrites, and then nitrates again.

NITROGEN FIXATION

Process of combining nitrogen of the atmosphere into any of the various stable chemical compounds valuable to the manufacture of fertilizers, and ammonia, among others.

NITROGLYCERIN

Glyceryl trinitrate, a powerful and sensitive explosive.

NITROUS OXIDE (NO_2)

A colorless gas of sweetish odor and taste; used as an anesthetic. Also called laughing gas.

NONELECTROLYTE

A compound whose water solution does not conduct electric current. NONMETALS
Elements that are usually poor conductors of heat and electricity and are electro-negative.

NORMAL SALT

A salt containing neither replaceable hydrogen nor hydroxyl.

NORMAL SOLUTION

A solution that contains one gram-equivalent of a substance dissolved in enough solvent to make one liter of solution.

NUCLEONS

The fundamental constituents of atomic nuclei(protons and neutrons).

O

OCCLUSION

The adsorption of gases by solids.

OCTANE RATING

A number indicating how a gasoline behaves with regard to knocking when compared with a test fuel given an arbitrary rating of 100.

OCTET

The term applied to a group of eight electrons in the highest energy levels of atoms.

ONE ATMOSPHERE

The average pressure of the atmosphere at sea level, equal to 760 mm. of mercury.

OPEN-HEARTH PROCESS

A process for making steel in a large, shallow pool.

ORBIT

The path of an electron about the nucleus of an atom.

ORGANIC

Term used to designate that group of chemicals that contain carbon. Approximately 300,000 such compounds have been identified, many occurring in nature, others produced by chemical synthesis. Sources: petroleum and coal tar by fractional distillation; soft coal and wood by destructive distillation; wood by chemical treatment; grains and fruits by fermentation; grains, vegetables and fruit by mechanical and chemical separation of starch and sugar; cotton by mechanical and chemical treatment; animals, seeds and nuts, by mechanical extraction of fats and oils.

ORLON

One of the synthetic fibers.

OSMOSIS

The passage of liquids and gases through porous membranes.

OXIDATION

Process of combining oxygen with some other substance.

OXYGEN-CARBON DIOXIDE CYCLE
The cycle of events whereby plants take in carbon dioxide and give off oxygen in photosynthesis, whereas animals take in oxygen and give off carbon dioxide in respiration.

OZONE
An allotropic form of oxygen containing three atoms per molecule.

P

PAINT BASE
The particles suspended in the oil of a paint.

PAINT VEHICLE
A quick drying oil that forms a flexible horn-like film. The paint base is suspended in this oil.

PARAFFINS, PARAFFIN SERIES (From parun affinis-small affinity)
Those hydrocarbon components of crude oil and natural gas whose molecules are saturated (i.e., carbon atoms attached to each other by single bonds) and therefore very stable. Examples: methane, ethane.

PARKERIZED
Dipped into a hot alkaline solution of sodium phosphate.

PARKES PROCESS
A method of separating silver from molten, crude lead by adding zinc.

PEPTIZATION
A breaking up of coarse particles into a finer state of subdivision.

PERIODIC TABLE
An arrangement of the elements in the order of their atomic numbers.

PH
A numerical scale that indicates the concentration of hydrogen ions in a solution; 7 is neutral, less than 7 is acid, and greater than 7 is basic.

PHENOL (C_6H_5OH)
Popularly known as carbolic acid. Important chemical intermediate intermediate derived primarily from coal tar and produced by chemical synthesis. Base for plastics, Pharmaceuticals, explosives, anti-septics, and many other end products.

PHENOLPHTHALEIN
An indicator which turns red in the presence of an excess of hydroxyl ions.

PHOSPHORS
Compounds that fluoresce under ultraviolet light.

PHOSPHORESCENCE
A faint glow similar in appearance to that emitted by phosphorus when it is exposed to the air in a dark room.

PHOTON
A unit of light (a particle of light).

PHOTOSYNTHESIS
The process by which plants build carbohydrate foods with the aid of sunlight, using carbon dioxide and water as the raw materials and chlorophyll as the catalyst.

PHYSICAL CHANGE
A change in color, size of particle, temperature, or other physical property that does not produce a new substance.

PHYSICAL EQUILIBRIUM
A condition of balance when the rate of a physical change in one direction is equal to an opposite physical change.

PICKLING
Treating a metal with acid to remove surface coatings of oxide.

PIGMENT
A substance that adds color to a mixture.

PLASTICIZERS
Organic chemicals used in modifying plastics, synthetic rubber and similar materials to give such special properties as elongation, flexibility and toughness as may be essential to their end uses.

PLASTICS
Officially defined as any one of a large and varied group of materials which consists of, or contains as an essential ingredient, an organic substance of large molecular weight; and which, while solid in the finished state, at some stage in its manufacture has been or can be formed (cast calendered, extruded, molded, etc.) into various shapes by flow - usually through application of heat and pressure singly or together. Each plastic has individual physical, chemical and electrical properties. Two basic types: thermosetting and thermoplastic. Prior to processing, plastic materials often are referred to as resins. Final form may be as film, sheet, solid, or foam; flexible or rigid.

POLAR MOLECULE
A molecule with an unsymmetrical electron distribution.

POLING
The use of green wood in the refining of copper ore to reduce the traces of copper oxide present.

POLYMER
A high molecular weight material containing a large number of repeating units. These may be hundreds or even thousands of the original molecules (monomers) which have linked together end to end. Rubber and cellulose are naturally occurring polymers. Most resins are chemically produced polymers. Polymers may be formed by polymerization or condensation. For instance, the polymer, polyethylene, is polymerized from the monomer, ethylene. An example of condensation is the production of phenol formaldehyde resins with the incidental formation of water or some simple substance.

POLYMERIZATION
A physical reaction by which polymers are formed from the linkage of monomers.

POLYMORPHISM
The ability to exist in two or more crystalline forms.

PORCELAIN
A product made from pure, white clay mixed with powdered feldspar and usually fired twice in a kiln.

POSITRON
A unit charge of positive electricity of approximately the same mass as the electron.

POTASH
Source of potassium, essential plant nutrient (other two basic nutrients: nitrogen, phosphorus). Potash value in a fertilizer is expressed in terms of equivalent amount of potassium oxide K_2O.

PRECIPITATE
An insoluble solid formed by adding one solution to another.

PRODUCER GAS
A cheap fuel gas for industrial purposes made by blowing a blast of steam and air through red-hot coke.

PROPERTIES
The characteristics by which we identify materials.

PROTEINS
Complex organic compounds necessary for the growth of living things or the repair of worn-out tissue.

PROTON
A positively charged particle found in the atom.

Q

QUICKLIME
Calcium oxide, often called unslaked lime.

R

RADICAL
A group of atoms which acts like a single atom in forming compounds.

RADIOACTIVITY
Emission of energy in waves or moving particles from the nucleus of an atom. Always involves change of one kind of atom into a different kind. A few elements such as radium are naturally radioactive. Other radiactive forms are induced (see RADIOISOTOPE).

RADIOCHEMICALS
Any compound or mixture containing a sufficient portion of radioactive elements to be detected by Geiger counter.

RADIOISOTOPE
An isotopic form of an element that exhibits radioactivity, whether naturally found or produced by fission and other induced nuclear changes. The latter are used in biological tracer work and industrial control operations. More than 500 radioactive substances have been produced.

RADON
A gaseous element produced by the disintegration of radium atoms.

REACTANTS
The elements or compounds entering into a chemical reaction.

REAGENT
Any substance used in a chemical reaction to produce another substance or to detect its composition.

REDOX REACTION
A reaction in which oxidation and reduction take place.

REDUCING AGENT
An agent that removes oxygen from a material.

REDUCTION
(1) Removal of oxygen. (2) The gain in electrons by an element.

REFRACTORY
Pertaining to a substance that is not easily melted.

REGENERATIVE HEATING
A system whereby the heat of outgoing flue gases is used to preheat incoming fuel gas and air.

RELATIVE HUMIDITY
The amount of moisture present in the air as a vapor compared with the total amount of moisture the air could hold at that temperature.

REPLACEMENT SERIES
The arrangement of the metals in the order of their decreasing chemical activity.

RESIN
A solid or semisolid amorphous organic compound or mixture of such compounds with no definite melting point and no tendency to crystallize. Resins may be of vegetable, animal or synthetic origin. Natural resins may be distinguished from gums in that they are insoluble in water. However, certain synthetic water soluble materials are referred to as resins or resin

stages. There are many types, each with distinctive physical and chemical properties. Some types of resin materials may be molded, cast, or extruded. Others are used for adhesives, for the treatment of textiles and paper, and for protective coatings. Still others are rolled or extruded into continuous sheets and films of various thicknesses. All, broadly speaking, have plastic use.

RHOMBIC
Referring to crystals having equilateral edges and oblique angles.

RIFFLES
Grooves in a sluice for catching gold in hydraulic mining operations.

S

SACRIFICIAL METAL
The more active of a pair of metals which is oxidized by an electric cell action.

SALTS
Crystalline compounds made up of metals and non-metals. Example: table salt is sodium and chlorine.

SAPONIFICATION
The process of making soap by adding lye to a glyceryl ester.

SARAN
One of the synthetic fibers.

SATURATED SOLUTION
A solution in which the solute in solution is in equilibrium with undissolved solute.

SEDIMENTARY
A term applied to rocks formed from sediment that has been deposited in layers.

SHELL-FILLER
An explosive that requires a severe shock to set it off.

SHERARDIZING
Coating with zinc by allowing zinc vapor to condense on the object.

SILICONES
Unique new group of polymers made by molecular combination of the inorganic chemical, silicone dioxide, with organic chemicals. Produced in variety of forms including silicone fluids, resins and rubber. Silicones have special properties, such as water-repellensy, wide temperature resistance, durability and dielectric property

SILT
A soil which is coarser than clay but finer than sand.

SINGLE REPLACEMENT REACTION
One in which an element replaces another in a compound.

SINTERING
Heating until fusion just begins.

SLAG
A by-product of smelting. It is formed by the action of low melting material (flux) on impurities in the ore. Slags contain calcium and aluminum silicates.

SLAKED LIME
Calcium hydroxide, or calcium oxide, that has united with water.

SMOKELESS POWDER
A nitrocellulose explosive.

SOAP
The sodium or potassium salts of a fatty acid, e.g., $NaC_{18}H_{35}O_2$.

SOLDER
An easily melted alloy, especially one of tin and lead.

SOLUBILITY PRODUCT CONSTANT

The product of the concentrations of the ions of slightly soluble salt at saturation.

SOLUTION

Mixture in which the identities of components are lost as such.

SOLVENT

A substance, usually an organic compound, which dissolves another substance.

SPECIFIC GRAVITY (GASES)

The ratio of the weight of one liter of air to the weight of one liter of the gas.

SPECIFIC GRAVITY (SOLID OR LIQUID)

The ratio of the weight of a unit volume of a substance to the weight of the same volume of water.

SPECIFIC HEAT

The heat required to raise the temperature of one gram of a substance one degree centigrade.

SPECIFIC VOLUME

The volume of one gram of a substance.

SPINNERETS

Thimble-like plates with tiny holes for extruding synthetic fibers.

STALACTITES

Icicle-like masses of calcium carbonate hanging from the roof of limestone caves.

STALAGMITES

Masses of calcium carbonate rising from the floor of limestone caves, formed by dripping of calcium bicarbonate solution from the cave roof.

STANDARD CONDITIONS

$0°$ C. and 1 atmosphere pressure (760 mm.).

STANDARD PRESSURE

A pressure equal to that furnished by a column of mercury 760 mm. high.

STANDARD TEMPERATURE

Zero degrees Centigrade.

STERLING

Containing 92.5% silver, or 925 fine.

S.T.P.

Abbreviation for "standard temperature and pressure."

STRONG ACID

One which is completely ionized in water solutions.

STRONG ELECTROLYTE

One which is ionized almost completely.

STRUCTURE FORMULAS

Formulas that tell how the atoms are joined in the molecules.

SUBLIMATION

A process in which a solid is vaporized and condensed to a solid without passing through the liquid state.

SUPERHEATED WATER

Water heated under pressure to a temperature above the normal boiling point.

SUPERPHOSPHATE

Phosphorus-bearing material made by action or sulfuric acid on phosphate rock to make phosphorus available as a plant nutrient. Phosphorus in soluble form is one of the three essential plant nutrients. (Other two: nitrogen, potassium.)

SUPERSATURATED

Pertaining to a solution saturated at a high temperature which retains the solute in solution as it cools.

SURFACE-ACTIVE AGENT
Any of a group of compounds added to a liquid to modify surface or interface tension. In the case of synthetic detergents, best known surface-active agent, reduction of tension provides cleansing action. Term also includes dispersing, emulsifying, foaming, penetrating and wetting agents. Usually synthetic organic in origin.

SURFACE COATINGS
Term used to cover paint, lacquer, varnish and other chemical compositions used for protecting and/or decorating surfaces.

SURFACTANT
A coined word which means "surface-active agent."

SYNCHROTRON
One of the "atom-smashing" machines for bombarding atomic nuclei.

SYNERGIST
A material which, in combination with another, improves the effectiveness of the combination to a degree in excess of the sum of the effects of the two materials taken independently.

SYNTHESIS
The reaction, or series of reactions, by which a complex compound is obtained from simpler compounds or elements.

SYNTHETIC DETERGENTS
Chemically-tailored cleaning agents soluble in water. Originally developed as soap substitute. Because they do not form insoluble precipitates, they are especially valuable in hard water. See SURFACE-ACTIVE AGENT.

SYNTHETIC RUBBER
Nab-made polymeric chemical with rubber-like attributes. Various types with varying composition and properties. Major types designated as S-type, butyl, neoprene (chloroprene polymers), and N-type.

T

TALL OIL
(Name derived from Swedish TALLOLJA; material first investigated in Sweden-not synonymous with our pine oil.)

Natural mixture of rosin acids, fatty acids, sterols, high molecular weight alcohols and other materials, derived primarily from waste liquors of wood pulp manufacture. Dark brown, viscous, oily liquid often called liquid rosin. Recent encyclopedia lists 38 major industry uses.

TANKAGE
A fertilizer made from slaughter house scraps.

TAR CRUDE
Basic organic raw material derived from distillation of coal tar and used for chemical manufacture.

TEMPERING
Regulation of the iron carbide, and thus the hardness of a piece of steel, by heating and sudden cooling.

TERNARY
Composed of three elements.

TERNE PLATE
Sheet iron coated with an alloy of tin and lead.

THERMITE REACTION
The replacement reaction between a metal, such as aluminum, and an oxide, such as ferric oxide, which liberates much heat.

THERMOPLASTIC TYPE OF PLASTICS
Those that can repeatedly melt or soften with heat and harden on cooling. Examples: vinyls, acrylics, polyethylene.

THERMOSETTING TYPE OF PLASTICS
Those that are heat-set in their final processing to a permanently hard state. Examples: phenolics, ureas and melamines.

THINNER
A liquid, such as turpentine, used in paint to make it spread more easily and penetrate better

TINCTURE
A solution the solvent of which is alcohol, e.g., tincture of iodine.

TITRATION
Determination of the concentration of a solution by comparing it with a standard solution, usually employing burettes for the operation.

TOLUENE ($CH_3C_6H_5$)
Hydrocarbon derived mainly from petroleum but also from coal. Base for TNT, lacquers, saccharin and many other chemicals.

TRIADS
Group of three elements in the same vertical column of the periodic table.

TRIBASIC ACID
An acid containing three replaceable hydrogen atoms per molecule.

TRIPLE SUPERPHOSPHATE
Phosphorus fertilizer of higher phosphorus content than in superphosphate; produced by addition of phosphoric acid to phosphate rock.

TUYERES
The nozzles of the blowpipes of a blast furnace.

TYNDALL EFFECT
The dispersion of a beam of light as it passes through a colloidal solution.

U

ULTRAVIOLET RAYS
Invisible radiations having a shorter wave length than violet light.

UNSLAKED LIME
Calcium oxide, or line to which water has not been added.

U.S.P.
Abbreviation for United States Pharmacopoeia, an official book that specifies strengths and degrees of purity of official remedies.

V

VALENCE
The number of electrons gained, lost, or shared in forming a chemical bond.

VALENCE ELECTRONS
Electrons in the outermost orbit which may be gained or lost in chemical reactions.

VAPOR
A gas that can be converted into a liquid at that temperature by pressure alone.

VAPOR DENSITY
The ratio of the weight of a gas to the weight of an equal volume of hydrogen measured under the same conditions.

VAPOR PRESSURE
The (partial) pressure exerted by a vapor.

VAPOR TENSION
The pressure which a vapor exerts on a liquid when the liquid and vapor are in equilibrium at a given temperature (the maximum vapor pressure for the given temperature).

VAT DYES
Water-insoluble, complex coal tar dyes that can be chemically reduced in a heated solution to a soluble form that will impregnate fibers. Subsequent oxidation then produces insoluble colored dye-stuff remarkably fast to washing, light and chemicals.

VEHICLE
The liquid portion of paint, such as linseed oil, used to hold the paint base in suspension.

VERMICULITE
Mica that has bean expanded with steam to make a light, porous material.

VISCOSITY
(1) The resistance to flow of a liquid.
(2) The internal friction of a liquid.

VITRIFIED
Heated to the point where melting just begins, thus closing pores.

VITRIOL
An acid substance.

VOLUME-VOLUME PROBLEMS
Those in which a known volume of one material is given and the volume of another material involved in the reaction is sought.

VOLT
The electrical pressure required to make a current of one ampere through a resistance of one ohm.

VULCANIZATION
Process of combining rubber (natural, synthetic, or latex) with sulfur and various other additives usually under heat and pressure, in order to eliminate tackiness when warm and brittleness when cool, and to change permanently the material from a thermoplastic to a thermosetting composition. Finally to otherwise improve strength, elasticity, and abrasive resistance.

W

WARFARIN
A new kind of rat poison.

WATER GAS
A fuel gas made by blowing a bast of steam through a bed of red-hot coke.

WATER GLASS
A syrupy solution of sodium silicate.

WATER OF HYDRATION
Water that has united with some chemicals as they form crystals called hydrates.

WEAK ACID
An acid which is but slightly ionized in water solutions.

WEAK ELECTROLYTE
One that is but slightly ionized.

WEIGHTED SILK
Silk that has been dipped in solutions of certain tin salts.

WEIGHT-WEIGHT PROBLEMS
Those in which a known quantity of one material is given and the amount of another material involved in the reaction is sought.

WEIGHT-VOLUME PROBLEMS
Those in which the weight or volume of one material is given and either the weight or volume of another material involved in the reaction is sought

WETTING AGENTS
Materials that reduce the surface tension of a liquid, causing it to spread out better.

X

X-RAYS
Light radiations of high frequency and very short wave length.

Z

ZEOLITES
Naturally occurring minerals, such as an aluminate of either sodium or potassium.

ZIRCONIUM
A metallic element with an exceedingly high melting point.

CHEMICAL LAWS

1. AVOGADRO'S HYPOTHESIS
Equal volumes of gases, under the same conditions of temperature and pressure, contain the same number of molecules.

A liter of oxygen contains the same number of molecules as a liter of hydrogen measured under the same conditions of temperature and pressure.

2. BOYLE'S LAW
If the temperature remains constant, the volume of a given mass of gas is inversely proportional to the pressure.

$$\frac{V_1}{V_2} = \frac{P_2}{P_1}$$

Example: If the pressure on a gas is doubled and the temperature is constant, the new volume is one-half the original volume.

3. CHARLES' LAW
If the pressure remains constant, the volume of a gas caries directly with the Absolute temperature.

$$\frac{V_1}{V_2} \quad \frac{T_1}{T_2}$$

Example: If the Absolute temperature of a gas is doubled, the volume is also doubled.

4. GAY-LUSSAC'S LAW OF COMBINING VOLUMES OF GASES
The relative combining volumes of gases and their products, if gaseous, may be expressed by small whole numbers.
Example: One volume of chlorine combines with one volume of hydrogen forming two volumes of hydrogen chloride.

5. HENRY'S LAW OF GAS SOLUBILITY
If the temperature is held constant, the weight of a gas which dissolves in a given volume is proportional to the pressure.
Example: The greater the pressure, the larger the volume of gas which can be dissolved. Suppose that one liter of water can dissolve 2 grams of carbon dioxide at 1 atmosphere of pressure. If the temperature remains the same, 4 grams can be dissolved if the pressure is increased to 2 atmospheres.

6. LAW OF CONSERVATION OF ENERGY
Energy can neither be created nor destroyed; it may, however, be changed from one form to another.

Example: When coal is burned, stored chemical energy is converted and released as heat energy.

7. LAW OF CONSERVATION OF MATTER (MASS)

   Matter can neither be created nor destroyed. If the matter is changed from one form to another, the new products produced have the same mass as the original substances.

8. LAW OF MASS ENERGY

   This law expresses the equivalence of mass and energy. It states that energy (E) is equal to mass (m) times the square of the velocity of light (c) in centimeters per second.

   $$E = mc^2$$

9. LAW OF DEFINITE PROPORTIONS

   Every chemical compound has a definite composition of weight.
   Example: If pure water is analyzed its composition will never vary.
   There will always be eight times as much oxygen by weight as hydrogen.

10. LAW OF MASS ACTION

    The speed of a chemical reaction is proportional to the product of the molecular concentration of the reacting substances.
    Example: Mass action refers to the changing of the equilibrium of a reaction by varying the concentration of one or more of the reactants. Thus, the law states that in a reversible reaction the speed at which it occurs depends on the concentration of the reactants.

11. LAW OF MULTIPLE PROPORTIONS

    When two elements unite to form more than one compound, the weights of one element which combine with a fixed weight of the other are in the ratio of small whole numbers.
    Example: In the compound carbon monoxide (CO), there are 12 grams of carbon and 16 grams of oxygen. In the compound carbon dioxide (CO_2), there are 12 grams of carbon and 16 grams of oxygen. Therefore,

    $$\frac{\text{weight of oxygen in CO}}{\text{weight of oxygen in CO}_2} = \frac{1}{2}$$

12. LE CHATELIER'S PRINCIPLE

    If a system which is in equilibrium is affected by a change in temperature or pressure, it will adjust itself so that the effect of the change will be reduced to a minimum.
    Example: If the pressure on a system in equilibrium is increased, the system will adjust itself so that it will occupy less volume.

13. PERIODIC LAW (MOSELEY'S)

    The chemical properties of the elements are a periodic function of their atomic numbers.

GLOSSARY OF COMMON SUBSTANCE

A

COMMON NAME	CHEMICAL NAME	FORMULA
Alum	Potassium aluminum sulfate	$K_2SO_4 \cdot Al_2(SO_4)_3 \cdot 24H_2O$
Alumina	Aluminum oxide	Al_2O_3
Alundum	Fused aluminum oxide	Al_2O_3
Ammonia water	Ammonium hydroxide	NH_4OH
Aniline	Phenyl amine	$C_6H_5NH_2$
Aqua ammonia	A solution of NH_3 in H_2O	NH_4OH
Aqua fortis	Nitric acid	HNO_3
Aqua regia	Hydrochloric and nitric acids	$3 HCl + HNO_3$
Asbestos (principal form)	Hydrated magnesium silicate	$3 MgO \cdot 2 SiO_2 \cdot 2H_2O$
Aspirin	Acetylsalicylic acid	$C_6H_4(COOH)OCOCH_3$

B

Babbitt	Alloy of Sn, Sb, and Cu	
Bakelite	Resin from phenol and formaldehyde	
Baking powder	A mixture of $NaHCO_3$, an acid ingredient, and starch	
Baking soda	Sodium bicarbonate	$NaHCO$
Bauxite	Hydrated aluminum oxide	$Al_2O_3 \cdot 3H_2O$ and $Al_2O_3 \cdot H_2O$
Bleaching powder	Calcium oxychloride	$CaOCl_2$
Blue vitriol	Cupric sulfate	$CuSO_4$
Bluestone	Cupric sulfate	$CuSO_4$
Bone ash	Calcium phosphate (impure)	$Ca_3(PO_4)_2$
Bone black	Animal charcoal	C
Boracic acid	Boric acid	H_3BO_3
Borax	Sodium tetraborate	$Na_2B_4O_7 \cdot 10 H_2O$
Brass	Alloy of Cu and Zn	
Brimstone	Volcanic sulfur	Impure S
Brine	Sodium chloride solution	NaCl and H_2O
Bronze	Alloy of Cu, Sn, and Zn	

C

Cadium yellow	Cadmium sulfide	CdS
Calcite	Calcium carbonate	$CaCO_3$
Calich	Sodium nitrate (impure)	$NaNO_3$
Calomel	Mercurous chloride	HgCl
Camphor, artificial	Pinene chloride	$C_{10}H_{17}Cl$
Cane sugar	Sucrose	$C_{12}H_{22}O_{11}$
Carbolic acid	Phenol	C_6H_5OH
Carbonic acid gas	Carbon dioxide	CO_2

GLOSSARY OF COMMON SUBSTANCES (CONT'D)

COMMON NAME	CHEMICAL NAME	FORMULA
Caustic potash	Potassium hydroxide	KOH
Caustic soda	Sodium hydroxide	$NaOH$
Ceruse	Basic lead carbonate	$2\, PbCo_3 \cdot Pb(OH)_2$
Chalk	Calcium carbonate (impure)	$CaCO_3$
Chile saltpeter	Sodium nitrate (impure)	$NaNO_3$
China clay	Aluminum silicate	$Al_2O_3 \cdot 2SiO_2 \cdot 2H_2O$
Chloride of lime	Calcium oxychloride	$CaOCl_2$
Chrome alum	Potassium chromium sulfate	$K_2SO_4 \cdot Cr_2(SO_4)_3 \cdot 24\, H_2O$
Cinnabar	Mercuric sulfide	HgS
Coke	Carbon (impure)	C
Common salt	Sodium chloride	$NaCl$
Copperas	Ferrous sulfate	$FeSO_4 \cdot 7H_2O$
Corrosive sublimate	Mercuric chloride	$HgCl_2$
Corundum	Aluminum oxide	$Al2O_3$
Cream of tartar	Potassium hydrogen tartrate	$KHC_4H_4O_6$

D

Dextrose	Glucose	$C_6H_{12}O_6$
Diamond	Carbon	C
Dry ice	Solid carbon dioxide	CO_2

E

Epsom salts	Magnesium sulfate	$MgSO_4$

F

Feldspar (one form)	Potassium aluminum silicate	$KalSi_3O_8$
Firedamp	Methane	CH_4
Flowers of sulfur	Sulfur	S
Fluorspar	Calcium fluoride	CaF_2
Fool1 s gold	Iron pyrite	FeS_2

G

Galena	Lead sulfide	PbS
Glass	A solid solution containing a mixture of silicates	
Glauber's salt	Sodium sulfate	$Na_2SO_4 \cdot 10H_2O$
Glucose	Dextrose	$C_6H_{12}O_6$
Glycerin	Glycerol	$C_3H_5(OH)_3$
Grain alcohol	Ethyl alcohol	C_2H_5OH
Graphite	Carbon	C
Green vitriol	Ferrous sulfate	$FeSO_4$
Gypsum	Calcium sulfate	$CaSO_4 \cdot 2H_2O$

H

Horn silver	Silver chloride	$AgCl$
Household ammonia	Ammonium hydroxide	NH_4OH
Hypo	Sodium thiosulfate	$Na_2S_2O_3 \cdot 5H_2O$

GLOSSARY OF COMMON SUBSTANCES (CONT'D)

COMMON NAME	CHEMICAL NAME	FORMULA
K		
Kaolin	Hydrogen aluminum silicate	$H_2Al_2(SiO_4)_2 \cdot H_2O$
L		
Lampblack	Carbon (impure)	C
Lanolin	Cholesterol	$C_{27}H_{46}O$
Laughing gas	Nitrous oxide	N_2O
Levulose	Fructose	$C_6H_{12}O_6$
Lime, hydrated	Calcium hydroxide	$Ca(OH)_2$
Lime, quick	Calcium oxide	CaO
Lime, slaked	Calcium hydroxide	$Ca(OH)_2$
Limestone	Calcium carbonate	$CaCO_3$
Limewater	Calcium hydroxide solution	$Ca(OH)_2$
Litharge	Lead oxide	PbO
Lithopone	Zinc sulfide and barium sulfate	ZnS and $BaSO_4$
Lunar caustic	Silver nitrate	$AgNO_3$
Lye	Sodium hydroxide	$NaOH$
Magnesia	Magnesium oxide	MgO
Magnesite	Magnesium carbonate	$MgCO_3$
Malachite	Basic copper carbonate	$CuCO_3 \cdot Cu(OH)_2$
Marble	Calcium carbonate (impure)	$CaCO_3$
Marsh gas	Methane	CH_4
Methanol	Methyl alcohol	CH_3OH
Minium	Lead tetroxide	Pb_3O_4
Moth balls	Naphthalene	$C_{10}H_8$
Muriate of potash	Potassium chloride	KCl
Muriatic acid	Hydrochloric acid	HCl
N		
Niter	Potassium nitrate	KNO_3
O		
Oil of bitter almonds	Benzaldehyde	C_6H_5CHO
Oil of vitriol	Sulfuric acid	H_3SO_4
Oil of wintergreen	Methyl salicylate	$CH_3COOC_6H_4OH$
Oileum	Fuming sulfuric acid	$H_2SO_4 \cdot SO_3$
P		
Pearl	Calcium carbonate	$CaCO_3$
Phosgene	Carbonyl chloride	$COCl_2$
Plaster of Paris	Calcium sulfate	$2CaSO_4 \cdot H_2O$
Potash	Potassium carbonate or potassium hydroxide	K_2CO_3 or KOH
Pyrolusite	Manganese dioxide	MnO_2
Q		
Quicklime	Calcium oxide	CaO
Quicksilver	Mercury	Hg

GLOSSARY OF COMMON SUBSTANCES (CONT'D)

COMMON NAME	CHEMICAL NAME	FORMULA
R		
Rochelle salt	Potassium sodium tartrate	$KNaC_4H_4O_6$
Route	Ferric oxide	Fe_2O_3
S		
Sal ammoniac	Ammonium chloride	NH_4Cl
Sal soda	Sodium carbonate	Na_2CO_3
Salt of sorrell	Potassium acid oxalate	$KHC_2O_4 \cdot H_2O$
Saltpeter	Sodium nitrate	$NaNO_3$
Sand	Silicon dioxide	SiO_2
Silica	Silicon dioxide	SiO_2
Slaked lime	Calcium hydroxide	$Ca(OH)_2$
Soda lime	Calcium oxide & sodium hydroxide	CaO and NaOH
Soap (one kind)	Sodium stearate	$C_{17}H_{35}COONa$
Spirit of hartshorn	Ammonium hydroxide	NH_4OH
Spirit of wine	Ethyl alcohol	C_2H_5OH
Sugar	Sucrose	$C_{12}H_{22}O_{11}$
Sugar of lead	Lead acetate	$Pb(C_2H_3O_2)$
Superphosphate	Calcium sulfate & calcium acid phosphate	$CaSO_4$ and $Ca(H_2PO_4)_2$
T		
TABLE SALT	Sodium chloride	NaCl
TALC	Hydrated magnesium silicate	$3MgO \cdot 4SiO_2 \cdot H_2O$
TARTAR EMETIC	Potassium antimonyl tartrate	$2K(SbO)C_4H_4O_6 \cdot H_2O$
V		
Vinegar	Acetic acid, dilute	$HC_2H_3O_2$
W		
Water glass	Sodium silicate	Na_2SiO_3
White lead	Basic lead carbonate	$2PbCO_3 \cdot Pb(OH)_2$
White vitriol	Zinc sulfate	$ZnSO_4$
Whiting	Calcium carbonate	$CaCO_3$
Wood alcohol	Methyl alcohol	CH_3OH
Z		
Zinc blende	Zinc sulfide	ZnS
Zinc white	Zinc oxide	ZnO

CHEMICAL ELEMENTS AND SYMBOLS

NAME OF ELEMENT	SYMBOL	ATOMIC NUMBER	ATOMIC WEIGHT
		A	
Actinium	Ac	89	227.0
Aluminum	Al	13	26.98
Americium	Am	95	[243]
Antimony	Sb	51	121.76
Argon	A	18	39.944
Arsenic	As	33	74.91
Astatine	At	85	[210]
		B	
Barium	Ba	56	137.36
Berkelium	Bk	97	[245]
Beryllium	Be	4	9.013
Bismuth	Bi	83	209.00
Boron	B	5	10.82
Bromine	Br	35	79.916
		C	
Cadmium	Cd	48	112.41
Calcium	Ca	20	40.08
Californium	Cf	98	[246]
Carbon	C	6	12.011
Cerium	Ce	58	140.13
Cesium	Cs	55	132.91
Chlorine	Cl	17	35.457
Chromium	Cr	24	52.01
Cobalt	Co	27	58.94
Copper	Cu	29	63.54
Curium	Cm	96	[243]
		D	
Dysprosium	Dy	66	162.46
		E	
Erbium	Er	68	167.2
Europium	Eu	63	152.0
		F	
Fluorine	F	9	19.00
Francium	Fr	87	[223]
		G	
Gadolinium	Gd	64	156.9
Gallium	Ga	31	69.72
Germanium	Ge	32	72.60
Gold	Au	79	197.0
		H	
Hafnium	Hf	72	178.6
Helium	He	2	4.003
Holmium	Ho	67	164.94
Hydrogen	H	1	1.0080
		I	
Indium	In	49	114.76
Iodine	I	53	126.91
Iridium	Ir	77	192.2
Iron	Fe	26	55.85
		K	
Krypton	Kr	36	83.80
		L	
Lanthanum	La	57	138.92

CHEMICAL ELEMENTS AND SYMBOLS (CONT'D)

NAME OF ELEMENT	SYMBOL	ATOMIC NUMBER	ATOMIC WEIGHT
Lead	Pb	82	207.21
Lithium	Li	3	6.940
Lutetium	Lu	71	174.99
M			
Magnesium	Mg	12	24.32
Manganese	Mn	25	54.94
Mercury	Hg	80	200.61
Molybdenum	Mo	42	95.95
N			
Neodymium	Nd	60	144.27
Neon	Ne	10	20.183
Neptunium	Np	93	[2373]
Nickel	Ni	28	58.69
Niobium	Nb	41	92.91
Nitrogen	N	7	14.008
O			
Osmium	Os	76	190.2
Oxygen	O	8	16.0000
P			
Palladium	Pd	46	106.7
Phosphorus	P	15	30.975
Platinum	Pt	78	195.23
Plutonium	Pu	94	[242]
Polonium	Po	84	210.0
Potassium	K	19	39.100
Praseodymium	Pr	59	140.92
Promethium	Pm	61	[145]
Protactinium	Pa	91	231.
R			
Radium	Ra	88	226.05
Radon	Rn	86	222.
Rhenium	Re	75	186.31
Rhodium	Rh	45	102.91
Rubidium	Rb	37	85.48
Ruthenium	Ru	44	101.1
S			
Samarium	Sm	62	150.43
Scandium	Sc	21	44.96
Selenium	Se	34	78.96
Silicon	Si	14	28.09
Silver	Ag	47	107.880
Sodium	Na	11	22.991
Strontium	Sr	38	87.63
Sulfur	S	16	32.066
T			
Tantalum	Ta	73	180.95
Technetium	Tc	43	[99]
Tellurium	Te	52	127.61
Terbium	Tb	65	158.93
Thallium	Tl	81	204.39
Thorium	Th	90	232.05
Thulium	Tm	69	168.94
Tin	Sn	50	118.70
Titanium	Ti	22	47.90
Tungsten	W	74	183.92

		U	
Uranium	U	92	238.07
		V	
Vanadium	V	23	50.95
		X	
Xenon	Xe	54	131.3
		Y	
Ytterbium	Yb	70	173.04
Yttrium	Y	39	88.92
		Z	
Zinc	Zn	30	65.38
Zirconium	Zr	40	91.22

(NOTE: Brackets indicate the isotope of longest known half-life.)

PERIODIC TABLE OF THE ELEMENTS

IA	IIA	IIIB	IVB	VB	VIB	VIIB	VIIIB			IB	IIB	IIIA	IVA	VA	VIA	VIIA	Noble gases
1 H 1.008																	2 He 4.003
3 Li 6.941	4 Be 9.012											5 B 10.81	6 C 12.011	7 N 14.007	8 O 15.999	9 F 18.998	10 Ne 20.179
11 Na 22.990	12 Mg 24.305											13 Al 26.982	14 Si 28.086	15 P 30.974	16 S 32.06	17 Cl 35.453	18 Ar 39.948
19 K 39.102	20 Ca 40.08	21 Sc 44.956	22 Ti 47.90	23 V 50.941	24 Cr 51.996	25 Mn 54.938	26 Fe 55.847	27 Co 58.933	28 Ni 58.71	29 Cu 63.546	30 Zn 65.37	31 Ga 69.72	32 Ge 72.59	33 As 74.922	34 Se 78.96	35 Br 79.904	36 Kr 83.80
37 Rb 85.468	38 Sr 87.62	39 Y 88.906	40 Zr 91.22	41 Nb 92.906	42 Mo 95.94	43 Tc 98.602	44 Ru 101.07	45 Rh 102.905	46 Pd 106.4	47 Ag 107.868	48 Cd 112.40	49 In 114.82	50 Sn 118.69	51 Sb 121.75	52 Te 127.60	53 I 126.905	54 Xe 131.30
55 Cs 132.905	56 Ba 137.34	57 La 138.905	72 Hf 178.49	73 Ta 180.948	74 W 183.85	75 Re 186.2	76 Os 190.2	77 Ir 192.22	78 Pt 195.09	79 Au 196.966	80 Hg 200.59	81 Tl 204.37	82 Pb 207.19	83 Bi 208.2	84 Po (~210)	85 At ~210	86 Rn (~222)
87 Fr (223)	88 Ra 226.02	89 Ac (227)	104	105													

58 Ce 140.12	59 Pr 140.907	60 Nd 144.24	61 Pm (145)	62 Sm 150.4	63 Eu 151.96	64 Gd 157.25	65 Tb 158.925	66 Dy 162.50	67 Ho 164.930	68 Er 167.26	69 Tm 168.934	70 Yb 173.04	71 Lu 174.97
90 Th 232.038	91 Pa 231.036	92 U 238.029	93 Np 237.048	94 Pu (244)	95 Am (243)	96 Cm (247)	97 Bk (247)	98 Cf (251)	99 Es (254)	100 Fm (257)	101 Md (256)	102 No (254)	103 Lr (257)

www.ingramcontent.com/pod-product-compliance
Lightning Source LLC
Chambersburg PA
CBHW081757300426
44116CB00014B/2154